Opioids in Anesthesia

Opioids in Anesthesia

Edited by
F. G. Estafanous, M.D.

Chairman, Department of Cardio-Thoracic Anesthesia,
The Cleveland Clinic Foundation, Cleveland, Ohio

With 79 Contributing Authors

Butterworth Publishers
Boston • London
Sydney • Wellington • Durban • Toronto

Every effort has been made to ensure that the drug dosage schedules within this text are accurate and conform to standards accepted at time of publication. However, as treatment recommendations vary in light of continuing research and clinical experience, the reader is advised to verify drug dosage schedules herein with information found on product information sheets. This is especially true in cases of new or infrequently used drugs.

Library of Congress Cataloging in Publication Data
Main entry under title:

Opioids in anesthesia.

   Includes bibliographical references and index.
   1. Narcotics—Physiological effect. 2. Anesthesia.
I. Estafanous, F. G. (Fawzy G.) [DNLM:
1. Anesthetics. 2. Narcotics. QV 89 0618]
RD86.064065 1984   615′.781   84–11040
ISBN 0–409–95183–8

Butterworth Publishers
80 Montvale Avenue
Stoneham, MA 02180

10 9 8 7 6 5 4 3 2

Printed in the United States of America

To my wife, Samiha, and my sons, Marcus and John,
for their love and understanding

Contents

Contributing Authors

Paul G. Barash, M.D.
Professor and Chairman, Department of
Anesthesiology, Yale University School
of Medicine, New Haven, Connecticut

Richard R. Bartkowski, M.D., Ph.D.
Assistant Professor of Anesthesia,
University of Pennsylvania School of
Medicine, Philadelphia, Pennsylvania

Michael G. Bazaral, M.D.
Staff Anesthesiologist, Department of
Cardio-Thoracic Anesthesia, The
Cleveland Clinic, Cleveland, Ohio

Byron C. Bloor, Ph.D.
Assistant Professor of Anesthesiology,
UCLA School of Medicine, Los Angeles,
California

James G. Bovill, M.B., F.F.A.R.C.S.I.
Consultant Anaesthetist, Department of
Anaesthesia, Academisch Ziekenhuis,
University of Amsterdam, Amsterdam,
The Netherlands

Eli M. Brown, M.D.
Chairman, Department of Anesthesiology,
Sinai Hospital of Detroit, Detroit,
Michigan

Daniel B. Carr, M.D.
Assistant Professor of Medicine
(Endocrinology), Harvard Medical School,
Boston, Massachusetts

J. G. Collins, Ph.D.
Assistant Professor of Anesthesiology and
Pharmacology, Yale University School of
Medicine, New Haven, Connecticut

Michael D'Ambra, M.D.
Instructor in Anesthesia, Harvard Medical
School at the Massachusetts General
Hospital, Boston, Massachusetts

David A. Davis, M.D.
Professor of Anesthesiology, Duke
University School of Medicine, Durham,
North Carolina

Holly Dec-Silver, R.N.
Research Associate, Department of
Anesthesia, University of California, San
Diego, School of Medicine, San Diego,
California

**Simon de Lange, M.B.B.S., Ph.D.,
F.F.A.R.C.S.**
Chef de Clinique Cardio-thoracic Surgery,
Academisch Ziekenhuis Leiden, Leiden,
The Netherlands

Philippe A. Durant, M.D.
Research Fellow, Department of
Neurosurgery, Mayo Clinic, Rochester,
Minnesota

John H. Eisele, Jr., M.D.
Professor of Anesthesiology, University of
California, Sacramento Medical Center,
Davis, California

Norig Ellison, M.D.
Professor of Anesthesiology, University of
Pennsylvania School of Medicine,
Philadelphia, Pennsylvania

Adel Ahmed El-Etr, M.D.
Professor and Chairman, Department of
Anesthesiology, Loyola University Stritch
School of Medicine, Maywood, Illinois

Burton S. Epstein, M.D.
Professor of Anesthesiology, The George
Washington University School of Medicine,
Washington, D.C.

Fawzy G. Estafanous, M.D.
Chairman, Department of Cardio-Thoracic
Anesthesia, The Cleveland Clinic,
Cleveland, Ohio

Nabil R. Fahmy, M.D.
Associate Professor of Anesthesiology,
Harvard Medical School at the
Massachusetts General Hospital, Boston,
Massachusetts

John E. Fisher, B.S.
Endocrine Unit, Massachusetts General
Hospital, Boston, Massachusetts

Joan W. Flacke, M.D.
Professor of Anesthesiology, UCLA School
of Medicine, Los Angeles, California

Werner E. Flacke, M.D.
Professor of Anesthesiology and
Pharmacology, UCLA School of Medicine,
Los Angeles, California

Edmond S. Freis, M.D.
Instructor in Anesthesia, Harvard Medical
School at the Massachusetts General
Hospital, Boston, Massachusetts

Elizabeth A. M. Frost, M.B., Ch.B.
Professor of Anesthesiology, Albert
Einstein College of Medicine, Bronx, New
York

M. M. Ghoneim, M.D.
Professor of Anesthesia, The University of
Iowa School of Medicine, Iowa City, Iowa

Paul R. Hickey, M.D.
Assistant Professor of Anaesthesia,
Harvard Medical School, Boston,
Massachusetts

Otto Hilfiker, M.D.
Lecturer in Anesthesiology, University of
Goettingen, West Germany

Martine H. Hoeneveld, R.N.
Department of Anaesthesia, Academisch
Ziekenhuis, University of Amsterdam,
Amsterdam, The Netherlands

Michael B. Howie, M.D.
Associate Professor of Anesthesiology and
Pharmacy, The Ohio State University
College of Medicine, Columbus, Ohio

Carl C. Hug, Jr., M.D., Ph.D.
Professor of Anesthesiology and
Pharmacology, Emory University School of
Medicine, Atlanta, Georgia

**C. J. Hull, M.B., B.S., D.A. (Eng.),
F.F.A.R.C.S.**
Professor of Anaesthesia, The University
of Newcastle upon Tyne; Honorary
Consultant Anaesthetist, Royal Victoria
Infirmary, Newcastle upon Tyne, England

Paul A. J. Janssen, M.D.
President, n.v. Janssen Pharmaceutica,
Beerse, Belgium

Joel A. Kaplan, M.D.
Professor and Chairman, Department of
Anesthesiology, Mt. Sinai School of
Medicine, New York, New York

Patricia A. Kapur, M.D.
Assistant Professor of Anesthesiology,
UCLA School of Medicine, Los Angeles,
California

Christine R. Keegan, M.A.
Research Assistant, Department of
Anesthesia, Massachusetts General
Hospital, Boston, Massachusetts

Dietrich Kettler, M.D.
Professor of Anesthesiology and Chairman,
Department of Anesthesiology, University
of Goettingen, West Germany

Luke M. Kitahata, M.D., Ph.D.
Professor of Anesthesiology, Yale
University School of Medicine, New
Haven, Connecticut

Fritz Klein, M.D.
Assistant Medical Research Professor,
Duke University School of Medicine,
Durham, North Carolina

Benjamin J. Kripke, M.D.
Clinical Professor of Anesthesiology,
UCLA School of Medicine, Los Angeles,
California

Demetrios G. Lappas, M.D.
Associate Professor of Anaesthesia,
Harvard Medical School at the
Massachusetts General Hospital, Boston,
Massachusetts

William B. Latta, M.D.
Instructor in Anesthesiology, Harvard
Medical School at the Massachusetts
General Hospital, Boston, Massachusetts

Wen Shin Liu, M.D.
Assistant Professor of Anesthesiology, The
University of Utah School of Medicine,
Salt Lake City, Utah

Edward Lowenstein, M.D.
Professor of Anaesthesia, Harvard Medical
School at the Massachusetts General
Hospital, Boston, Massachusetts

Maki Matsumoto, M.D.
Postdoctoral Fellow, Department of
Anesthesiology, Yale University School of
Medicine, New Haven, Connecticut

Thomas McDonnell, M.D.
Assistant Professor of Anesthesia,
University of Pennsylvania School of
Medicine, Philadelphia, Pennsylvania

Robert D. McKay, M.D.
Associate Professor of Anesthesiology,
University of Alabama in Birmingham
School of Medicine, Birmingham, Alabama

Charles H. McLeskey, M.D.
Associate Professor of Anesthesia,
Bowman Gray School of Medicine of
Wake Forest University, Winston-Salem,
North Carolina

Ira Michaels, M.D.
Assistant Professor of Anesthesiology, Yale
University School of Medicine, New
Haven, Connecticut

Ronald D. Miller, M.D.
Professor and Vice Chairman, Department
of Anesthesia, University of California,
San Francisco, School of Medicine, San
Francisco, California

Michael R. Murphy, M.D.
Associate Professor of Anesthesiology,
Emory University School of Medicine,
Atlanta, Georgia

Rabiah Noueihed, M.D.
Research Fellow, Department of
Neurosurgery, Mayo Clinic, Rochester,
Minnesota

Gerard W. Ostheimer, M.D.
Associate Professor of Anaesthesia,
Harvard Medical School, Boston,
Massachusetts

Tsutomu Oyama, M.D.
Professor and Chairman, Department of
Anesthesiology, Hirosaki University School
of Medicine, Hirosaki, Japan

Nathan L. Pace, M.D.
Associate Professor of Anesthesiology, The
University of Utah School of Medicine,
Salt Lake City, Utah

Daniel M. Philbin, M.D.
Associate Professor of Anaesthesia,
Harvard Medical School at the
Massachusetts General Hospital, Boston,
Massachusetts

Michael L. Quinn, Ph.D.
Systems Analyst, Department of
Anesthesia, Veterans Administration
Hospital, La Jolla, California

J. G. Reves, M.D.
Professor of Anesthesiology, The
University of Alabama in Birmingham
School of Medicine, Birmingham, Alabama

Sandra L. Roberts, M.D.
Resident in Anesthesia, The University of
Iowa Hospitals and Clinics, Iowa City,
Iowa

Michael F. Roizen, M.D.
Associate Professor of Anesthesia, Medicine, and Pharmacology, University of California, San Francisco, School of Medicine, San Francisco, California

Carl E. Rosow, M.D.
Assistant Professor of Anaesthesia, Harvard Medical School at the Massachusetts General Hospital, Boston, Massachusetts

Theodore J. Sanford, Jr., M.D.
Assistant Clinical Professor in Anesthesia, University of California, San Diego, School of Medicine, San Diego, California

John J. Savarese, M.D.
Associate Professor of Anaesthesia, Harvard Medical School at the Massachusetts General Hospital, Boston, Massachusetts

Robert C. Schneider, M.D.
Assistant Professor of Anaesthesia, Harvard Medical School at the Massachusetts General Hospital, Boston, Massachusetts

Peter S. Sebel, M.B. B.S., Ph.D., F.F.A.R.C.S.I.
Senior Lecturer and Consultant, Anaesthetics Unit, The London Hospital Medical College, Whitechapel, London, England

Theodore C. Smith, M.D.
Professor of Pharmacology and Anesthesiology, Loyola University Stritch School of Medicine, Maywood, Illinois

N. Ty Smith, M.D.
Professor of Anesthesiology, University of California, San Diego, School of Medicine, San Diego, California

Hans Sonntag, M.D.
Professor of Anesthesiology, University of Goettingen, West Germany

Theodore H. Stanley, M.D.
Professor of Anesthesiology, The University of Utah School of Medicine, Salt Lake City, Utah

Robert K. Stoelting, M.D.
Professor and Chairman, Department of Anesthesia, Indiana University School of Medicine, Indianapolis, Indiana

Stephen J. Thomas, M.D.
Associate Professor of Anesthesiology, New York University School of Medicine, New York, New York

John H. Tinker, M.D.
Professor and Head, Department of Anesthesia, The University of Iowa School of Medicine, Iowa City, Iowa

J. Richard Trout, Ph.D.
Associate Professor of Biostatistics, Yale University School of Medicine, New Haven, Connecticut

Joost van der Maaten
Visiting Medical Student in Anesthesiology Research, University of Utah, The University of Leiden, The Netherlands

Harry B. van Wezel, M.D.
Resident, Department of Anaesthesia, Academisch Ziekenhuis, University of Amsterdam, Amsterdam, The Netherlands

Patrick J. Warren, M.D.
Department of Anaesthesia, Academisch Ziekenhuis, University of Amsterdam, Amsterdam, The Netherlands

Charles J. Westover, Jr., M.D.
Clinical Instructor of Anesthesia, University of California, San Diego, School of Medicine, San Diego, California

J. Earl Wynands, M.D.
Professor of Anaesthesia and Surgery, Faculty of Medicine, McGill University, Montreal, Quebec, Canada

Tony L. Yaksh, Ph.D.
Associate Professor of Pharmacology, Mayo Medical School, Rochester, Minnesota

Andrew M. Zurick, M.D.
Staff, Cardio-Thoracic Anesthesiologist, The Cleveland Clinic, Cleveland, Ohio

Additional Participants and Invited Guests

Adel Abadir, M.D.
Brooklyn, New York

Hassan Ali, M.D.
Boston, Massachusetts

Anthony Ascioti, M.D.
Syracuse, New York

John Bentley, M.D.
Tucson, Arizona

Lawrence Berman, M.D.
Nashville, Tennessee

James Bodine
Piscataway, New Jersey

Judy Bonfiglio, CRNA
Piscataway, New Jersey

Azmy Boutros, M.D.
Cleveland, Ohio

Edward Brunner, M.D.
Chicago, Illinois

Mary Cantrell, M.D.
Detroit, Michigan

Robert Capps, M.D.
Portland, Oregon

Helmut Cascorbi, M.D.
Cleveland, Ohio

Charles Christian, M.D.
Durham, North Carolina

Ron Cookson, Ph.D.
Marlow, Bucks, England

Paul Dauchot, M.D.
Cleveland, Ohio

David Davis, M.D.
Durham, North Carolina

Joris de Castro, M.D.
La Louviere, Belgium

Terence Downer
Piscataway, New Jersey

Nancy Drake
Piscataway, New Jersey

Edmond I. Eger II, M.D.
San Francisco, California

Robert Epstein, M.D.
Charlottesville, Virginia

Robert Fragen, M.D.
Chicago, Illinois

George Griffiths
Piscataway, New Jersey

William Hamilton, M.D.
San Francisco, California

James Harp, M.D.
Philadelphia, Pennsylvania

Gunter Hempelmann, M.D.
Giessen, Germany

Ann Hill, M.D.
Ann Arbor, Michigan

Anthony Ivankovich, M.D.
Chicago, Illinois

Edward Johnson, M.D.
Dallas, Texas

Carol Karp
Piscataway, New Jersey

Arthur Keats, M.D.
Houston, Texas

David Kirk
Piscataway, New Jersey

William Kiser, M.D.
Cleveland, Ohio

Jean Guy Maille, M.D.
Montreal, Canada

Kenneth Mailloux
Piscataway, New Jersey

James Mann, M.D.
Rockville, Maryland

Toni Marina
West Orange, New Jersey

Robert Marino, M.D.
New Orleans, Louisiana

Thomas McDonnell, M.D.
Philadelphia, Pennsylvania

Stanley Mogelnicki, M.D.
Atlanta, Georgia

Craig Moldenhauer, M.D.
Atlanta, Georgia

Roger Moore, M.D.
Browns Mills, New Jersey

Michael Nugent, M.D.
Rochester, Minnesota

Yasu Oka, M.D.
Bronx, New York

Robert Paulissian, M.D.
Chicago, Illinois

Ellison Pierce, M.D.
Boston, Massachusetts

Kenneth Potter, M.D.
Cleveland, Ohio

Steven Prevoznik, M.D.
Philadelphia, Pennsylvania

Rose Rogan, M.D.
West Orange, New Jersey

Patricia Russell, M.D.
Rockville, Maryland

Amira Safwat, M.D.
Davis, California

Paul Samuelson, M.D.
Birmingham, Alabama

Brant Sankey, M.D.
Cleveland, Ohio

Stephen Schlossberg
Piscataway, New Jersey

Juergen Scheuttler, M.D.
Venusberg, West Germany

John Schweiss, M.D.
St. Louis, Missouri

Dhun Sethna, M.D.
Cleveland, Ohio

Harvey Shapiro, M.D.
La Jolla, California

Lee Shepard, M.D.
Cleveland, Ohio

Kinichi Shibutani, M.D.
Chappaqua, New York

George Silvay, M.D.
New York, New York

Donald Stanski, M.D.
Stanford, California

Stephen Steen, M.D.
Los Angeles, California

Linda Stehling, M.D.
Syracuse, New York

Wendell Stevens, M.D.
Portland, Oregon

Sharon Storey, M.D.
Houston, Texas

Leo Strunin, M.D.
Calgary, Canada

Jorge Urzua, M.D.
Santiago, Chile

Leroy Vandam, M.D.
Boston, Massachusetts

Gabriel Vanden Bussche, M.D.
Beerse, Belgium

Robert Watson, M.D.
Washington, D.C.

Paul White, M.D.
Stanford, California

Richard Wildnauer, Ph.D.
Piscataway, New Jersey

Carolyn Wilkinson, M.D.
Chicago, Illinois

John Youngberg, M.D.
New Orleans, Louisiana

Howard Zauder, M.D.
Syracuse, New York

Elmer Zsigmond, M.D.
Chicago, Illinois

Preface

The last two decades have seen the development of synthetic opioids, agents much more potent than morphine and free from many of its side effects. These new drugs have helped to refine anesthetic management for many patients; inevitably, their use also raises many questions. We are indebted to the scientists whose brilliance and dedication contributed to the development of such potent opioids and to one man, Dr. Paul Janssen, who developed the family of very potent short-acting and ultra-short-acting opioids that have effectively established their place in the everyday practice of anesthesia.

I am privileged to present this book to my colleagues. It is the product of a two-day symposium organized in 1983 by the Cleveland Clinic Foundation and sponsored by Janssen Pharmaceutica. The well-recognized scientists and clinicians who contributed to the symposium shared their results and experiences, and they and prominent guests participated actively in open and stimulating discussions. This publication reviews the historical role of opioids, evaluates their current status, and predicts their future role in anesthesia practice. The extensive discussions point to several challenging issues that need further research, such as the selectivity of the various opioids to their receptors, their effects on other central receptors, and the interaction of opioids with muscle relaxants and other drugs used during surgery.

My appreciation goes to my colleagues in the Department of Cardio-Thoracic Anesthesia at the Cleveland Clinic and to my secretary, Joanne Stoddard. My special gratitude to Ms. Nancy Megley, editor in the Medical Division of Butterworth Publishers, who worked tirelessly and patiently to achieve the publication of this book.

F. G. E.

Opioids in Anesthesia

I BACKGROUND AND CONCEPTS

1 NARCOTICS IN ANESTHESIA: PAST, PRESENT, AND FUTURE

Edward Lowenstein

If, in 1965, an anesthetist had been asked to predict the future of narcotics in anesthesia practice, he might have talked about a minor role in premedication and balanced anesthesia, spoken of a major role in management of postoperative pain, and perhaps remarked about neuroleptanalgesia. Narcotics were not considered an exciting subject for investigation or an appropriate area for innovation. After all, they had "been around" for millenia. In the 120 years since an anesthetic was first used in a surgical procedure, narcotics had assumed a rather mundane position. Certainly, few or none would have predicted the dramatic developments that have occurred in the subsequent nineteen years.

EARLY CHALLENGES

Cardiac surgery was in its infancy in the 1960s. Challenges generated by patients with end-stage valvular heart disease who required surgical correction of their anatomic lesion combined to change drastically the status of narcotics. The necessity for safely providing anesthesia for such patients was one challenge; maintaining life after a "successful" operation was a second. In those days, many patients survived the operation only to succumb to respiratory failure. This led initially to the practice of prophylactic tracheostomy and mechanical ventilation. The indications were so inexact, however, that many patients who required respiratory support were denied it, and others received it unnecessarily. Therefore postoperative retention of the endotracheal tube, a practice formerly deemed cruel or abhorrent, was initiated.

This started a cascade which, among other events, led to the initiation of narcotic "anesthesia." To allow patients to retain an oral or nasal endotracheal tube with only acceptable discomfort and avoid catastrophic straining and "bucking," intravenous morphine was administered. This was done with great trepidation due to fear of circulatory deterioration, but it quickly became apparent that patients tolerated the narcotics without harm. Gradually, increasing incremental doses of morphine beyond those considered allowable were administered so as to achieve the above objectives. We soon realized that the cumulative doses exceeded any reported

3

in recent medical literature. Since the patients were being ventilated, they did not sustain hypoxemia or hypercapnia, and detectable circulatory effects appeared to be rare.

OPIOID ANESTHESIA

These observations led to the conceptual leap of administering large intravenous doses of morphine concurrently with, and then as, the anesthetic [1]. In timid and then bold steps, the total dose of morphine increased from approximately 0.5 to 3 mg per kilogram body weight. The most striking aspect of this anesthetic regimen was the lack of apparent circulatory effect. This contrasted dramatically with previous experiences in these very ill candidates for cardiac surgery, and led to rapid acceptance, first at the Massachusetts General Hospital and subsequently throughout the world.

The concept of narcotic anesthesia provided a stimulus for conduct of basic research of opioid pharmacology, biochemistry, and structure-function relationships, and continuing study of clinical responses. Virtually no area of anesthesiology has remained untouched. Since subsequent experience has indicated that narcotics used as anesthetics have limitations and disadvantages as well as advantages, the search for more suitable narcotics has continued.

In 1971 we published a list of limitations [2]. This included:

1. Awareness during anesthesia and recall of intraoperative events.
2. Circulatory depression when adjuvants were administered.
3. Liberation of catecholamines and incomplete attenuation of circulatory responses to anesthetic and surgical stimuli. Both were associated with increase in myocardial oxygen demand.
4. Hypotension.
5. Liberation of antidiuretic hormone.

6. Permanent neurologic damage.
   The list did not include an increased blood volume requirement in patients receiving 3 to 11 mg/kg morphine [3], and expiratory grunting [4], an apparent analog of the chest wall stiffness observed with some synthetic narcotics.

Each of these apparent disadvantages has received a great deal of attention. With the exception of permanent neurologic damage, which has not been substantiated, each is still an issue of investigation and concern.

SYNTHETIC NARCOTICS

The search for a better narcotic without the important disadvantage of the increased blood volume requirement attendant upon ultra-high-dose morphine administration led Stanley [5,6] to use the synthetic narcotic fentanyl as an anesthetic for patients undergoing surgical correction of valvular and coronary heart disease. The subsequent acceptance of fentanyl as narcotic of choice for critically ill surgical patients has led to a more intense search for narcotics free of unwanted side effects.

Anesthetists now have a growing family of synthetic narcotics, with friendly names like Al [7] and Su [8], narcotic agonist/antagonist drugs, and effective narcotic antagonists. Endogenous opioids have been identified and their existence substantiated [9]. Narcotic receptors have been identified, located, and classified [10–12]. Narcotics are being administered intradurally and extradurally [13,14]. Truly, the area is virtually bursting with activity.

At present, high-dose synthetic narcotic anesthesia, the equivalent of 5 to 20 mg/kg morphine, has found its most ardent advocates among cardiac anesthetists. When this technique works well, it makes anesthetic management of extremely ill patients uncannily easy. The "railroad track" strip charts only dreamed about in the past have become a frequent reality; however, the opposite is also true. The need for increasingly higher doses, uncontrolled hemodynamics [15], and metabolic and electrocardiographic evidence of myocardial ischemia [16] are well documented. Thus cardiac anesthetists also compose the most skeptical and unconvinced group.

Will more potent compounds prove to provide superior anesthesia? As stated previously [17], we believe that similarities among opiates are greater than differences. To expect each new opiate to possess dramatically different characteristics has been and almost certainly will continue to be unrealistic.

To my way of thinking, the two greatest drawbacks to sole dependence upon narcotics as universal anesthetics are inevitable production of muscular rigidity and unreliability of producing amnesia [18,19]. Why occupancy of opiate receptors causes muscle rigidity is teleologically inexplicable. That analgesia should be accompanied by amnesia also is not necessarily logical. The consequence of these two limitations is the necessity of administering other drugs to compensate for these characteristics. In essence, this means that every narcotic anesthetic requires administration of a neuromuscular blocking drug and an anesthetic adjuvant. Since every intervention has predictable and unpredictable complications (side effects), we must question whether narcotics will continue to grow in importance or decline to a lesser role.

CONCLUSION

While prediction is fraught with hazard, I will take that risk. I believe narcotic anesthesia will continue to thrive for a number of reasons. First, the scientific body of knowledge has expanded sufficiently to give us a rational basis for pursuing the practice of using large doses of narcotics as primary anesthetics. I believe that increased understanding of endorphins, enkephalins, and narcotic receptors will lead to more specific analgesics with a decreased frequency of undesirable effects. Another factor is that the discipline of pharmocokinetics has developed and become widely appreciated [20]. Synthetic narcotics are known to have differing pharmacokinetic properties that make them appropriate for operations of varying stimulation and length.

From a more practical standpoint, blood level ranges will be established for anesthetic action [21]. Rapid measurement of blood levels in patients will permit precise adjustment of dosage. On-line electroencephalographic analysis will provide a noninvasive alternative to direct measurement of blood levels [22]. Controlled infusion based on pharmacokinetic properties will permit rapid resumption of respiratory competence with analgesia postoperatively.

Muscle rigidity will continue to mandate muscle relaxant administration in virtually all narcotic anesthetics. Recall will continue to be a concern with so-called pure narcotic anesthesia. Intrathecal and epidural narcotics will continue to increase in importance, and low- and medium-dose narcotics as a component of balanced anesthesia and neuroleptanalgesia will continue to achieve wide acceptance. Inhalation anesthetics will retain their importance as adjuncts to high-dose narcotic anesthetics when additional inhibition of responses is required.

Last but not least, economics will constitute a major determinant of whether new and expensive synthetic narcotics will realize their potential as anesthetics. Advantages will have to be documented by cost-benefit analysis to achieve the widespread acceptance that is necessary to justify continuing development and manufacture.

REFERENCES

1. Lowenstein E, Hallowell P, Levine FH, et al. Cardiovascular response to large doses of intravenous morphine in man. N Engl J Med 1969;281:1389–93.

2. Lowenstein E. Morphine "anesthesia"—a perspective. Anesthesiology 1971;35:563–5.

3. Stanley TH, Gray NH, Stanford DW, et al. The effects of high-dose morphine on fluid and blood requirements in open-heart operation. Anesthesiology 1973;38:536–41.

4. Freund FG, Martin WE, Wong KC, Hornbein TF. Abdominal muscle rigidity induced by morphine and nitrous oxide. Anesthesiology 1973;38:358–62.

5. Stanley TH, Webster LR. Anesthetic requirements and cardiovascular effects of fentanyl-oxygen and fentanyl-diazepam-oxygen anesthetic in man. Anesth Analg (Cleve) 1978;57:411–16.

6. Stanley TH, Philbin DM, Coggins CH. Fentanyl-oxygen anesthesia for coronary artery surgery. Cardiovascular and antidiuretic hormone responses. Can Anaesth Soc J 1979;26:168–72.

7. Kay B, Stephenson DK. Alfentanil (R39209): initial clinical experience with a new narcotic analgesia. Anesthesia 1980; 35:1197–1201.

8. de Lange S, Boscoe MJ, Stanley TH, Pace N. Comparison of sufentanil-O_2 and fentanyl-O_2 for coronary artery surgery. Anesthesiology 1982;56:112–18.

9. Hughes J, Smith TW, Kosterlitz HW, et al. Identification of two related pentapeptides from the brain with potent opiate agonist activity. Nature 1975;258:577–9.

10. Pert CB, Snyder SH. Opiate receptor: its demonstration in nervous tissue. Science 1973;179:1101–14.

11. Lord JAH, Waterfield AA, Hughes J, et al. Endogenous spinal peptides: multiple agonists and receptors. Nature 1977;267:495–500.

12. LaMotte C, Snowman A, Pert CB, et al. Opiate receptor binding in rhesus monkey brain: association with limbic circuits. Brain Res 1978;155:374–9.

13. Behar M, Magora F, Olshwang D. Epidural morphine in treatment of pain. Lancet 1979;1:527–8.

14. Yaksh TL, Rudy TA. Analgesia mediated by a direct spinal action of narcotics. Science 1976;192:1357–8.

15. Waller JL, Hug CC Jr, Nagle DM, Craver JM. Fentanyl-oxygen "anesthesia" and coronary bypass surgery. Anesth Analg (Cleve) 1980;59:562–3.

16. Sonntag H, Larsen R, Hilfiker O, Kettler D, Brockschnieder B. Myocardial blood flow and oxygen consumption during high-dose fentanyl anesthesia in patients with coronary artery disease. Anesthesiology 1982; 56:417–22.

17. Lowenstein E, Philbin DM. Narcotic "anesthesia" in the eighties. Anesthesiology 1981;55:195–7.

18. Hilgenberg JC. Intraoperative awareness during high-dose fentanyl-oxygen anesthesia. Anesthesiology 1981;54:341–3.

19. Mummaneni N, Rao TLK, Montoya A. Awareness and recall with high-dose fentanyl-oxygen anesthesia. Anesth Analg (Cleve) 1980;59:948–9.

20. Hug CC Jr. Pharmacokinetics of drugs administered intravenously. Anesth Analg (Cleve) 1978;57:704–23.

21. Austin KL, Stapleton JV, Mather LE. Relationship between blood meperidine concentrations and analgesic response. Anesthesiology 1980;53:460–6.

22. Sebel PS, Bovill JG, Wauquier A, Rog P. Effects of high-dose fentanyl anesthesia on the electroencephalogram. Anesthesiology 1981;55:203–11.

2 NARCOTIC ANESTHESIA?

C. J. Hull

When in 1941 Langton Hewer popularized the use of trichloroethylene, it became common practice to control the accompanying tachypnea with small intravenous doses of meperidine, which also reduced the required concentration of trichloroethylene.

Narcotic supplementation of inhalational anesthesia has remained popular in England. Since opioids are effective in suppressing the excitatory characteristics of methohexitone, althesin, and etomidate, they have also found wide use in the induction sequence. These low-dose techniques rarely require more than 150 μg of fentanyl. There is no doubt that narcotic-supplemented anesthesia with spontaneous ventilation requires careful technique, and it can be difficult to distinguish breath holding from frank respiratory depression. I anticipate that alfentanil, having rapid onset and recovery characteristics, will find favor in this method of anesthesia for very short procedures.

PROBLEMS WITH FENTANYL

In a moderate-dose method, patients first are given fentanyl at the 200- to 400-μg level before induction, then further supplements as necessary during anesthesia with oxygen, nitrous oxide, and minimal halothane or enflurane. They may be expected to breathe spontaneously after one hour or more of anesthesia.

At higher doses than this, postoperative controlled ventilation may be necessary, and the level of provision of postoperative care becomes a critical factor. As Dr. Lowenstein has indicated, very high doses of narcotics can take on some of the characteristics of anesthetic agents. However, I regard the ability to induce both unconsciousness and a state of physical unresponsiveness to surgical stimuli as important characteristics of an anesthetic agent, and therefore I have some difficulty in regarding opioids as anesthetic agents.

Unconsciousness is very difficult to guarantee, however much fentanyl is given. Moreover, Murphy and Hug [1] have shown very recently that the minimum alveolar concentration (MAC) value for enflurane can be reduced only by some 65% at any dose of morphine or fentanyl in dogs. Halsey (Halsey MJ, personal communication) failed to demonstrate pressure reversal of opioid narcosis in small mammals; opioids differ in this respect from all other classes of anesthetic agents, for which pressure reversal is both predictable and complete. While in no way minimizing the value of opioids, we would mislead ourselves or others if we equated opioid narcosis with anesthesia.

If the spontaneously breathing patient is inadequately anesthetized, the problem will be very clear to all concerned so that awareness is unlikely to be a problem. Once we paralyze and ventilate the patient with non-anesthetic gases, however, the problem of awareness becomes paramount. Dr. Lowenstein anticipates that electroencephalographic analysis may resolve this problem— I remain skeptical.

We must exercise particular care when describing newer opioids such as alfentanil as "short-acting." While the effects of a single dose are without question evanescent, the kinetic profile predicts a degree of cumulation with repeated doses. Although the elimination half-life is much shorter than that of fentanyl, we should not become too ecstatic about a drug with a value no less than that of pancuronium.

ONSET OF TOLERANCE

The rapid onset of tolerance is an unwelcome nettle that we must not shrink from grasping. While acquired tolerance to opioids is well known, it is not well recognized that its onset may be very rapid. In one study [2], volleys of supramaximal electrical stimuli were intermittently applied to the radial nerves of six anesthetized dogs with chloral hydrate, and the changes in heart rate and mean arterial pressure were observed. After a single 100 μg per kilogram dose of fentanyl, the response was seen to be suppressed almost totally, with recovery as the plasma concentration declined. A mean kinetic model was derived from the serial plasma concentrations. In a second series of dogs, ten incremental doses of fentanyl (predicted by the model as those required to raise the plasma concentration logarithmically) were given at 20-minute intervals, the last of these being, as before, 100 μg/kg. The response to stimulation was now suppressed by less than 10% despite the much higher concentration, and it was concluded that the concentration-response relationship was heavily modified

by the conditioning procedure. Clearly, these results tell us nothing about tolerance to fentanyl analgesia in humans, but they do suggest that the rapid onset of tolerance should be regarded as a real phenomenon that should be neither discounted nor ignored.

CONCLUSION

Now we come to the serious business of historical accuracy. The concept of narcotic anesthesia *was* introduced in Boston, but not by Dr. Lowenstein and his colleagues and certainly not in 1969. On referring to the *Boston Medical and Surgical Journal* of November 18, 1846, one finds the first scientific paper on ether anesthesia by H. J. Bigelow, which relates Morton's successful demonstration at Dr. Lowenstein's own hospital.

On October 28, however, a letter was written by E. R. Smilie [3] and published three weeks before Bigelow's celebrated paper:

As it is frequently found desirable to produce insensibility in persons requiring painful operations, I have made use of a . . . solution of opium for that purpose, with excellent success. When reduced to vapor by gentle heat, regulating the amount inhaled according to the length of time required for the operation, and for the entire absence of symptoms induced by pain, and those which usually result from the use of opium, I have thought the method of preparation and exhibition invaluable.

He continues with a description of the preparation and its administration to the patient:

. . . into a glass retort, and by causing a slow evaporation with moderate heat, the patient being permitted to breathe the gaseous vapour from an elastic tube affixed to the mouth of the retort. The judgment of the physician is to be exercised with regard to the quantity inspired, which must be regulated according to the character of the disease and the duration of the required operation.

[Signed] E. R. Smilie, 22 School Street, Boston

There can be no doubt that Dr. Smilie published a scientific paper on narcotic anesthesia in 1846, and what is more, claimed successful use of the inhalational route!

Unfortunately, there were two things that Dr. Smilie did not know—first, morphine crystals sublime at 197°C, so that gentle warming of an opium solution would not yield any useful quantity of morphine vapor. Second, as may be adduced from the title of his paper, Dr. Smilie was not to know for some weeks that, unlike morphine, diethyl ether is a most effective anesthetic agent.

REFERENCES

1. Murphy MR, Hug CC Jr. The anesthetic potency of fentanyl in terms of its reduction of enflurane MAC. Anesthesiology 1982;57: 485–8.
2. Askitopoulou H, Whitwam JG, Chakrabarti MK, Al-Khudhairi D, Hull CJ, Bower S. Acute tolerance of cardiovascular reflexes to fentanyl in the dog. Br J Anaesth 1982; 54:226P.
3. Smilie ER. Insensibility produced by the inhalation of the vapor of the ethereal solution of opium. Boston Med Surg J 1846;35 (October 28).

3 OPIATE RECEPTORS, ENDOGENOUS LIGANDS, AND ANESTHESIA: A SYNOPSIS

Daniel B. Carr and John E. Fisher

Recently, it has become possible to describe mechanisms of analgesia in detail sufficient to give a provisional account of how nociceptive stimuli may be amplified or attenuated within pain pathways, and of the mechanisms by which narcotic analgesics influence this process. This brief review summarizes the development of the concept of multiple opiate receptors, the recognition of endogenous peptide ligands for these subtypes, and the relevance of this basic work for clinical anesthesiology.

MULTIPLE OPIATE RECEPTORS IN VIVO

The concept that distinct, complementary opiate receptors may be activated or blocked in vivo by selective pharmacologic administration emerged most clearly from work by Martin and colleagues [1,2]. They identified three distinct behavioral syndromes produced by morphine congeners in the chronic spinal dog, and attributed each syndrome to the action of a prototypical agonist upon a separate receptor. Morphine, acting upon a μ receptor, produces miosis, bradycardia, hypothermia, antinociception, and indiffer- ence to environmental stimuli. Ketocyclaz- ocine, like morphine, produces miosis and depresses the flexor reflex but, unlike mor- phine, produces sedation rather than indif- ference and has little effect on the skin twitch reflex, heart rate, or temperature. Ketocy- clazocine neither suppresses nor precipitates abstinence in the morphine-dependent dog, indicating that its interaction with the puta- tive μ receptor is minimal and suggesting that its effects are due to selective action upon a distinct receptor, termed κ. In contrast to both morphine and ketocyclazocine, N-allyl- normetazocine (SKF 10,047) causes pupil- lary dilation, tachypnea, tachycardia, and canine mania. The agent SKF 10,047 is struc- turally related to ketocyclazocine in that both compounds are benzomorphans but, unlike the latter, SKF 10,047 precipitates absti- nence in the morphine-dependent dog and hence can act at least partially as a μ antag- onist. The unique hallucinogenic (in hu- mans) and adverse effects of SKF 10,047 ar- gue for an agonist interaction between it and a third opiate receptor subtype, termed σ. Consonant with their role as agonists, all three prototypic drugs are reversed in their effects by the pure antagonist naltrexone.

Three other strategies have also confirmed the presence in vivo of multiple opiate receptor subtypes with prototypical agonists as described on preceding page [3]. First is the detailed observation of behavior of rats placed in the novel environment of a Y-maze after pretreatment with putative agonists. For example, cyclazocine and SKF 10,047—both σ receptor agonists—cause naloxone-insensitive behavioral arousal and bizarre behavior reminiscent of hallucinosis, but μ and κ agonists produce behavioral depression. Second, seizure thresholds of rats exposed to fluothyl, a volatile convulsant, permit construction of dose-response curves and testing of naloxone antagonism, as well as tolerance and cross-tolerance among putative opiate receptor agonists. Third is a subject's ability to discriminate between or generalize from one narcotic's stimulus effects to those of a second drug. Such techniques have been described as animal models of subjective effects in humans. In their simplest form, such tests are based on rewards (e.g., by training a rat to press one bar for food after it has been pretreated with a narcotic, and a different bar after saline pretreatment) or punishments (e.g., to turn right in a maze after drug injection and left after saline to avoid an electric shock). This type of approach has further validated the concept that three principal receptors, operationally equivalent to μ, κ, and σ, determine the discriminative effects of narcotic compounds in mammals.

OPIATE RECEPTORS: ISOLATION AND ENDOGENOUS LIGANDS

The explosion of interest in opiates during the 1970s can be traced to the purification of brain opiate receptors by several groups [4–7] in 1972–1973 and the isolation of two brain peptides with opiate bioactivity in 1975 [8]. These synergistic advances facilitated in vitro studies, such as quantification of peptide fragment affinity for opiate receptors, in a field in which advances had heretofore resulted from an approach based upon in vivo responses to alkaloids, benzomorphans, and phenylpiperidine analogs. Moreover, the recognition of endogenous opioid receptors and agonists enlarged the scope of opiate research by attracting to it many investigators studying normal physiology, in contrast to the smaller number previously working on problems of drug abuse or analgesic pharmacology.

The first identification of brain opiate receptors quantified the binding of tritiated narcotics or narcotic antagonists to brain homogenates or synaptosomal fractions. Such binding was stereospecific, saturable, reversible, and of high affinity. For the most part, binding affinity of ligands appeared to correlate with analgesic potency [9]. Opiate receptors were demonstrated in areas of the nervous system important for nociception and affect [10]. Sodium chloride at physiologic concentrations increased the binding of opiate antagonists but decreased the binding of opiate agonists [11]. This effect was specific for sodium, not a general property of cations or high ionic strength, and was indicative of a change of receptor conformation in the presence of sodium and, more speculatively, of an effect upon sodium channels due to opiate agonist-receptor interaction in vivo.

While other groups performed in vitro analyses of the opiate receptor, the Aberdeen group tracked the purification of opiate activity in brain extracts by screening putative opiate agonists for their ability to inhibit electrically induced contractions of guinea pig ileum or mouse vas deferens, two complementary bioassays that these same authors had standardized earlier [12]. Not only did this approach culminate in the isolation of two opioid pentapeptides, leucine and methionine enkephalin [8], it led directly to the observation that the rank order of potency of the enkephalins compared to another endogenous opioid peptide, β-endorphin, differed between the two bioassays. The conclusion that the enkephalins and β-endorphin acted upon a receptor in mouse vas deferens differently than on the receptor in guinea pig ileum was strengthened by findings on inhibition of binding of radiolabeled naloxone or leucine enkephalin in guinea pig brain homogenates [13]. For the enkephalins, β-endorphin, and other narcotic agonists including peptide analogs and benzomorphans, activity in guinea pig ileum correlated more with inhibition of brain ^{3}H-naloxone binding then with inhibition of brain ^{3}H-leu-enkephalin binding. Naloxone antagonized activity in guinea pig ileum at lower doses than in mouse vas deferens. Bioactivity of agonists in the latter organ seemed to parallel their ability to inhibit ^{3}H-leu-enkephalin binding rather than to inhibit ^{3}H-naloxone binding. The group therefore invoked the existence of a novel receptor, termed δ, to account for the differences in rank order of potency in the two bioassay and two binding assay systems. In keeping with Martin's earlier nomenclature, they called the receptor in guinea pig ileum the μ receptor.

Numerous studies, many of which employ peptide analogs of the enkephalins or β-endorphin, have confirmed and extended these results of Lord et al [12]. Among more recent biochemical evidence in support of multiple opioid receptor types are: (a) receptor affinities cluster into groups consisting of morphine, enkephalin, and benzomorphan types when probed by a number of synthetic ligands or native peptide sequences [14]; (b) structure-activity relationships [15,16] derived from selective μ or δ analogs indicate different spatial requirements for binding to each receptor; (c) regional differences occur in the brain distribution of distinct receptor sites [17]; (d) site-specific protection of receptors from irreversible inactivation is accomplished by use of selective μ or δ ligands; and (e) cultured clonal neural cell lines contain the δ opiate receptor only [15]. A high-affinity μ receptor subtype has also been identified through studies employing naloxazone, a specific antagonist at this site [18]. Other detailed studies of the guanosine triphosphate (GTP) sensitivity of ligand binding to opiate receptors have revealed a GTP-sensitive type with selectivity resembling that of the μ category and a GTP-insensitive type

whose selectivity resembles that of the δ category.

In Martin's description of distinct opiate-induced syndromes in the chronic spinal dog, he noted differences in the potency of varied ligands, including the recently isolated enkephalins, and speculated that "perhaps these apparent disparate results can be reconciled by postulating that a naturally occurring brain polypeptide may interact with a receptor more related to the κ than the μ receptor" [1]. Pursuit of this idea was hindered by the fact that benzomorphan drugs bind to both μ and κ receptors, particularly the former. Nonetheless, several laboratories did identify a brain membrane receptor whose binding to benzomorphans such as ethylketocyclazocine was minimally affected by competition with μ or δ agonists [19], but readily displaceable by κ-receptor-specific ligands such as bremazocine. Moreover, quantification of the relative proportion of κ receptors in different species indicated that previous inconsistencies were due to marked interspecies divergence in the content of brain κ receptor sites [20].

Identification of the endogenous ligand for the κ receptor was accomplished not as the result of bioassay or receptor approaches, but rather as a consequence of microsequencing of pituitary opioid peptides. Biosynthetic studies, which have recently been reviewed [21], identified three separate precursors for the three related families of opioid peptides: first, the precursor to adrenocorticotropic hormone and β-endorphin; second, the prohormone for leu- and met-enkephalin; and third, that for α-neoendorphin and dynorphin. All known opioid peptides have an amino terminus tyrosine, followed by glycine, phenylalanine, and then either methionine or leucine. Differences in the carboxy terminal extensions underlie the marked differences in actions of individual sequences. Audigier and co-workers found that met-enkephalin [Arg^6, Phe^7], a heptapeptide from adrenal medulla, interacted with κ receptors in guinea pig ileum [22]. When the sequence of dynorphin was delineated, tests of longer segments of the molecule succeeded in confirming its κ agonism [23]; however, such studies proved that the presence of a basic residue (e.g., Arg) at position 7 was a requirement for κ receptor specificity, in contrast to the report of Audigier. Immunohistochemical studies have shown that the distribution of dynorphin neurons is separable from that of enkephalin neurons, but it will be some time before the numerous interactions between endogenous κ receptor agonists and overlapping peptide systems will be fully elucidated.

It is not yet possible to specify an endogenous agonist for σ receptors, although the availability of phencyclidine, a psychotomimetic analgesic that appears to bind in vitro to σ receptors [15], to share discriminative effects in vivo with σ agonists such as SKF 10,047 [3], and which may be tritiated to a high specific activity, may facilitate such an isolation. Phencyclidine may also produce effects mediated by opiate receptors besides the σ type, however [24].

OPIATE RECEPTORS AND PAIN

Clearly, the physiology of opiate receptors and their ligands is at an early stage of study but is already complex. Important nonopioid analgesia systems have also been defined. While certain areas of consensus are clear, many observations defy unification in a coherent model of opiate receptor modulation of pain [25].

Of the four receptor types described, only the σ receptor does not appear to have potential for development of clinically useful analgesics. At the other extreme is the μ receptor, which may be activated by morphine, β-endorphin, met-enkephalin, or enkephalin analogs with enhanced μ receptor selectivity, to produce a marked antinociceptive effect clinically and in animal models [26,27] employing heat, pressure, chemical noxia, or tooth pulp stimulation. Agonists with δ receptor specificity, such as leu-enkephalin or certain analogs, possess analgesic activity, especially against heat or chemical noxia, in many but not all studies, yet they are less potent than μ receptor agonists. The anatomic distribution of μ versus δ receptors suggests a more clear-cut involvement of the former receptor type in analgesia [17,18].

The mechanisms by which binding of μ receptor agonists to their receptor culminate in analgesia remain cloudy. Only for certain μ receptor ligands is there a good correlation between receptor binding affinity and analgesic potency. Also, evidence has recently appeared to indicate a low fractional occupancy of opiate receptors at analgesic doses of the nonspecific agonist etorphine [28]. This effect may be relevant to Pasternak's finding that opiate analgesia is correlated with activation of a subpopulation of high-affinity μ receptors, while low-affinity μ receptors mediate other opiate effects such as respiratory depression [29].

Another issue of practical significance is the likely cross-reactivity in vivo between μ and δ receptor agonism of "selective" ligands. Even without invoking such nonselectivity of ligand binding, in vivo interactions between μ and δ ligand-receptor complexes may take place. Allosteric coupling between separate δ and μ receptors [30] has been suggested by the reduction in number of ^{3}H-naloxone binding sites by leucine enkephalin and the potentiation of morphine analgesia by δ-selective peptides. Other perennial questions that further complicate evaluation of the analgesic properties of the opioids include their bioavailability within the brain and synaptosomes, their catabolism, and their interactions with other neurotransmitter systems.

As for the κ receptor, there is little question that it too can mediate clinical antinociception, and that it does so through pathways independent of μ or δ receptor subtypes [12,27]. Pentazocine, for example, is predominantly a κ receptor agonist. It is interesting that in animal models, κ receptor agonists are active in writhing, paw pressure, and teeth pulp stimulation tests—in all of

TABLE 3.1. Opiate receptors: major types, synthetic and endogenous agonists, and nociceptive importance

Receptor	Synthetic Agonists	Endogenous Agonists	Antinociceptive Effect
μ	Morphine Tyr-Pro-Phe-ProCONH$_2$ (morphiceptin) Tyr-DAla-Gly-MePhe-Met(O)-ol (FK 33,824) Tyr-DAla-Gly-MePhe-Gly-ol (DAGO)	β-Endorphin Methionine enkephalin	+ + + +
δ	Tyr-DAla-Gly-Phe-DLeu (DADLE) Tyr-DAla-Gly-Phe-NMeMetAc (Metkephamid)	Leucine enkephalin Methionine enkephalin β-Endorphin	+ + to + + +
κ	Bremazocine Ethylketazocine Ketocyclazocine	Dynorphin	+ + +
σ	N-Allylnormetazocine (SKF 10,047) Phencyclidine	?	0 to +

which μ agonists are also active. Unlike μ receptor agonists, κ receptor agonists are ineffective against thermal pain except at doses producing sedation and motor impairment [31]. This observation forms the basis for a combined method in which heat and pressure noxia are tested sequentially in individual animals in order to assess whether compounds are more μ or κ receptor-like in vivo and their respective potencies [32]. (Table 3.1)

CONCLUSION

It is likely that multiple opiate receptors normally are activated during noxious stimuli and contribute to the complex subjective effects that ensue. Recognition of receptor subtypes and their in vitro analyses, often employing analogs of endogenous opioids, has already produced analgesic drugs of clinical usefulness. Although it still is difficult to predict in vivo consequences of drug administration from in vitro studies, promising new avenues of opiate physiology and drug design have been opened up by studies of opiate receptors and their endogenous ligands. As newer, more selective reagents become available, we may expect to see clinical application of agents with fewer side effects [33], diminished addiction liability, and possibly, greater specificity for the particular cause of pain.

Preparation of this manuscript was supported in part by grants from the National Institutes of Health (AM-07028 and RR-1066 to D. B. C.). D. B. C. is a Daland Fellow of the American Philosophical Society. The authors thank Mrs. Mary Douvadjian for expert secretarial assistance.

REFERENCES

1. Martin WR, Eades CG, Thompson JA, Huppler RE, Gilbert PE. The effects of morphine- and nalorphine-like drugs in the nondependent and morphine-dependent chronic spinal dog. J Pharmacol Exp Ther 1976;197:517–32.
2. Gilbert PE, Martin WR. The effects of morphine- and nalorphine-like drugs in the nondependent, morphine-dependent and

cyclazocine-dependent spinal dog. J Pharmacol Exp Ther 1976;198:66–82.

3. Adler AW. The in vivo differentiation of opiate receptors: introduction. Life Sci 1981;28:1543–5.

4. Pert CV, Snyder SH. Opiate receptor: demonstration in nervous tissue. Science 1973;1979:1011–14.

5. Terenius L. Characteristics of the "receptor" for narcotic analgesics in synaptic plasma membrane fraction from rat brain. Acta Pharmacol Toxicol 1973;33:377–84.

6. Simon EJ, Hiller JM, Edelman I. Stereospecific binding of the potent narcotic analgesic [³H] etorphine to rat-brain homogenate. Proc Natl Acad Sci USA 1973; 70:1947–9.

7. Wong DT, Horng JS. Stereospecific interaction of opiate narcotics in binding of ³H-dihydromorphine to membranes of rat brain. Life Sci 1973;13:1543–56.

8. Hughes J, Smith TW, Kosterlitz HW, Fothergill LA, Morgan BA, Morris HR. Identification of two related pentapeptides from the brain with potent opiate agonist activity. Nature 1975;258:577–9.

9. Stahl KD, van Bever W, Janssen P, Simon EJ. Receptor affinity and pharmacological potency of a series of narcotic analgesic, antidiarrheal and neuroleptic drugs. Eur J Pharmacol 1977;46:199–205.

10. Kuhar MJ, Pert CB, Snyder SH. Regional distribution of opiate receptor binding in human and monkey brain. Nature 1973; 245:447–50.

11. Simon EJ, Hiller JM, Groth J, Edelman I. Further properties of stereospecific opiate-binding sites in rat brain: on the nature of the sodium effect. J. Pharmacol Exp Ther 1975;192:531–7.

12. Lord JAH, Waterfield AA, Hughes J, Kosterlitz HW. Endogenous opioid peptides: multiple agonists and receptors. Nature 1977;267:495–9.

13. Hutchinson M, Kosterlitz HW, Leslie FM, Waterfield AA. Assessment in the guinea-pig ileum and mouse vas deferens of benzomorphans which have strong antinociceptive activity but do not substitute for morphine in the dependent monkey. Br J Pharmacol 1975;55:541–6.

14. Chang K-J, Cuatrecasas P. Heterogeneity and properties of opiate receptors. Fed Proc 1981;40:2729–34.

15. Zukin RS, Zukin SR. Multiple opiate receptors: emerging concepts. Life Sci 1981; 29:2681–90.

16. Janssen PAJ. Stereochemical anatomy of morphinomimetics. In: Loh HH, Ross DH, eds. Neurochemical mechanisms of opiates and endorphins. 1979;20:103–29.

17. Goodman RR, Synder SH, Kuhar MJ, Young WS III. Differentiation of delta and mu receptor localizations by light microscopic autoradiography. Proc Natl Acad Sci USA 1980;77:6239–43.

18. Zhang A-Z, Pasternak GW. μ- and δ-opiate receptors: correlation with high- and low-affinity opiate binding sites. Eur J Pharmacol 1980;67:322–4.

19. Pfeiffer A, Herz A. Demonstration and distribution of an opiate-binding site in rat brain with high affinity for ethylketocyclazocine and SKF 10,047. Biochem Biophys Res Commun 1981;101:38–44.

20. Maurer R. Multiplicity of opiate receptors in different species. Neurosci Lett 1982; 30:303–7.

21. Cox BM. Endogenous opioid peptides: a guide to structures and terminology. Life Sci 1982;31:1645–58.

22. Audigier Y, Mazarguil H, Rossier J, Cros J. Met-enkephalin [Arg⁶, Phe⁷] interacts with the κ-receptors on guinea-pig ileum. Eur J Pharmacol 1980;68:237–8.

23. Chavkin C, James IF, Goldstein A. Dynorphin is a specific endogenous ligand of the κ opioid receptor. Science 1982;215:413–15.

24. Glick SD, Guido RA. Naloxone antagonism of the thermoregulatory effects of phencyclidine. Science 1982;217:1272–3.

25. Carr DB, Carr JM. Mechanisms of bone pain and the role of brain opiates in its relief. In: Stoll BA, Parbhoo SP, eds. Bone metastasis and its treatment. New York: Raven Press, 1982:375–93.

26. Gacel G, Fournie-Zaluski MC, Fellion E, Roques B. Evidence of the preferential involvement of μ receptors in analgesia using enkephalins highly selective for peripheral μ or δ receptors. J Med Chem 1981;24:1119–24.

27. Skingle M, Tyers MB. Further studies on opiate receptors that mediate antinociception: tooth pulp stimulation in the dog. Br J Pharmacol 1980;70:323–7.

28. Perry DC, Rosenbaum JS, Kurowski M, Sadee W. [³H] Etorphine receptor binding in

vivo: small fractional occupancy elicits analgesia. Mol Pharmacol 1982;21:272–9.

29. Pasternak GW. Opiate, enkephalin, and endorphin analgesia: relation to a single population of opiate receptors. Neurology (NY) 1981;31:1311–5.

30. Vaught JL, Rothman RB, Westfall TC. Mu and delta receptors: their role in analgesia and in the differential effects of opioid peptides on analgesia. Life Sci 1982;30:1443–55.

31. Tyers MB. A classification of opiate receptors that mediate antinociception in animals. Br J Pharmacol 1980;69:503–12.

32. Upton N, Sewell RDE, Spencer PSJ. Differentiation of potent μ- and κ-opiate agonists using heat and pressure antinociceptive profiles and combined potency analysis. Eur J Pharmacol 1982;78:421–9.

33. Holaday JW, Ruvio BA, Robles LE, Johnson CE, D'Amato RJ. M 154,129, a putative delta antagonist, reverses endotoxic shock without altering morphine analgesia. Life Sci 1982;31:2209–12.

4 OPIATE RECEPTORS: CLASSIFICATION AND ACTION

Robert K. Stoelting

This chapter is limited to a brief review of the classification of opiate receptors, which Dr. Carr introduced in Chapter 3, and speculation on how knowledge of these receptors may have future application to us as anesthesiologists. I also wish to speak briefly about a new concept that has been proposed with respect to the opiate receptors, namely, the dual-receptor complex.

THE OPIATE RECEPTORS

Table 4.1, which is similar to Table 3.1 (p. 14), summarizes the classification of the opiate receptors proposed by Martin [1]. Review of the literature that references this classification shows that different effects are often attributed to the same receptor. Nevertheless, currently it appears valid to

TABLE 4.1. Classification of opiate receptors*

Receptor	Effect	Agonist	Antagonist
μ (morphine)	Supraspinal analgesia Depression of ventilation Euphoria Physical dependence	β-Endorphin Morphine	Naloxone Pentazocine
δ (enkephalin)	Modulation of μ receptor activity Supraspinal analgesia	Leu-enkephalin β-Endorphin Pentazocine?	Naloxone Met-enkephalin
κ	Spinal analgesia Depression of ventilation Sedation Miosis	Dynorphin Morphine Pentazocine Nalbuphine Butorphanol	Naloxone
σ	Vasomotor stimulation Stimulation of ventilation Hallucinations Dysphoria	Not identified Pentazocine? Ketamine?	Naloxone

*According to Martin [1].

think in terms of four specific types: μ, δ, κ, and σ. By far the most studied receptor types are the μ, or morphine-preferring, and the δ, or enkephalin-preferring, receptors. As Dr. Carr pointed out, there may be subpopulations of the various opiate receptor sites with different affinities for the same agonist or antagonist. Eventually we may be able to design or select a drug that produces a specific effect without undesirable side effects. From our standpoint now, the effect to be anticipated when an agonist interacts with any of these receptors is analgesia, which is invariably associated with some undesirable side effects, such as ventilatory depression.

The endogenous agonist that probably interacts with the μ receptor is β-endorphin. A substance chemically indistinguishable from morphine has been isolated from human milk, however, suggesting that morphine or a morphine-like substance may also be an endogenous agonist for the μ receptor [2].

The main role of δ receptors is apparently that of modulating μ receptor activity. The agonist for the δ receptor appears to be leu-enkephalin. In addition, pentazocine or other agonist/antagonists may be examples of drugs that act preferentially at the δ receptors. The circulatory effects produced by shock have been blocked in animals by administering a specific δ receptor antagonist that left intact the μ receptors [3]. These observations suggest, again, that in the future we may be able to administer an opiate that selectively produces desirable effects without concomitant adverse responses.

The κ receptor also plays some role in analgesia. According to Martin's classification, this receptor is associated with some undesirable effects, such as depression of ventilation. Nevertheless, one report has described bremazocine as an agonist at the κ receptor that has analgesic potency twice that of morphine and is totally devoid of any depression of ventilation [4]. This observation again suggests that there may be drugs on the horizon that we can use to produce specific effects without achieving undesirable side effects.

THE DUAL-RECEPTOR COMPLEX

The proposed dual-receptor complex theory (Figure 4.1) [5] is the type of concept that will in the future help anesthesiologists to appreciate and pharmacologists to design drugs that produce specific effects. The theory proposes that morphine and delta receptors exist as a complex. When morphine or an agonist for the μ receptor interacts with

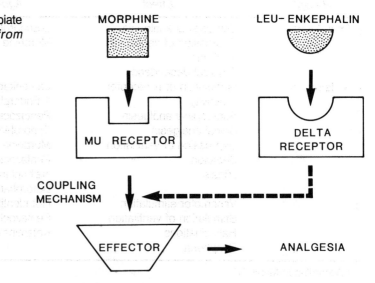

FIGURE 4.1. The proposed opiate receptor complex. *Redrawn from Vaught et al [5].*

that receptor, the result is coupling of the μ receptor with the effector, which ultimately produces analgesia. This mechanism is analogous, if you will, to the activity of the β receptor by which a catecholamine activates the adenylate cyclase system, ultimately producing a biologic response [6]. The role of the δ receptor in this complex is not to produce analgesia, but rather to modulate the activity of the coupling mechanism. Conceptually, leu-enkephalin, an agonist for the δ receptor, interacts with that receptor and facilitates the coupling mechanism of the μ receptor with its effector, producing analgesia. As a result, one may be able to potentiate analgesia produced by the μ receptor by administering a drug that facilitates the coupling mechanism. The ultimate goal when we potentiate analgesia through this mechanism—if indeed it is there—will be to do it without producing additional ventilatory depression or other adverse side effects.

CONCLUSION

An understanding of opiate receptors and their subpopulations may make available to us in the future opiates that are more specific in achieving the effects for which they are administered.

REFERENCES

1. Martin WR. History and development of mixed opioid agonists, partial agonists and antagonists. Br J Clin Pharmacol 1979; 7:273S–9S.
2. Hazum E, Sabatka JJ, Chang K-J, Brent DA, Findlay JWA, Cuatrecasas P. Morphine in cow and human milk: could dietary morphine constitute a ligand for specific morphine (mu) receptors? Science 1981;213:1010–2.
3. Holiday JW, Ruvio BA, Robles LE, Johnson ČE, D'Amato RJ. M154-129, a putative delta antagonist, reverses endotoxic shock without altering morphine analgesia. Life Sci 1982; 31:2209–12.
4. Freye E, Hartung E, Schenk GK. Bremazocine: an opiate that induces sedation and analgesia without respiratory depression. Anesth Analg (NY) 1983;62:483–8.
5. Vaught JL, Rothman RB, Westfall TC. Mu and delta receptors: their role in analgesia and in the differential effects of opioid peptides on analgesia. Life Sci 1982;30:1443–55.
6. Maze M. Clinical implications of membrane receptor function in anesthesia. Anesthesiology 1981;51:160–71.

5 AGONIST/ANTAGONIST OPIOID ANALGESICS: NALBUPHINE HYDROCHLORIDE

Nabil R. Fahmy

Nalbuphine hydrochloride (Nubain, DuPont Pharmaceuticals) is an agonist/antagonist analgesic that was synthesized in 1965 by Endo Laboratories. Chemically, it is (—)-17-(cyclobutylmethyl)-5,5α-epoxymorphinan-3, 6α,14-triol hydrochloride (Figure 5.1). The empiric formula of the base is $C_{21}H_{27}NO_4$ (molecular weight, 357) and it is structurally related to the pure opioid agonist oxymorphone and the pure antagonist naloxone.

ANIMAL PHARMACOLOGY

Opioid Agonist Activity

Subcutaneous nalbuphine was found to be (on a weight basis) about equally as or slightly more potent than morphine, at least twice as potent as pentazocine, and five times as potent as codeine in the phenylquinone writhing test in mice and rats [1]. Like other agonist/antagonist analgesics, nalbuphine shows little or no analgesic effect in the hot-plate test in mice and does not induce the Straub tail in mice or narcosis in rats [1]. These actions are specific to morphine and other agonist analgesics. Intrathecal nalbuphine, however, was about 35 times less potent than morphine in inhibiting acetic acid-induced writhing in rats [2]. It was about half as potent as morphine and about twice as potent as pentazocine in antagonizing contractions of the longitudinal muscles of the isolated guinea pig ileum [3]. Nalbuphine decreased the minimum alveolar concentration (MAC) of cyclopropane by 22% in rats [4]. No additional reduction in anesthetic requirements occurred with increasing doses. In comparison, subcutaneous morphine reduced MAC by 54%. In dogs, nalbuphine or butorphanol decreased enflurane MAC to a lesser extent than morphine [5]. The agonist/antagonist drugs, however, showed a ceiling effect at a much lower maximum extent of MAC reduction (8% to 11%) than was achievable with morphine (63%). The reason for the large discrepancy between the studies is not clear. It might be related to species differences, to different effects of the two anesthetics, or to other unknown factors.

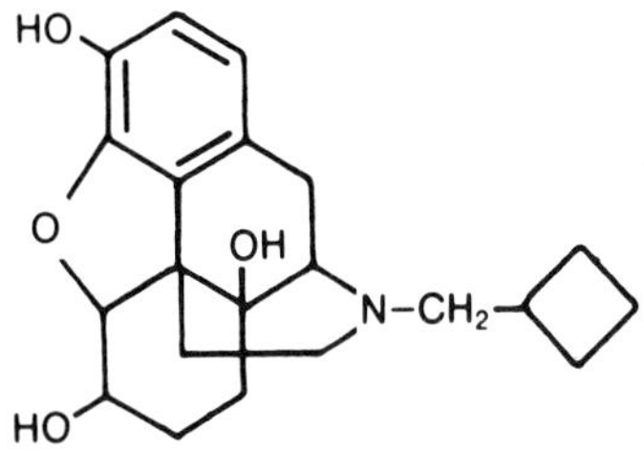

HO

OH

N–CH$_2$–

Nalbuphine

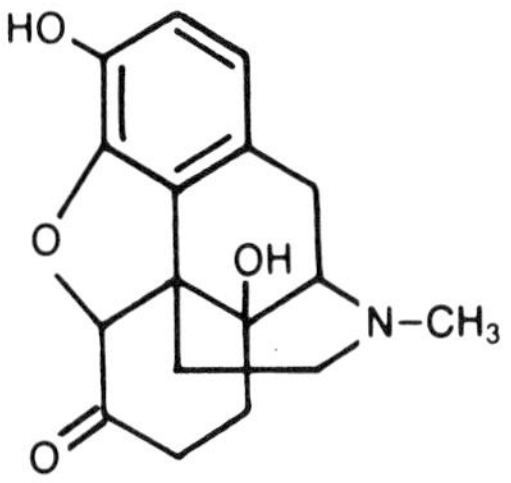

HO

OH

N–CH$_3$

O

Oxymorphone

HO

OH

N–CH$_2$–CH=CH$_2$

O

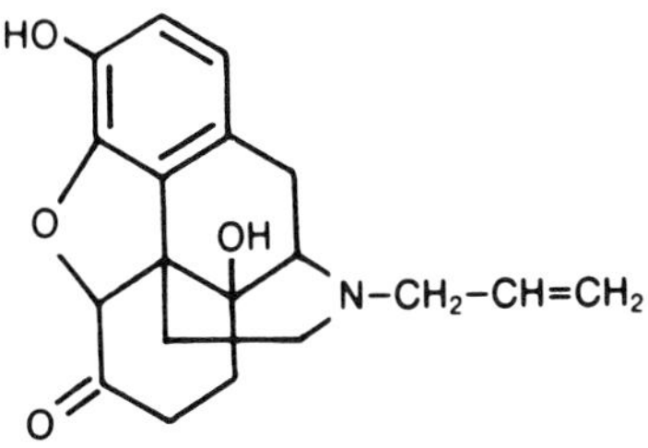

Naloxone

FIGURE 5.1. Structural formulas for nalbuphine, oxymorphone, and naloxone.

Opioid Antagonist Activity

The opioid antagonist activity of nalbuphine has been demonstrated in mice, rats, rabbits, and monkeys. In mice, nalbuphine was 11 times as potent as pentazocine, 0.26 times as potent as nalorphine, and 0.04 times as potent as naloxone in blocking induction of the Straub tail by morphine [1]. Oxymorphone-induced loss of righting reflex in rats and respiratory depression in rabbits were also counteracted by nalbuphine [1]. In morphine-dependent rhesus monkeys, nalbuphine precipitated abstinence signs [6]. The drug was about three times more potent a narcotic antagonist than pentazocine, and about four times less potent than nalorphine, in the mouse jumping test [7].

Other Effects in Animals

The behavioral and autonomic effects (including those on blood pressure, respiration, and temperature) of nalbuphine are minimal in several animal species. It produces electroencephalographic patterns in the monkey that are distinguishable from those of pure agonists and pure antagonists [8].

CLINICAL PHARMACOLOGY

Nalbuphine probably acts at the μ and κ receptors. In human beings, the observation that the drug produces very few dysphoric effects suggests that, unlike other agonist/antagonist opioids, it does not act to a significant extent on σ receptors.

Opiate Effects and Analgesic Potency in Humans

The safety and efficacy of nalbuphine as an analgesic for the management of moderate to severe pain have been documented by several studies. The drug acts within 2 to 3 minutes after intravenous administration and in less than 15 minutes after subcutaneous or intramuscular injection. The duration of analgesic effects ranges from 3 to 6 hours.

When intravenously administered nalbuphine and morphine were compared in experimentally induced tourniquet pain in six healthy volunteers, doses of 0.15 mg per kilogram of body weight of either drug resulted in equivalent pain tolerance [9]. Successive 0.15 mg/kg doses of either agent caused a steady increase in pain tolerance only with morphine. Use of nalbuphine in (acute) postoperative pain showed that the drug was as potent as or only slightly less potent than morphine; nalbuphine at 11 to

13 mg equaled morphine at 10 mg [10]. In another study [11] in which intravenous nalbuphine and pentazocine were compared in 100 patients with postoperative pain, nalbuphine was found to be about three times as potent as pentazocine, and had a slightly longer duration of action.

As preoperative medications, nalbuphine and morphine in doses of 0.1 and 0.15 mg/kg were equianalgesic, and both drugs were more effective at the higher dose level [12]. In chronic pain studies in orthopedic and cancer patients, the analgesic effect of nalbuphine was comparable to that of morphine on a weight basis without overt evidence of development of physical tolerance [13].

In analgesic-supplemented (balanced) anesthesia, nalbuphine offers several advantages over morphine [14], including cardiovascular stability, adequate postoperative ventilation, rapid recovery of wakefulness, lower frequency of nausea and vomiting, and a shorter stay in the recovery room. Mean total dose requirements are usually 1 mg/kg (compared with 0.5 mg/kg of morphine) with a range of 0.5 to 3 mg/kg.

Opioid Antagonist Activity in Humans

The opioid antagonist properties of nalbuphine and nalorphine were compared in healthy subjects who were physically dependent upon 60 mg of morphine per day. It was found that nalbuphine-induced abstinence syndrome was indistinguishable from that produced by nalorphine; nalbuphine was about 25% as potent an antagonist as nalorphine on a weight basis [15].

Intravenous nalbuphine, 0.1 mg/kg, effectively reduced the respiratory depression induced by oxymorphone, 1.5 mg, in healthy volunteers [16]. A modest additional reduction occurred when naloxone, 0.4 mg, was then given. Opioid-induced respiratory depression was reversed with nalbuphine in other studies [4,17]. Administration of nalbuphine to patients receiving chronic treatment with potent opioids or to drug addicts can precipitate withdrawal symptoms [18].

Respiratory Effects

Premedication with intramuscular or intravenous nalbuphine or morphine was associated with a similar degree of respiratory depression [12,19]. Furthermore, intravenous administration of either drug to persons who were healthy or patients who had had myocardial infarction produced similar degrees of respiratory depression in doses up to 0.15 mg/kg [9,20,21].

Depression of ventilation by nalbuphine, however (unlike morphine and other opioid analgesics), appears to reach a level beyond which additional depression does not readily occur. Studies in rats indicate that the arterial carbon dioxide tension ($PaCO_2$) reached a plateau at doses between 20 and 50 μg/kg/min [4]. It then remained unchanged until the infusion rate increased to 200 μg/kg/min, where further increments of $PaCO_2$ occurred. Similarly, in nine healthy volunteers, intravenous nalbuphine, 0.1 mg/kg, produced a modest degree of respiratory depression that did not increase when the dose was increased to 0.5 or 1 mg/kg [16]. Romagnoli and Keats [20] reported that a single 10-mg/70 kg intravenous dose of either nalbuphine or morphine produced similar onset, degree, and duration of respiratory depression in 23 healthy subjects. Administration of incremental doses of 10 mg/70 kg at hourly intervals resulted in significantly greater depression with morphine. Respiratory depression with nalbuphine reached a ceiling in the 30- to 60-mg/70 kg dose range, beyond which further increases in dose did not cause additional depression of ventilation [20].

Hemodynamic Effects

Nalbuphine does not produce important alterations in hemodynamic variables. Administration of the drug to relieve the pain of acute myocardial infarction was associated with minimal effects on cardiovascular function [21]. Similarly, no significant change in hemodynamics was observed after intravenous administration of 10 mg of either morphine or nalbuphine to patients undergoing cardiac catheterization [22]. Intravenous nalbuphine was associated with hemodynamic stability when used as an adjunct to nitrous oxide–relaxant anesthesia [14]. A stable circulation may be partly related to minimal histamine release by nalbuphine [23]. This is in contrast to morphine, which liberates measurable amounts of histamine [24]. The adminstration of higher incremental doses of nalbuphine (up to 2 or 3 mg/kg intravenously) to patients with coronary or valvular heart disease as part of balanced anesthesia did not result in significant hemodynamic alterations [25]. The hemodynamic effects of nalbuphine differ from those of pentazocine and butorphanol, which increase pulmonary artery pressure and cardiac workload [26].

Dependence Liability

The long-term administration of agonist/antagonist opioid analgesics produces physical dependence that is qualitatively different from that observed with the pure agonist (morphine-like) analgesics [27,28]. The withdrawal symptoms are milder and there is less drug-seeking behavior. Nalbuphine is less likely than opioid agonists to produce euphoria in the usual analgesic doses; it precipitated moderate to severe abstinence symptoms in morphine-dependent mice.

Its abuse potential was evaluated in eight previous opiate users in whom increasing single doses were administered [15]. The subjects were given 8, 24, and 72 mg/70 kg of nalbuphine with 10 and 30 mg/70 kg of morphine and placebo, subcutaneously, in a double-blind crossover study. Drug administrations were separated by at least one week. Nalbuphine at the 8- and 24-mg/70 kg levels was identified as "opiate-like" but the subjects indicated it to be "barbiturate-like" at the 72-mg/70 kg level. In another study [15], six individuals were given increasing doses of nalbuphine over a maximum of 51 days. Total daily doses in excess of 142 mg/70 kg caused headaches, difficulty in concentration, bizarre thoughts, irritability, nervousness, blurring of vision, depression, and strange dreams. Two subjects had psychotomimetic symptoms at daily doses above 147 mg/70 kg and refused further drug until the symptoms subsided. The authors estimated the abuse potential of nalbuphine to be similar to that of pentazocine but less than that of codeine or propoxyphene. Studies with long-term (up to six months) administration of oral nalbuphine (alone or in combination with aspirin or paracetamol) revealed that withdrawal symptoms occurred only rarely after abrupt discontinuation of drug administration (DuPont Pharmaceuticals; data on file). It is noteworthy that, unlike buprenorphine, the effects of nalbuphine can be reversed by naloxone [1].

Toxicity Studies

Acute toxicity with nalbuphine is relatively low in animals, and death occurs when very large multiples of the usual human analgesic dose are used. Chronic subcutaneous administration to rats and dogs may cause reversible hair loss at body sites distant from injection sites (DuPont Pharmaceuticals; data on file). This has not been reported in humans at doses as high as 4 mg/kg/day for up to 51 days. Chronic administration of nalbuphine to rats and rabbits does not impair fertility and general reproductive performance, and there is no evidence of embryotoxicity or teratogenesis (DuPont Pharmaceuticals; data on file).

Pharmacokinetics

Very few data are available on the pharmacokinetic properties of nalbuphine, particularly in humans.

It is rapidly absorbed after subcutaneous administration to rats and dogs. Plasma half-life values for these animals are 12 minutes and 8.3 hours respectively. The significantly shorter half-life of nalbuphine in the rat is due primarily to a more rapid rate of metabolism. The pharmacokinetic profile and peak plasma levels after five daily subcutaneous doses in dogs do not differ from those observed after a single dose, suggesting that this agent does not accumulate in tissues and that enzyme induction and saturation do not occur. In human beings, peak plasma levels of 48 ng/ml occur 30 minutes after an intramuscular dose of 10 mg. Although studies with other routes of administration have not been reported, delayed absorption after subcutaneous or oral administration in humans is unlikely, based on the reported onset of analgesic effects [29–31].

The elimination half-life is about 5 hours in healthy subjects and 3 to 3.5 hours after incremental intravenous doses to a total dose of 2 to 3 mg/kg in patients undergoing cardiac surgery. There are no data on elimination of nalbuphine in the presence of hepatic or renal disease.

The ratio of parenteral to oral nalbuphine in equianalgesic doses (about 1:5 or 1:6) suggests substantial first-pass biotransformation [29].

Nalbuphine and its metabolites are excreted in both urine and feces; fecal excretion is the major route of elimination and results largely from biliary excretion. In humans, 7% of administered nalbuphine is excreted in urine as unchanged drug, its conjugates, and two metabolic products, namely, 14-hydroxy-7,8-dihydronormorphine and 14-hydroxy-7, 8-dihydro-N-cyclobutylmethyl-nor-morphine.

THERAPEUTIC USES

Anesthesia

Intramuscular nalbuphine for premedication was compared with a placebo in a double-blind study in pediatric patients [32]. Significant improvement in the children's emotional state was found at induction of anesthesia and in the postoperative period. In adult patients, preoperative use of nalbuphine or morphine produced comparable degrees of analgesia and sedation [12,19].

A dose of 1 mg/kg of nalbuphine is usually adequate as a supplement to nitrous oxide-relaxant (balanced) anesthesia [14]. Nalbuphine was evaluated in an open study in 150 patients as a component of balanced anesthesia [33]. Patients received 3 to 5 mg/kg of sodium thiopental, 2.5 to 7.5 mg of droperidol, muscle relaxants, and nitrous oxide, 50%. An initial dose of 0.5 to 0.75 mg/kg nalbuphine was given, followed by an additional dose of 0.25 mg/kg prior to surgical incision. In procedures lasting longer than 90 minutes, an additional 0.25 mg/kg was given every 30 minutes. The authors noted adequate suppression of reflex activity during the operation, stable cardiovascular values, and minimal respiratory depression.

Use of a combination of nalbuphine and lorazepam prior to ophthalmic procedures performed under local anesthesia was well tolerated by most patients, with lack of recall of operative events in 20 of 30 cases [34].

Reversal of Respiratory Depression

Nalbuphine, 0.1 mg/kg, was given as a single intravenous dose to reverse postoperative respiratory depression after oxymorphone or hydromorphone balanced anesthesia. Respiratory depression was rapidly reversed without apparent reversal of analgesia. Renarcotization did not occur [17].

Pain Relief

In a comparison of intramuscular morphine and nalbuphine for relief of postoperative pain, peak analgesia obtained with nalbuphine was slightly less than that with morphine, nalbuphine being about 0.7 to 0.8 times as potent as morphine when analgesia was calculated [10]. Comparison of the two using parallel study groups of postoperative pediatric patients showed comparable degrees of analgesia [35].

In a double-blind crossover study of patients with postoperative pain, nalbuphine was about three times as potent as pentazocine on a weight basis after intramuscular or intravenous administration. Peak effects (60 minutes after intramuscular administration and 30 minutes after intravenous injection) were similar for both drugs [11,13].

Subcutaneously administered nalbuphine and morphine were compared in a multiple-dose, double-blind parallel group study in patients with pain of advanced malignancy. The author concluded that the analgesic potency of nalbuphine was comparable to that of subcutaneous morphine [18].

Waye and Braunfeld [36] reported that nalbuphine was less effective than meperidine in patients undergoing colonoscopy.

Parenteral nalbuphine is also effective in pain relief during labor, acute myocardial infarction, and a variety of medical conditions including renal and biliary colic.

Oral Nalbuphine

Oral nalbuphine, 15 and 45 mg, was compared with intramuscular nalbuphine, 3 and 9 mg, in 104 patients with postoperative pain [29]. The authors believe the oral drug to be one-fourth to one-third as potent as intramuscular drug in total analgesic effect and 10% as potent in peak analgesic effect. In another study in patients with postoperative pain, the oral agent was about three times as potent as oral codeine [30].

Side Effects

Sedation is the most frequently observed adverse effect during nalbuphine administration. Its overall incidence is about 36%. Nausea and vomiting are experienced by about 6% of patients and are less frequent than with morphine, meperidine, or pentazocine. Therapeutic doses of nalbuphine produce respiratory depression similar in degree to that observed with usual doses of morphine. The ceiling observed on depression of respiration may limit the respiratory

depressant liability of large analgesic doses for severe pain. Psychotomimetic reactions (hallucinations, dysphoria, feeling of unreality, distorted body image, and depersonalization) are of low frequency, in marked contrast to the situation with pentazocine. In a comparative double-blind crossover study, 52% of patients (14 of 27) receiving 60 mg of pentazocine intramuscularly experienced psychotomimetic reactions as compared with 7% (4 of 56) receiving 10 or 20 mg of nalbuphine intramuscularly [13]. Other reactions encountered in 5% or fewer of patients included sweaty and clammy sensations, dizziness and vertigo, dry mouth, and headache. No data are available on acute or chronic toxicity in humans. Tissue damage at injection sites has not been described. Subjects receiving 40 mg of intramuscular nalbuphine per day for seven days had elevated values on liver function tests [37]. The significance of this study is questionable, however, because the study group consisted of previous narcotic users who had elevated predrug values in most cases. There are no reported cases of nalbuphine overdosage.

CONCLUSIONS

Nalbuphine is an effective analgesic with opioid agonist and antagonist properties. It is effective in alleviating moderate to severe postoperative pain, pain of malignancies, and pain associated with some medical disorders. It is a useful analgesic adjunct in balanced anesthesia provided adequate doses (0.5 to 3 mg/kg) are used. It can reverse respiratory depression after balanced anesthesia with opioid agonists.

In equianalgesic doses, nalbuphine has about the same onset, peak, and duration of action as morphine. Distinct advantages over morphine include minimal histamine release, hemodynamic stability, lower abuse potential, a ceiling effect for respiratory depression, and less prevalence of nausea and vomiting. Nalbuphine is superior to pentazocine in that it is associated with a lower incidence of psychotomimetic reactions, maintains circulatory homeostasis, and has a longer duration of action. Compared with butorphanol, it does not increase pulmonary arterial pressure and has a lower frequency of psychotomimetic effects. Buprenorphine, an agonist/antagonist opioid analgesic, produces prolonged respiratory depression that cannot be reversed by naloxone. Nalbuphine does not cause chest wall rigidity even in very high doses.

Further studies are required to determine the use of nalbuphine in labor and its potential effects on the fetus. Also, reports of clinical experience are needed to establish clearly the drug's usefulness for long-term administration in patients with chronic pain.

REFERENCES

1. Blumberg H, Dayton HB, Wolf PS. Analgesic properties of the narcotic antagonist EN-2234A. Pharmacologist 1968;10:201.
2. Schmauss C, Doherty C, Yaksh TL. The analgesic effects of an intrathecally administered partial opiate agonist, nalbuphine hydrochloride. Eur J Pharmacol 1983;86:1–7.
3. Kosterlitz HW, Waterfield AA, Berthoud V. Assessment of the agonist and antagonist properties of narcotic analgesic drugs by their actions on the morphine receptor in the guinea pig ileum. In: Braude MC, Harris LS, May EL, et al, eds. Narcotic antagonists. New York: Raven Press, 1973:319–34.
4. DiFazio CA, Moscicki JC, Magruder MR. Anesthetic potency of nalbuphine and interaction with morphine in rats. Anesth Analg (Cleve) 1981;60:629–33.
5. Murphy MR, Hug CC Jr. The enflurane-sparing effect of morphine, butorphanol, and nalbuphine. Anesthesiology 1982;57:489–92.
6. Villarreal JE, Karbowski MG. The actions of narcotic antagonists in morphine-dependent rhesus monkeys. Adv Biochem Psychopharmacol 1974;8:273–89.
7. Cowan A. Use of the mouse jumping test for estimating antagonistic potencies of morphine antagonists. J Pharmacol Pharmacodyn 1976;28:177–82.
8. Gehrmann JE, Killam KF Jr. Assessment of CNS drug activity in rhesus monkeys by analysis of the EEG. Fed Proc 1976;35:2258–63.
9. Gal TJ, DiFazio CA, Moscicki JC. Analgesic and respiratory depressant activity of nalbuphine: a comparison with morphine. Anesthesiology 1982;57:367–74.
10. Beaver WT, Feise GA. A comparison of the analgesic effect of intramuscular nalbuphine and morphine in patients with postoperative pain. J Pharmacol Exp Ther 1978;204:487–96.
11. Tammisto T, Tigerstedt I. Comparison of the analgesic effects of intravenous nalbuphine and pentazocine in patients with postoperative pain. Acta Anaesthesiol Scand 1977;21:390–4.
12. Fahmy NR. Nalbuphine as a premedicant drug. A clinical evaluation. Abstracts of scientific papers, Annual Meeting of the American Society of Anesthesiologists 1977:53–4.
13. Houde RW, Wallenstein SL, Rogers A, Kaiko RF. Annual report of the analgesic studies section of the Memorial Sloan-Kettering Cancer Center. Problems of Drug Dependency Committee Proceedings 1976;149–68.
14. Fahmy NR. Nalbuphine in "balanced" anesthesia: its analgesic efficacy and hemodynamic effects. Anesthesiology 1980;53:S66.
15. Jasinski DR, Mansky PA. Evaluation of nalbuphine for abuse potential. Clin Pharmacol Ther 1972;13:78–90.
16. Julien RM. Effects of nalbuphine on normal and oxymorphone-depressed ventilatory responses to carbon dioxide challenge. Anesthesiology 1982;57:A320.
17. Magruder MR, Delaney RD, DiFazio CA. Reversal of narcotic-induced respiratory depression with nalbuphine hydrochloride. Anesthesiol Rev 1982;9:34–7.
18. Stambaugh JE. Evaluation of nalbuphine. Efficacy and safety in the management of chronic pain associated with advanced malignancy. Curr Ther Res 1982;31:393–401.
19. Fragen RJ, Caldwell N. Acute intravenous premedication with nalbuphine. Anesth Analg (Cleve) 1977;56:808–12.
20. Romagnoli A, Keats AS. Ceiling effect for respiratory depression by nalbuphine. Clin Pharmacol Ther 1980;27:478–85.

21. Lee G, Low RI, Amsterdam EA, et al. Hemodynamic effects of morphine and nalbuphine in acute myocardial infarction. Clin Pharmacol Ther 1981;29:576–81.

22. Romagnoli A, Keats AS. Comparative hemodynamic effects of nalbuphine and morphine in patients with coronary artery disease. Bull Texas Heart Inst 1978;5:19–24.

23. Fahmy NR, Sunder N, Soter NA. A comparison of histamine-releasing properties and hemodynamic effects of morphine and nalbuphine in humans. Anesth Analg (NY) 1984;64:210.

24. Fahmy NR, Sunder N, Soter NA. Role of histamine in the hemodynamic and plasma catecholamine responses to morphine. Clin Pharmacol Ther 1983;33:615–20.

25. Lake CL, Duckworth EN, DiFazio CA, Durbin CG, Magruder MR. Cardiovascular effects of nalbuphine in patients with coronary or valvular heart disease. Anesthesiology 1982;57:498–503.

26. Heel RC, Brogden RN, Speight TM, Avery GS. Butorphanol: a review of its pharmacological properties and therapeutic efficacy. Drugs 1978;16:473–505.

27. Isbell H. The search for the nonaddicting analgesic: has it been worth it? Clin Pharmacol Ther 1977;22:377–84.

28. Jasinski DR. Human pharmacology of narcotic antagonists. Br J Clin Pharmacol 1979;7:287S–90S.

29. Beaver WT, Feise GA, Robb D. Analgesic effect of intramuscular and oral nalbuphine in postoperative pain. Clin Pharmacol Ther 1981;29:174–80.

30. Okun R. Analgesic effects of oral nalbuphine and codeine in patients with postoperative pain. Clin Pharmacol Ther 1982;32:517–24.

31. Sunshine A, Zighelboim I, de Sarrazin C, de Castro A, Olson NZ, Laska E. A study of the analgesic efficacy of nalbuphine hydrochloride in patients with postpartum pain. Curr Ther Res 1983;33:108–14.

32. Rita L, Seleny F, Goodarzi M. Comparison of the calming and sedative effects of nalbuphine and pentazocine for paediatric premedication. Can Anaesth Soc J 1980;27:546–9.

33. Magruder MR, Christofforetti R, DiFazio CA. Balanced anesthesia with nalbuphine hydrochloride. Anesthesiol Rev 1980;7:25–9.

34. Hofmann RF, Weiler HH. Lorazepam and nalbuphine as local anesthetic ophthalmic surgery premedications. Ann Ophthalmol 1983;15:64–6.

35. Bikhazi GB. Comparison of morphine and nalbuphine in postoperative pediatric patients. Anesthesiol Rev 1978;5:34–6.

36. Waye JD, Braunfeld SF. A randomized double-blind study of nalbuphine as an analgesic for colonoscopy. Gastrointest Endosc 1982;28:86–7.

37. Elliott HW, Navarro G, Nomof M. A double-blind controlled study of the pharmacological effects of nalbuphine (EN-2234A). J Med 1970;1:74–89.

6 CLINICAL APPLICATIONS OF A NARCOTIC ANTAGONIST: NALBUPHINE

Carl C. Hug, Jr.

Nalbuphine, a narcotic antagonist analgesic, has had limited but promising application as a supplement to other agents in producing general anesthesia and postoperatively in reducing ventilatory depression and pain. This chapter reviews clinical experience and what it suggests about the potential and limitations of nalbuphine in anesthesia practice.

INTRAOPERATIVE APPLICATIONS

Dr. Fahmy has reviewed the clinical experience showing that nalbuphine can substitute for morphine as an analgesic (see Chapter 5). With a combination of drugs, including nalbuphine, hemodynamic stability was achieved and the patients appeared to recover somewhat more rapidly after nalbuphine than after morphine.

One might raise the question whether nalbuphine alone could be used in place of a pure agonist such as fentanyl to achieve the anesthetic objectives of unconsciousness or profound analgesia and suppression of somatic, autonomic, and hemodynamic responses to noxious stimulation. I think the answer is no. The data that support this negative response to the question are as follows.

Murphy and I [1] showed that the ability of nalbuphine (and also of butorphanol) to reduce the anesthetic requirements for enflurane (i.e., the minimal alveolar concentration, MAC, of enflurane) was much more limited than that of pure agonists. That is, maximum reductions of enflurane MAC were less than 10% to 15%. In other words, there was a very low ceiling on the anesthetic actions of the agonist/antagonists.

The limited effectiveness of nalbuphine and butorphanol as primary anesthetic agents was also evident in patients undergoing anesthesia for coronary artery surgery. Lake and colleagues [2] administered nalbuphine in doses as high as 2 mg per kilogram of body weight. Although the patients exhibited fairly stable hemodynamics during and after the administration of nalbuphine, not all were asleep after this dose. Even after the addition of diazepam and nitrous oxide, changes in hemodynamics were evident in some patients in response to surgical incision.

Some of my colleagues at Emory University Hospital examined butorphanol as a primary anesthetic agent for patients about to undergo coronary artery surgery [3]. After doses as high as 0.3 mg/kg (equivalent to a 1.5-mg/kg dose of morphine in terms of relative analgesic potencies), none of the patients was asleep and all remained capable of following commands correctly. To render the patients unconscious, they were given hypnotic drugs (diazepam, thiopental, and nitrous oxide). Even after this combination there were increases in systemic blood pressure and in pulmonary capillary wedge pressure in response to noxious stimulation. It appeared that butorphanol in large doses and in combination with other drugs was unable to suppress the autonomic and cardiovascular responses to noxious stimulation.

Thus it appears that moderate doses of the agonist/antagonist analgesics can be used successfully to supplement other drugs in producing general anesthesia, but they cannot serve as primary anesthetic agents.

POSTOPERATIVE APPLICATIONS

An additional application of agonist/antagonists currently under investigation involves the use of these agents in the postoperative period. This application does not represent a new concept; in fact, Bellville and Fleishli [4] first demonstrated the interaction of a pure agonist (morphine) and an agonist/antagonist (nalorphine) on human ventilation more than fifteen years ago.

The concept is that a narcotic agonist interacts with an opioid receptor to produce a response. The intensity of that response is related to the number of agonist-receptor complexes formed, which in turn is proportional to the concentration of agonist present at the receptor site. Similarly, an agonist/antagonist can interact with the same receptor, but the intensity of effects produced is limited, and further increases in the concentration of agonist/antagonist at the receptor site do not result in any greater degree of effect. If both types of drugs (agonist and agonist/antagonist) are present at the same time in the area of opioid receptors, the number of receptors occupied by either drug will be proportional to their relative concentrations. It is conceivable that if a sufficiently high

concentration of an agonist/antagonist were present, it would essentially occupy all of the receptors and exert its maximum ceiling effect, and at the same time exclude the pure agonist from associating with the opioid receptor.

We can conceive of an application of this concept in the postoperative period following high-dose narcotic anesthesia. For example, after very large doses of fentanyl, there is often prolonged ventilatory depression. We know that we can use a pure antagonist to restore spontaneous ventilation, but we also recognize that there are risks associated with the use of drugs such as naloxone. Perhaps we could use an agonist/antagonist type of analgesic to reduce the degree of ventilatory depression to an acceptable level while preserving analgesia and preventing adverse side effects such as hypertension, tachycardia, and the unmasking of pain.

Dr. Roach and some of our colleagues at Emory University Hospital have been examining this possible application of nalbuphine in patients after coronary artery surgery [5]. To date we have examined 21 patients in the intensive care unit. The first group of 11 patients received a total dose of fentanyl approximating 120 µg/kg and also received diazepam during the course of anesthesia and surgery. A second group of 10 patients received fentanyl alone in a dose approximating 100 µg/kg. After the patients were reasonably stable in terms of hemodynamics, body temperature, acid-base balance, and so on, they were examined for the possibility of discontinuing ventilatory support and against the criteria for extubation. If they were unable to maintain an arterial partial pressure of carbon dioxide (P_{CO_2}) less than 50 mm Hg, they received nalbuphine in incremental doses of 15 µg/kg.

In the first group of patients, a total nalbuphine dose of 66 µg/kg was required to allow the patients to maintain spontaneous ventilation with an arterial P_{CO_2} less than 48 mm Hg. In the second group of patients, who received only fentanyl, the average dose of nalbuphine required to restore acceptable spontaneous ventilation was 46 μg/kg. These preliminary results suggest the concept originally demonstrated by Bellville and Fleischli [4] may be applicable to patients receiving large doses of narcotic analgesics for anesthetic purposes. Incidentally, one other group of investigators has been examining the application of nalbuphine in the antagonism of ventilatory depression in the postoperative period after the use of narcotic analgesics for anesthesia [6].

Of concern in our study was the possibility that adverse hemodynamic and other side effects would be produced by the administration of this narcotic agonist/antagonist. All but 1 of the 21 patients had preservation of analgesia after the initial administration of nalbuphine. At a later time some of the patients complained of pain and additional doses of nalbuphine were administered with satisfactory relief of that pain. One of the patients did not achieve satisfactory pain relief with additional doses of nalbuphine, nor did he experience relief after the administration of morphine at any time during the remaining seven days of his hospital stay. One wonders whether or not any analgesic would have been successful in controlling his discomfort.

With regard to hemodynamic changes, four patients exhibited some elevation of blood pressure immediately after the administration of nalbuphine. In three cases the peak systolic blood pressure did not exceed the maximum systolic blood pressure recorded in the preoperative period. One of the patients exhibited a systolic blood pressure slightly higher than the preoperative level after nalbuphine, but the elevation was brief and readily controlled by the administration of a vasodilator.

CONCLUSION

It seems worthwhile undertaking an appropriately randomized and controlled study of the use of nalbuphine in the postoperative period to antagonize excessive ventilatory depressant effects from residual narcotics administered in high doses for anesthetic purposes. These preliminary data suggest that it is feasible to reduce the degree of ventilatory depression to an acceptable level while preserving adequate analgesia. Of course, even modest degrees of ventilatory depression may be unacceptable in some patients for whom any degree of hypercapnia is contraindicated.

It appears that the agonist/antagonist nalbuphine has two potential applications of interest to the anesthesiologist: (a) as a supplement to other anesthetic drugs and (b) in the postoperative period for the antagonism of excessive ventilatory depression due to narcotic analgesics while preserving adequate degrees of analgesia.

REFERENCES

1. Murphy MR, Hug CC Jr. The enflurane sparing effect of morphine, butorphanol, and nalbuphine. Anesthesiology 1982;57:489–92.
2. Lake CL, Duckworth EN, DiFazio CA, Durbin CG, Magruder MR. Cardiovascular effects of nalbuphine in patients with coronary or valvular heart disease. Anesthesiology 1982;57:498–503.
3. Moldenhauer CC, Hug CC Jr, Nagle DM, Youngberg JA. High-dose butorphanol in anesthesia for aortocoronary bypass surgery. Abstracts of the Third Annual Meeting of the Society of Cardiovascular Anesthesiologists, San Francisco, May 10–13, 1981:59–60.
4. Bellville JW, Fleischli G. The interaction of morphine and nalorphine on respiration. Clin Pharmacol Ther 1968;9:152–62.
5. Roach GW, Moldenhauer CC, Finlayson DC, Hug CC Jr, Kopel ME, Tobia V, Kelly S. Nalbuphine reversal of respiratory depression following high dose fentanyl anesthesia. Abstracts of the Fifth Annual Meeting of the Society of Cardiovascular Anesthesiologists, San Diego, April 24–27, 1983:140–1.
6. Magruder MR, Delaney RD, DiFazio CA. Reversal of narcotic-induced respiratory depression with nalbuphine hydrochloride. Anesthesiol Rev 1982;9:34–7.

Part I DISCUSSION

DR. J.G. REVES: I have two questions. First, when we discuss agonist/antagonist drugs, do we know the particular receptor sites where agonistic and antagonistic effects occur? My second concerns the ceiling effect, which is a very interesting phenomenon, particularly with regard to respiration. My question is, does one drug (agonist) occupy one type of receptor while another drug (antagonist) works at a different receptor?

DR. ROBERT K. STOELTING: It is my understanding that potent narcotics such as morphine and fentanyl act as pure agonists at the μ receptors. Agonist/antagonist drugs are thought to act at loci other than the μ receptors, specifically, at the δ, κ, and even σ receptors. It is not clear whether these drugs act specifically on just one receptor type, and it has been proposed that they may act at all three receptors in one way or another. For example, drugs such as pentazocine seem to exert their effects at the δ and κ receptors, and the goal of producing relatively pure analgesia with few or no respiratory side effects seems to involve stimulating the κ receptors.

DR. DANIEL B. CARR: Agonist/antagonist is a confusing term when we are speaking of a single compound acting upon one receptor subtype. As Dr. Stoelting indicated, these drugs are thought to act through different receptor subtypes, and I would say the rule rather than the exception is that several of these agents may act at the same receptors. Dr. Martin used what I think is a much clearer term in the review he published in 1967 entitled "Narcotic antagonists." His term was *partial agonist,* which indicates not that there is simultaneous antagonism and activation, but that the agent is only partly effective in activating the receptor complex.

DR. ARTHUR KEATS: Have you seen clinical effects with these drugs that correspond to activity in particular receptors?

DR. CARR: Yes, and as a rule we feel that the wide range of effects caused by partial agonists occurs because of their various spectra of action on different receptor subtypes rather than on one pure subtype.

DR. CARL E. ROSOW: Dr. Martin discussed what he called a dual-receptor hypothesis in the 1967 paper. At that time he was considering only two types of receptors. He stated that morphine-like drugs bind to morphine receptors. The nalorphine-like drugs also bind at morphine receptors but have no efficacy there; and by binding, and thus blocking, other substances from stimulating receptors at these sites, they act as antagonists. But then the nalorphine-like drugs also bind at a separate receptor where they produce their effect.

The clinical syndrome caused by agonist/antagonists produces a plateau effect in more than analgesia, MAC reduction, and respiratory depression. These agents also appear to cause plateauing of responses to smooth muscle stimulation and some pupillary effects. We can identify these clinical effects, but I think no one has gone so far as to identify the specific receptor sites responsible for them.

I have a question for Dr. Hug about the way we measure analgesic effects. In the laboratory, we usually use a tail-clip or hot-plate test and measure flexor withdrawal. When we calculate MAC, we also measure flexor withdrawal. The effects of nalorphine-like drugs are not detected by hot-plate or tail-plate tests, however, and likewise we cannot expect to get accurate data from a typical test of MAC. Therefore it may not be valid to measure the effects of the agents by these tests. We can observe that the drugs do not produce anesthesia in high doses, but for determining the ceiling effect, these tests may not have any relevance.

We have just completed a study on butorphenal using response to intubation as our measure. We checked for hypertension, tachycardia, and tearing, and we found no plateauing of drug effects up to 0.1 mg/kg.

DR. CARL C. HUG, JR.: Your comments are perfectly appropriate. The MAC is simply one end point, one way to quantify a drug's effects, and certainly is not representative of the spectrum of effects we hope to achieve with anesthetic drugs. By that one measurement we often can see a ceiling effect. As you mentioned, though, we cannot always achieve it to the degree possible with some of the other pure agonists.

I would like to pose a question in return. When you did the intubation response study, did you give your patients any other agents, either as premedication or administered concurrently?

DR. ROSOW: Yes. It was a double-blind comparison of morphine and butorphenal. Sleep was induced with a thiobarbiturate.

DR. HUG: The point I wanted to bring out is that since other agents were being used in these patients, drug interactions become an important consideration. For example, when a drug's effects on respiration are being studied, even such a simple change as falling asleep will alter the response dramatically. Sleep alone will depress respiration. If the two occur together there is a synergistic interaction. The same is true with drug interactions, and we haven't begun to touch the surface of that problem.

DR. PAUL F. WHITE: A question for Dr. Hug relates to the use of the agonist/antagonist compounds to reverse the residual respiratory depressant effects following high doses of narcotic analgesics. Three of ten patients developed some recurrence of narcotic effect. Could you comment on this apparent renarcotization in the light of what is known (or not known) about the pharmacokinetics of agonists/antagonists? If this is going to become an important role for the agonist/antagonist compounds, it would be useful to know what their elimination half-life values are relative to the commonly used opioid compounds.

DR. HUG: I can't comment precisely, only conceptually. The rather prolonged period of respiratory depression associated with fentanyl seems related to the rate at which the drug is eliminated from the body. Renarcotization occurred after a relatively small dose of nalbuphine. We know very little about the kinetics of that drug, but it appears that with a relatively small dose, the concentration of nalbuphine required to reverse the effects of fentanyl dropped off before enough fentanyl had been eliminated to reverse respiratory depression. With insufficient antagonist, the depressant effect returned. When additional doses of nalbuphine were given, we restored the antagonistic component of the response.

DR. THEODORE H. STANLEY: Drs. Hull and Hug have stimulated two of my irritant receptors, and I beg to disagree with some of their comments. The concept that opioids are unreliable in their ability to produce anesthesia is a distinct source of irritation. I believe this is a matter of dosage, and I would like to elicit comments on that score from the two discussants.

The second irritant receptor was activated by the correlation of studies in a way that suggests 100 µg/kg may be the same in the dog as it is in man. This is a big irritant, because we have worked with many species and found enormous differences. For instance, our studies have shown that 100 µg/kg of fentanyl is less than an ED_{10} in the dog, and that 200 µg/kg is an ED_{10} for about two minutes. The ED_{50} for unresponsiveness to a surgical (MAC-like) stimulus or something similar appears to be 750 to 1000 µg/kg in the dog. Therefore I think work involving this kind of stimulus in another species is really quite irrelevant to comparisons of the effects of similar doses in human beings.

DR. HUG: The dose of fentanyl we used produced 87% suppression of the change in heart rate and blood pressure, so I agree it was not a totally effective drug. We were not trying to produce total suppression, though. The purpose of the exercise was to demonstrate the presence or absence of tolerance. I would be the first to agree that results in the dog cannot be extrapolated to other species, and to extrapolate from anything other than the group of dogs we studied would be a mistake.

The point I'd like to make is that if we consider a graph that plots fentanyl concentration against MAC reduction, the result is a sigmoid dose curve. The implications of your statement, Dr. Stanley, are that if we discontinue fentanyl at about 100 ng/ml and continue to plot the curve far enough, we will see an upturn. That's possible, but until it is tested we don't know. Again, we are measuring only one aspect of MAC.

Most of the studies that have been done with fentanyl in very high doses have involved the presence of other drugs, however; we cannot ignore that. If we rely, for example, on the patient's recall of intraoperative events, we don't have a valid measure of the effect of fentanyl alone—we have measured the effect of fentanyl and another drug. This is an important distinction.

I agree with Dr. Stanley that we can produce unconsciousness and most of the objectives of anesthesia, although obviously not muscle relaxation, with drugs such as alfentanil and fentanyl. In practical terms, though, we need to look at the doses we are actually using and the effects we are trying to achieve, and distinguish between those we can attain with one drug alone and those that involve a drug interaction. Drug interaction is the area that really needs study and evaluation.

DR. EDMOND I. EGER, II: The sigmoid curve that Dr. Hug has just described, which perhaps explains Dr. Stanley's irritant receptor difficulties, is echoed by a study Dr. Munsen did informally several years ago. He observed that morphine and nitrous oxide each lowered the MAC for flurox-ene and other inhaled anesthetics. He thought if he could combine the two, he might achieve a suitable MAC with just nitrous oxide and mor-phine.

He tried his idea on five patients. First, he gave nitrous oxide alone and found that all five patients had a strong desire to leave the operating room when the incision was made. When he added a very low dose of morphine, 0.1 to 0.2 mg/kg, he found that only 40% to 60% of his patients had that desire. At 0.4 mg/kg, 40% to 60% of the patients still clearly wanted to leave the room. He doubled the dose once more, but still 40% to 60% of the patients wanted to escape. These re-sults are consistent with the first part of Dr. Hug's curve. Had Munsen gone farther, he might per-haps have reached an upturn in the curve.

We may be looking at two different effects of narcotics. One is an effect on opiate receptors, whereby we see an upswing in effect that then levels off as maximum activation (or inactivation) is achieved. The second is an inherent anesthetic effect completely independent of the opiate re-ceptors, similar to the effect we see with inhaled anesthetics. It occurs with all lipid-soluble drugs and perhaps with all the narcotics we are talking about—all, at least, that can enter a lipid domain in the brain. This concept bears further explora-tion.

To move to a second point, Dr. Carr suggested that we should think of the agonist/antagonists as partial agonists. Conceptually I find that very dif-ficult. We are told that a high dose of fentanyl can achieve anesthesia, but that this effect can be abolished or decreased by injection of what he would call a partial agonist. If it truly is a partial agonist, we should not see a decrease in the ago-nistic effect when it is added to another agonist. The fact that a reduction was seen would lead me to call these agents agonist/antagonists rather than partial agonists.

DR. KEATS: I have one comment related to the higher dose range of the dose-response curve: at that range, most of these drugs become convul-sants, not anesthetics. I think it's important to remember this.

DR. THEODORE C. SMITH: The concept of recep-tors is based on a number of studies with different drugs in different animals. We don't know that every animal has all the postulated receptors, and we must be cautious about assigning some theo-retical role to each drug based on a response in one species that cannot be demonstrated in an-other.

In answer to Dr. Eger's second point, it is pos-sible to conceive of a drug as being a partial ag-onist. Imagine a large number of drug molecules competing for a limited number of receptors, such that when a partial agonist is added to the system, it substitutes onto some of the receptors a ma-terial that is less efficacious at producing the re-sponse. With sufficient quantities of this drug, receptors could be occupied by very weak or in-effectual agents, which would prevent a more po-tent agonist from exerting an effect.

In fact, we have had a partial agonist in an-algesia for a long time. Codeine given to a person in pain can be a partial agonist since it may have limited efficacy in relieving the pain. Yet in a person who has received 3 to 4 mg/kg of mor-phine, the effects of morphine are diminished and the patient's ventilation improves with each sub-sequent dose of codeine.

Let me add a few words to Dr. Lowenstein's history of these agents. I believe the term *opioid* was coined by George Atcheson at the University of Cincinnati because of dissatisfaction with the usage at the time. *Opiates,* he thought, were com-pounds derived from the opium poppy, which would exclude drugs such as Demerol. *Narcotic* had long been used by pharmacologists to mean narcosis or loss of consciousness, but during the 1930s the lawyers had usurped the term to refer to drugs covered by the Harrison Narcotic Act, so *narcotic* was not a very good pharmacologic term either. Atcheson objected to the awkward-ness of saying "narcotic analgesics." So he intro-duced the term *opioid* to mean "those drugs of the family of morphine and morphine-like com-pounds."

DR. JOAN W. FLACKE: I would like to comment on Dr. Stanley's point about species differences. Al-though it is well known that dogs require much more narcotic—certainly more ketamine—and have a higher MAC for enflurane than humans do, it does not follow that, qualitatively, they act any differently. In fact, I don't believe there is any evidence that they do.

I also want to say that I think perhaps we worry too much about patients' recall of their anes-thesia. Surely it is not news to any of us that patients occasionally have recall during narcotic anesthesia, and that the frequency of recall is reduced if benzodiazepines are given concurrently. We worry about taking away the patient's ability to indicate responsiveness by moving. A recent article described a patient lightly anesthetized with halothane (no muscle relaxant) who did not move and yet had recall. Thus recall can occur with drugs other than narcotics as we administer lighter and lighter amounts of anesthesia. The difference here is that if patients receiving narcotics have recall, it is rare that they remember pain, although this too has been reported.

DR. TONY L. YAKSH: It is interesting that we speak about morphine and its action on some putative entity we call a receptor. The fact that we can ascribe an action to a receptor clearly depends upon the dosage of drug employed. Low receptor concentrations, of course, are the ones we use to define the nature of the receptor. As dosage increases, the likelihood of nonspecific action, that is, an action mediated by another receptor, increases astronomically. This again raises a question that came up earlier: what happens if there is a two-phase dose-response curve? Might it not suggest a separate site of action?

One of the ways we define receptors is by their pharmacologic profile, and so far at this conference no one has really discussed the profile of the high-dose opiates. If we were to define an opiate receptor, we would first look for cross-tolerance among a series of agents of like family and then look for the development of tolerance, as described earlier. Second, we would look for a systematic study of naloxone reversibility. If, as Dr. Eger suggested, this high-dose effect is nonspecific, that is, is not mediated by an opiate receptor, then its pharmacologic profile should indeed be distinctive.

Finally, we have very little clinical experience with agents that act at multiple sites, so it is hard to comment on their clinical significance. I would argue that, with the exception of the partial agonists, all the agents now in use act upon receptor sites similar to those identified for morphine.

DR. DHUN SETHNA: I have worked with β receptors in myocardial microsomes, and I want to ask people working with opiate receptors about the term *negative cooperation*. When a drug binds to a receptor in the myocardium, there is increased binding up to a limit. Eventually the binding of the drug to tissue levels off and may even diminish. This can be shown mathematically by a Scatchard plot. If the Scatchard plot is linear, affinity is constant. A curvilinear plot indicates changing affinities to the same receptor or else binding to a different receptor site that has a different binding affinity. I would like to know whether anyone working with opiate receptors has demonstrated so-called negative cooperation, or a curvilinear Scatchard plot. My question may have some relevance to the use of high-dose opiates.

DR. CARR: Your question is an incisive one. The term *negative cooperativity* has been applied repeatedly to try to explain what Dr. Stoelting referred to as an interaction between δ and μ receptors. Despite numerous studies and a great many data, very fundamental aspects of this interaction still are not understood. There are several intermediate processes between the binding of a ligand to its receptors and the physiologic effect, and in each process ceiling effects are found. We need not assume that negative cooperativity must play a role in each instance where ceiling effects occur. For example, the presence of biphasic Scatchard plots of binding μ agonists to their receptors provides evidence for the existence of separate high- and low-affinity μ receptors.

DR. LEROY VANDAM: The information and discussion presented at this session focus on receptors. Our knowledge of receptors is very much in transition now, and it will be interesting to look back on what we have said during this meeting.

In a sense, our discussions here are a recapitulation of what happened as we came to understand catecholamine receptors. We started from the concepts of sympathin E and sympathin I and tried to explain them on the basis of clinical phenomena. At this gathering we are again attempting to cause clinical phenomena to fit with concepts that are still theoretical. The catecholamine receptors were separated into several categories according to their molecular biology and pharmacology. What we once described as sympathin E and I are now understood to relate to two or three different kinds of receptors for each. We are in an early stage of knowledge about the opioid receptors, and I am certain that when we learn more about their molecular pharmacology the clinical phenomena will be explained.

II COMPOSITION, ACTION, AND PHYSIOLOGIC EFFECTS

7 THE DEVELOPMENT OF NEW SYNTHETIC NARCOTICS

Paul A. J. Janssen

More than 25 years of extensive research in the field of narcotic analgesics has led to the development of a series of potent analgesics that are tailor-made for different purposes. This chapter describes the stepwise discovery of their properties and the practical implications of their clinical use.

DEXTROMORAMIDE

Our interest in narcotic analgesics started in 1953 and was stimulated by the discovery of dextromoramide in 1956. Dextromoramide (Figure 7.1), like isomethadone a 3.3-diphenylpropylamine, was found to be several times more potent and longer acting than the available analgesics of that time [1].

When injected in rats, dextromoramide was several times more potent than reference drugs. The lowest median effective dose (ED_{50}) in the tail-withdrawal test was 0.1 mg per kilogram of body weight, compared with 0.8 mg/kg for methadone, 3.2 mg/kg for morphine, and 6.2 mg/kg for pethidine (Table 7.1). A peak analgesic effect was observed 6 minutes after administration.

Dextromoramide was also found to be relatively safe. Its safety margin after oral administration—that is to say, the ratio be-

tween the median lethal dose (LD_{50}) and the lowest ED_{50} for surgical analgesia—was 105; the safety margin for methadone, calculated in the same way, is 12, for morphine 71, and for pethidine 4.8.

Today, although dextromoramide is available in more than 50 countries for the parenteral and oral treatment of severe pain, it has become a compound of merely historical significance [2].

PIRITRAMIDE

Piritramide (Figure 7.1), synthesized in 1960, was introduced as an analgesic for postoperative pain [3]. Pharmacologically, it is approximately three times more potent than morphine, with a similar duration of action but faster onset (Table 7.1).

The first 4-aminopiperidine derivative among the narcotic analgesics, it has an unusual chemical structure for a morphinomimetic. The drug was selected to relieve postoperative pain because it is devoid of emetic activity. It is well known that morphine and morphine-like analgesics induce emesis in dogs. On injection of piritramide in dogs, vomiting was never observed. Since its introduction in our clinic, the drug has been de-

Dextromoramide	R 875	1956

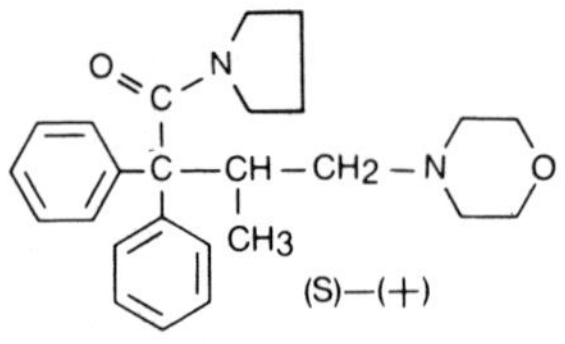

D-tartraat

Phenoperidine	R 1406	1957

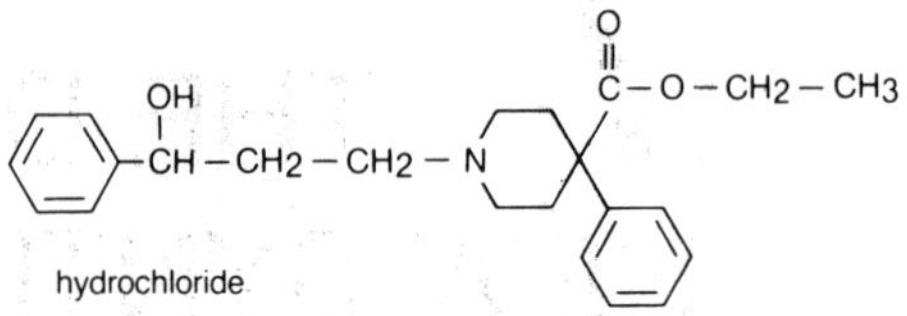

hydrochloride

Piritramide	R 3365	1960 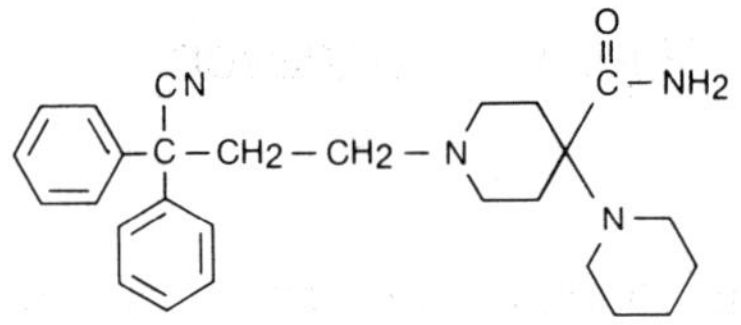

Fentanyl	R 4263	1960

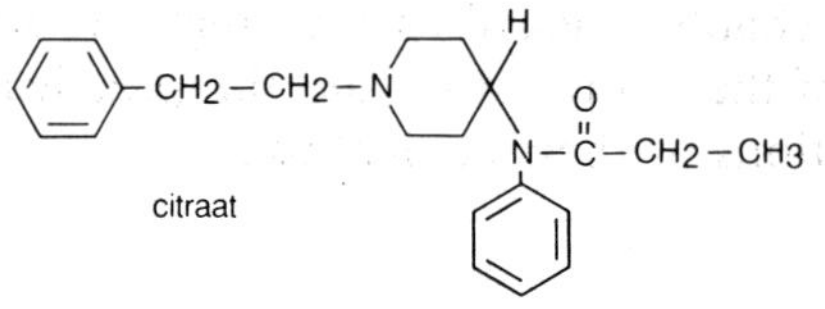

citraat

FIGURE 7.1.   Chemical structures and generic names of narcotic analgesics synthesized by Janssen Research Laboratories.

scribed to be a suitable analgesic for relief of postoperative pain [3,4]. In adults, 20 mg of piritramide is equivalent in analgesic effect to 15 mg of morphine and has a greater hypnotic effect. The frequency of other side effects, particularly nausea, vomiting, and hypotension, and to some extent also the respiratory depression, is less than with currently used analgesics.

PHENOPERIDINE AND FENTANYL

Phenoperidine, a derivative of norpethidine, was synthesized in 1957. Fentanyl, synthesized in 1960, is a 4-anilino-piperidine derivative [5,6].

With the development of these compounds the emphasis was put on potency and safety. When compared with pethidine, for example, the advantages are obvious (Table 7.1). The lowest ED_{50} of pethidine is 6.2 mg/kg and its LD_{50} is 29 mg/kg; thus the safety margin of intravenous pethidine is 4.8. With phenoperidine, the lowest ED_{50} is 0.1 mg/kg, which makes it 50 times more potent than pethidine. As its LD_{50} is 4.7 mg/kg, the safety margin increases to 39 [6].

Fentanyl was a further step in the right direction. With a lowest ED_{50} of 0.01 mg/kg, fentanyl is at least 560 times more potent than pethidine, and with an LD_{50} of 3.1 mg/kg, its safety margin increases to 277. This

Carfentanil	R 33 799	1974

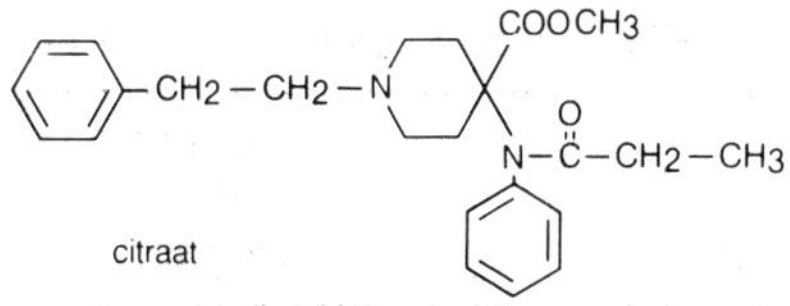

COOCH3

CH2—CH2—N

O
N—C—CH2—CH3

citraat

Sufentanil	R 33 800	1974

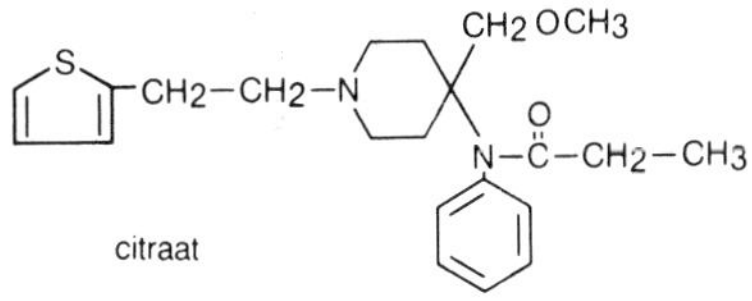

CH2OCH3

CH2—CH2—N

O
N—C—CH2—CH3

citraat

Lofentanil	R 34 995	1975

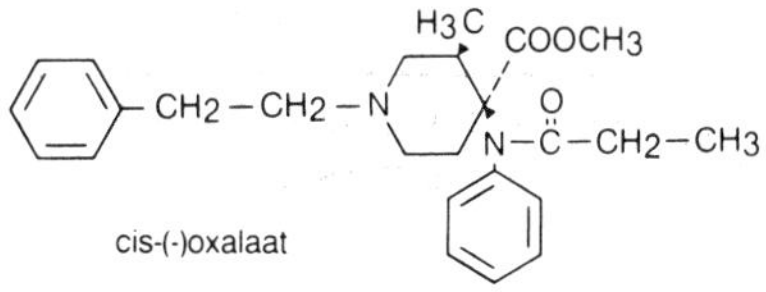

H3C   COOCH3

CH2—CH2—N

O
N—C—CH2—CH3

cis-(-)oxalaat

Alfentanil	R 39 209	1976

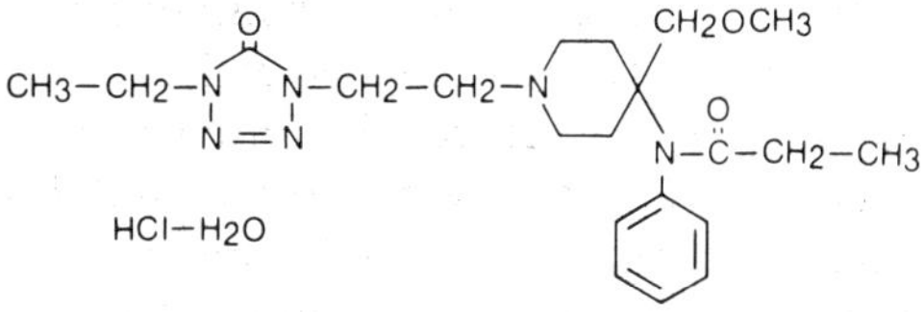

CH2OCH3

CH3—CH2—N   N—CH2—CH2—N

N = N

O
N—C—CH2—CH3

HCl—H2O

large safety margin of fentanyl has made it useful in a broad range of surgical applications. Thanks to its relatively short duration of action and ability to produce satisfactory anesthesia with minimal respiratory and cardiovascular depression, fentanyl has become widely accepted as the drug of choice in intravenous anesthesia. Several derivatives of fentanyl were developed between 1974 and 1976 to fit into new techniques of anesthesia and to fulfill needs in anesthesiology (Figure 7.1).

Advanced surgical techniques have indeed created the need for morphinomimetics with rapid onset of action, duration of analgesia adapted to the clinical situation, well-defined dose-response relationship, and maximal safety margin. To attain these objectives, a strategy was followed that was based on the importance of intrinsic potency amelioration, since specificity and safety seem to be directly related to potency. Indeed, at equianalgesic doses, the risk of side effects is minimized, since fewer molecules are available to affect sites other than the intended opiate receptors. On the other hand, cardiovascular stability increases with potency of the narcotics.

Chemical modification of fentanyl (Figure 7.2) at the C-4 position of the piperidine ring proved to be successful. Introduction of functional groups, for example, a carbome-

TABLE 7.1. Effectiveness and safety of the synthetic narcotics*

Compound	Lowest ED_{50} (mg/kg)	LD_{50} (mg/kg)	Safety Margin	Potency Ratio	Peak Effect (min)
Pethidine	6.2	29	4.8	1	4
Morphine	3.2	223	71	1.9	30
Piritramide	1.3	13	11	4.9	7
Methadone	0.8	9.4	12	7.9	6
Dextromoramide	0.1	10	105	65	6
Phenoperidine	0.1	4.7	39	51	8
Alfentanil	0.04	48	1,080	140	1
Fentanyl	0.01	3.1	277	560	4
Sufentanil	0.0007	18	26,716	9,200	8
Lofentanil	0.0006	0.07	112	10,400	8
Carfentanil	0.0004	3.1	8,460	16,600	10

*Lowest ED_{50} values in the tail-withdrawal test in rats, LD_{50} values, safety margins, and potency ratio of different analgesics after intravenous administration.

thoxy or methyleneoxy-methyl group, together with replacement of the phenyl ring in the nitrogen-phenethyl substituent by the isosteric 2-thienyl moiety respectively, led to carfentanil (structure II) and sufentanil (structure III), two very potent and long-lasting analgesics. A supplementary regio-stereoselective methyl substitution [cis-(-)] at the C-3 position of the piperidine ring in carfentanil resulted in the extremely potent and long-lasting lofentanil (structure IV).

Until then, structural modifications of fentanyl resulted in enhancement of analgesic potency and duration of action. At the same time—about 1975—preclinical and clinical experience with the aforementioned

FIGURE 7.2. Chemical structures of N-4-substituted (1-2-arylethyl)-4-piperidinyl-N-phenylpropanamides.

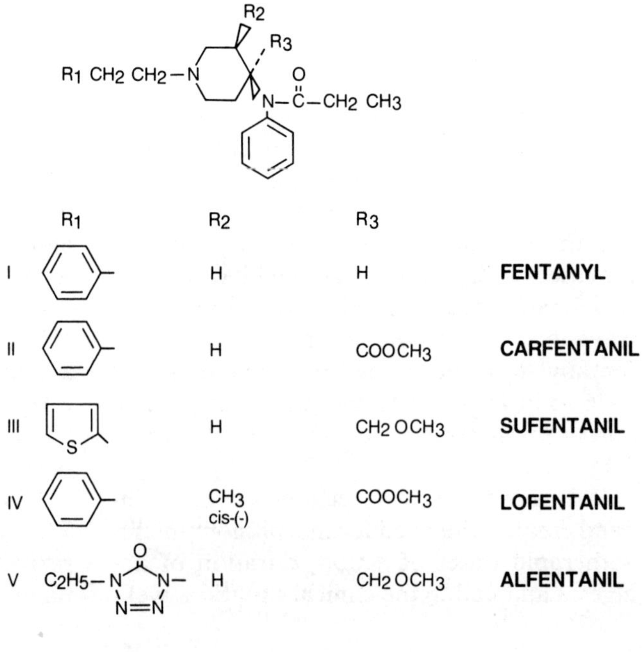

narcotics, together with the development of new surgical techniques in anesthesia, led to renewed insights in the required profile of narcotic analgesics. The idea soon became attractive that a safe narcotic analgesic with an extremely rapid onset of action and an ultra-short duration could offer unexpected possibilities. Intrinsic potency, although not without importance, no longer represented the main criterion for selection.

Alfentanil (structure V), the result of substituting a tetrazolinone ring for the thienyl group in sufentanil, gives concrete form to this new approach. The tetrazolinone ring represents a new pharmacophoric moiety in medicinal chemistry. With pethidine as reference, the potency ratios, measured at the lowest ED_{50} values for alfentanil, fentanyl, sufentanil, and carfentanil, are 140, 560, 9200, and 16,600 respectively (Table 7.1).

SUFENTANIL

Sufentanil and carfentanil thus combine very high potency with a broad safety margin. The lowest ED_{50} of sufentanil is 0.0007 mg/kg, so that it is approximately 9000 times more potent than pethidine (7). Its LD_{50} is extremely high: 18 mg/kg. Thus the safety margin in rats is 26,700, which is wider than that of other narcotics. The range between the analgesic dose and that producing convulsions in dogs is 1000-fold for sufentanil and 160-fold for fentanyl [8]. This difference becomes important when very large doses of narcotic analgesics are used in an attempt to produce anesthesia.

Clinical studies have shown sufentanil to have a more reliable action than fentanyl, with less variability in patient response to the same dosage. It appears to be very similar to fentanyl in terms of hemodynamic changes during induction, but provides greater hemodynamic stability during surgery [9,10]. Furthermore, sufentanil has been shown to provide better attenuation of the stress response to laryngoscopy, intubation, and incision than fentanyl [11,12].

CARFENTANIL

Carfentanil is about twice as potent as sufentanil. Up to now it has not been used in human anesthesia, but it has been extensively used for the immobilization of wild animals, to facilitate translocation, handling, or marking in various ecologic projects. Depending on dosage and weight of the animal, induction of immobilization is rapid (from 5 to 15 minutes) and reliable. Respiratory depression and side effects are surprisingly mild [13].

ALFENTANIL

When administered in high doses, powerful morphine-like analgesics such as fentanyl, sufentanil, and carfentanil share extended duration of analgesic action with long-lasting depression of the respiratory system. The use of these compounds in human anesthesia has always been limited by the inevitable occurrence of respiratory depression, which may last longer than the analgesic action. When high doses are given or when these compounds are used for relatively short operations, patients either need to be reversed when the procedure is completed or they require postoperative ventilation. First, this may be a problem in many hospitals with a limited recovery area and, second, as approximately 50% of all surgical interventions are short to very short procedures, lasting less than 30 minutes, there undoubtedly exists an urgent need for a powerful but short-acting analgesic. Alfentanil could be the first compound to fulfill this need [14].

In animals, alfentanil is three to four times less potent than fentanyl (Table 7.1) but its onset of action is more rapid, the peak effect being reached within 1 minute. Its duration is short: at twice the lowest ED_{50} alfentanil acts for 10 minutes compared with 30 minutes for fentanyl (Figure 7.3). Its effects on respiration are also shorter than those of fentanyl [15].

These characteristics suggest that alfen-

FIGURE 7.3. Time-effect curves in the tail-with-drawal reaction test in rats after intravenous administration of alfentanil, fentanyl, sufentanil, lofentanil, and carfentanil. ED_{50} values and confidence limits for surgical analgesia are expressed in mg/kg at various time intervals after administration. Lowest ED_{50} values at time of peak effect are indicated.

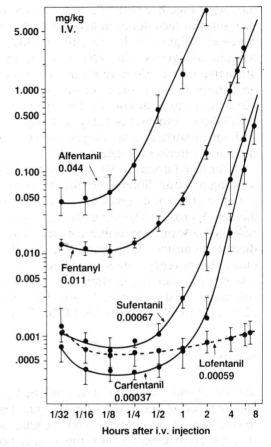

tanil is a particularly suitable analgesic for use in short interventions such as gynecologic, urologic, diagnostic, and short outpatient procedures [16–18]. It can also be used to provide surgical analgesia during interventions of moderate to long duration without substantial accumulation of the drug [19–21].

Alfentanil provides more rapid normalization of postoperative respiratory depression than fentanyl [18]. Furthermore, postoperative complications and side effects have been less frequent with alfentanil than with fentanyl. At doses of less than 12 μg/kg, spontaneous respiration can be maintained in most cases. When respiratory depression does occur, it is of relatively short duration and reversal is generally not required.

The long-lasting respiratory depression in some patients after large doses of fentanyl may be associated with accumulation and slow release of drug from its storage sites [22,23]. Alfentanil, however, seems to have very limited storage in the tissue compartment. Thus it should not only provide anesthesiologists with an alternative narcotic, but broaden their perspective on the use of narcotics.

LOFENTANIL

Lofentanil is approximately 20 times more potent than fentanyl and is by far the longest-acting analgesic known [8]. Its duration of action in the tail-withdrawal test at a dosage equal to twice the lowest ED_{50} is not less than 600 minutes, in comparison with 30 minutes for fentanyl, 34 minutes for sufentanil, and 60 minutes for carfentanil (Figure 7.3). Because of this, intravenous use of lofentanil can only be justified when respiration is assisted for longer periods, as in the intensive care unit.

This duration of action makes lofentanil a particularly interesting compound for long-term analgesia, such as in patients with cancer when it is administered by the peridural route. Because of its high lipid solubility (the log P of 4.2 is higher than for fentanyl) it penetrates the subarachnoid space rapidly and intense analgesia is reached in 5 to 10 minutes after epidural injection. The stability of the drug receptor complex prolongs its duration of action over more than 24 hours in many cases [24].

CONCLUSIONS

Anesthesia in general and the narcotic analgesic field in particular have in the past 25 years made impressive progress in at least three major aspects. The safe use of powerful narcotics has become possible thanks to the development of compounds with a greater dissociation between their analgesic and toxic doses. Intravenous anesthesia has become more manageable with the synthesis of shorter-acting substances such as fentanyl and, above all, alfentanil. When administered either as a bolus or as an infusion, these drugs show analgesic activities that can be turned on and off almost as easily as volatile anesthetics. Finally, newer, more potent, and more specific opiates are no longer dangerous for patients with cardiac insufficiency but, because of their stress-inhibiting effects, act protectively for high-risk patients.

REFERENCES

1. Janssen PAJ, Jageneau AH. A new series of potent analgesics. Dextro 2:2-diphenyl-3-methyl-4-morpholino-butyrylpyrrolidine and related amides. I. Chemical structure and pharmacological activity. J Pharm Pharmacol 1957;9:381–400.

2. Calesnick B. An evaluation of two new analgesics (dextromoramide and racemoramide) in healthy subjects and in patients with chronic pain. J Chron Dis 1959;10(1):58–66.

3. Saarne H. Clinical evaluation of the new analgesic piritramide. Acta Anaesthesiol Scand 1969;13:11–19.

4. Takkin S, Tammisto T. A comparison of pethidine, piritramide and oxycodone in patients with pain following cholecystectomy. Anaesthesist 1973;22:162–6.

5. Nilsson E, Janssen PAJ. Neurolept analgesia—an alternative to general anesthesia. Acta Anaesthesiol Scand 1961;5(2):73–84.

6. Janssen PAJ, Niemegeers CJE, Dony JGH. The inhibitory effect of fentanyl and other morphine-like analgesics in the warm water-induced tail-withdrawal reflex in rats. Arzneim Forsch 1963;13:502–7.

7. Niemegeers CJE, Schellekens KHL, van Bever WFM, Janssen PAJ. Sufentanil, a very potent and extremely safe intravenous morphine-like compound in mice, rats and dogs. Arzneim Forsch 1976;26:1551–6.

8. de Castro J, van de Water A, Wouters L, Xhonneux R, Reneman R, Kay B. Comparative study of cardiovascular neurological and metabolic side-effects of eight narcotics in dogs. Acta Anaesthesiol Belg 1979;30:5–99.

9. de Lange S, Boscoe MJ, Stanley TH. Comparison of sufentanil-O_2 and fentanyl-O_2 anaesthesia for coronary artery surgery. Anesthesiology 1982;56:112–18.

10. Sebel PS, Bovill JG. Cardiovascular effects of sufentanil anesthesia. Anesth Analg (Cleve) 1982;61:115–19.

11. Bovill JG, Sebel PS, Fiolet JWT, Touber JL, Kok K, Philbin DM. The influence of sufentanil on endocrine and metabolic responses to cardiac surgery. Anesth Analg (NY) 1983;62:391–7.

12. de Lange S, Boscoe MJ, Stanley TH, de Bruijin N, Philbin DM, Coggins CH. Antidiuretic and growth hormone responses during coronary artery surgery with sufentanil-oxygen and alfentanil-oxygen anesthesia in man. Anesth Analg (Cleve) 1982;61:434–8.

13. De Vos V. Immobilization of free-ranging

wild animals using a new drug. Vet Rec 1978;103:64–8.

14. Niemegeers CJE, Janssen PAJ. Alfentanil (R 39 209)—a particularly short-acting intravenous narcotic analgesic in rats. Drug Dev Res 1981;1:83–8.

15. Brown JH, Pleuvry BJ, Kay B. Respiratory effects of a new opiate analgesic, R 39 209, in the rabbit; comparison with fentanyl. Br J Anaesth 1980;52:1101–6.

16. van Leeuwen L, Deen L. Alfentanil, a new potent and very short-acting morphinomimetic for minor operative procedures. A pilot study. Anaesthesist 1981;30:115.

17. Kay B, Cohen AT. Intravenous anaesthesia for minor surgery. A comparison of etomidate or althesin with fentanyl and alfentanil. Br J Anaesth 1983 (in press).

18. Sinclair ME, Cooper GM. Alfentanil and recovery. Anaesthesia 1983;38:435–7.

19. Steegers P, Booij L, Pelgrom R. Continuous infusion of alfentanil. Acta Anaesthesiol Belg 1982;33:81–7.

20. Nauta J, Stanley TH, de Lange S, Koopman D, Spierdijk J, van Kleef J. Anaesthetic induction with alfentanil: comparison with thiopental, midazolam and etomidate. Can Anaesth Soc J 1983;30:53–60.

21. de Lange S, Stanley TH, Boscoe MJ. Alfentanil-oxygen anaesthesia for coronary artery surgery. Br J Anaesth 1981;53:1291–6.

22. Bovill JG, Sebel PS, Blackburn CL, Heykants J. The pharmacokinetics of alfentanil (R 39 209): a new opioid analgesic. Anesthesiology 1982;57:439–43.

23. Stanski DR, Hug CC Jr. Alfentanil—a kinetically predictable narcotic analgesic. Anesthesiology 1982;57:435–8.

24. Bilsback P, Rolly G. A double blind epidural administration of lofentanil, buprenorphine or saline for post-operative pain. 4th International Congress of the Belgian Society of Anesthesia and Resuscitation, Louvain-en-Woluwe-Brussels, Sept 7–10, 1983. Acta Anaesthesiol Belg 1983;34 [Suppl 1]:88.

8 CARDIOVASCULAR, METABOLIC, AND NEUROPHYSIOLOGIC EFFECTS OF OPIOIDS

Peter S. Sebel

Opioid anesthesia for cardiac surgery using morphine was first suggested by Lowenstein and colleagues [1]. Techniques using fentanyl have achieved extensive popularity since their description by Stanley and Webster [2]. Many anesthesiologists have a conceptual problem with such techniques, whereby massive doses of a potent opioid analgesic are administered to a point at which responsiveness is ablated for periods up to 24 hours. This is very different from conventional techniques of balanced anesthesia in which relatively small doses of different agents are used together to create a balanced whole. Opioid techniques have an advantage, however, in that, in most cases, excellent cardiovascular stability, particularly during the induction period, is obtained. There are problems with the use of opioids as sole anesthetic agents, and this chapter points to controversy in the areas of cardiovascular stability and suppression of metabolic and neurophysiologic responses.

CARDIOVASCULAR STABILITY

Figure 8.1A shows the cardiovascular stability that can be obtained using fentanyl at a dosage of 60 μg per kilogram of body weight. In this patient undergoing coronary artery surgery, there was no variation in arterial pressure, heart rate, or stroke volume in the period before cardiopulmonary bypass. In contrast, the patient whose recording is shown in Figure 8.1B became hypertensive after intubation. This settled without treatment, but a further hypertensive episode occurred after sternotomy and required vasodilator therapy. In unsupplemented opioid anesthesia, up to 50% of patients become hypertensive. Why do these hypertensive episodes, which are potentially dangerous to the damaged myocardium, occur?

Lowenstein [4] suggested that hypertension in patients anesthetized with morphine was due to light anesthesia. This appears an unlikely cause with fentanyl, because elec-

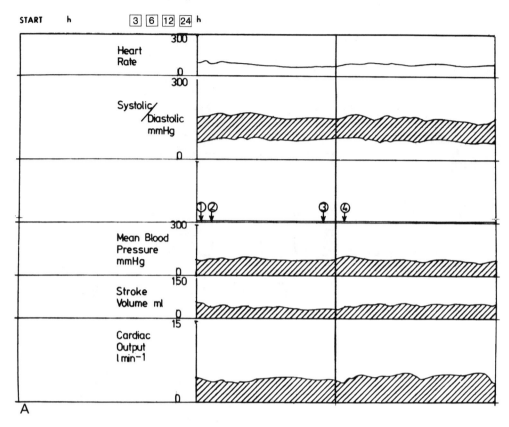

FIGURE 8.1.   The envelope of trend recordings from two patients anesthetized with fentanyl (60 μg/kg) and nitrous oxide–oxygen. The tracing in A is taken from a patient in whom good cardiovascular stability was obtained. The tracing in B shows a patient who became hypertensive on intubation. It resolved, but a further period of hypertension occurred after

troencephalographic (EEG) changes consistent with deep surgical anesthesia are present throughout surgery, including hypertensive episodes [5]. Furthermore, no frequency shifts indicative of decreasing anesthetic depth are seen during hypertensive episodes. It is also unlikely that increases in circulating catecholamines are the cause, as catecholamine levels do not increase before bypass in patients anesthetized with fentanyl [6]. It is a clinical impression that the most marked hypertensive response occurs after sternotomy, especially during pericardial traction and aortic root manipulation. It may be that this is caused by stimulation of a specific cardiac chemoreceptor. Such a receptor, sensitive to hypoxia and serotonin, has

been demonstrated in the region of the left main coronary artery [7].

Sonntag and colleagues [8] studied myocardial lactate production in patients with coronary artery disease who received fentanyl anesthesia. They found increased production of myocardial lactate after sternotomy in seven out of nine patients. Myocardial lactate production is a good indicator of ischemia, and these data, so far unconfirmed by other investigators, raise important questions about the use of opioid anesthesia.

Another possible explanation for the hypertensive episodes is that acute tolerance may be developing to the opioid. In a study correlating EEG changes with alfentanil

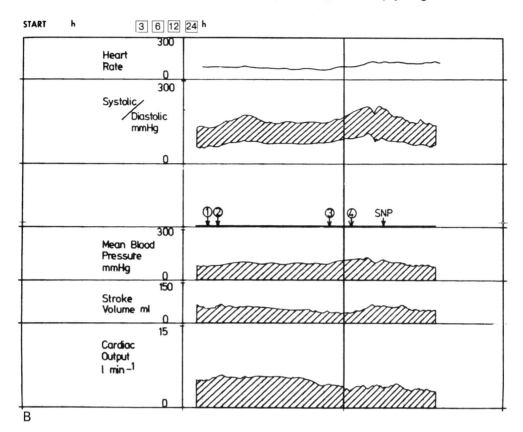

sternotomy and required treatment with sodium nitroprusside. Cardiac output was calculated on a beat-to-beat basis using pulse contour analysis. Point 1, induction of anesthesia; point 2, intubation; point 3, chest incision; point 4, sternotomy. SNP *(in B)* indicates the start of sodium nitroprusside administration. *From Sebel et al [3]. By permission.*

blood levels, Bovill and colleagues [9] found a strong positive correlation ($r = 0.94$) between the total dose of alfentanil used for surgery and the concentration of alfentanil at awakening. This positive correlation means that the more alfentanil a patient requires for surgery, the greater will be his plasma alfentanil concentration when he awakens, and thus acute tolerance to the agent occurs. Such a phenomenon may also be occurring in the cardiovascular control system. In Chapter 2, Professor Hull refers to this phenomenon occurring with fentanyl administered to dogs. Thus, although good cardiovascular stability is usually obtained with opioid anesthesia, the problem of breakthrough hypertension and the possible danger of an ischemic myocardium should be considered.

METABOLIC RESPONSES

One aspect of the use of large doses of opioids that has attracted much interest is their ability to suppress the hormonal and metabolic responses to surgical stress [10]. In comparison with halothane, fentanyl suppresses the catecholamine response to surgery but not to cardiopulmonary bypass [6]. Sufentanil has a similar effect, with marked increases in catecholamines occurring during bypass [11]. Walsh and colleagues [12] continued fentanyl administration into the postoperative period and also found marked increases in catecholamines on bypass. They were unable to detect any effect of fentanyl on postoperative nitrogen balance; that is, catabolism had not been decreased, an effect one would expect to find if stress responses had been suppressed. In contrast, epidural anesthesia suppressed metabolic responses associated with pelvic surgery and resulted in improved nitrogen balance [13]. Whether the suppression of metabolic responses by opioids is of any clinical importance to patients remains to be demonstrated.

NEUROPHYSIOLOGIC EFFECTS

There are two case reports in the literature of awareness during fentanyl anesthesia [14,15], but there is no information as to overall prevalence of awareness. Studies on EEG effects [5] showed that fentanyl anesthesia was associated with a marked increase in high-voltage slow delta activity. No frequency shifts in response to stimuli were seen and the EEG did not alter in the prebypass period. Similar results were obtained during sufentanil and alfentanil anesthesia [9,16]. It appears that awareness during opioid anesthesia is of low frequency and is generally a sporadic occurrence. It seems likely from our EEG studies that, when given in sufficient doses and combined with adequate premedication (e.g., lorazepam), opioids do, in fact, produce anesthesia.

Perhaps more serious is the report by Rao and colleagues [17] of convulsions following fentanyl administration. Unfortunately, these authors had no EEG documentation. Our own studies [5] demonstrated the occurrence of sharp wave activity after fentanyl administration, but these waves looked dissimilar to epileptic spikes and never became generalized. In over 1000 patients anesthetized with opioids who had continuous EEG monitoring, we have never seen EEG changes suggestive of epileptic activity. Rao and colleagues did not modify the effects of fentanyl with prior administration of a muscle relax-

ant, and it is possible that they saw the increase in muscle tone, the catatonic rigidity, that may occur when opioids are administered alone and in large doses.

CONCLUSION

Opioid anesthetic techniques provide stable anesthesia for cardiac surgery. Areas of unresolved controversy include hypertension and myocardial lactate production after sternotomy, the suppression of metabolic responses, and the possibility of awareness and convulsions during anesthesia.

REFERENCES

1. Lowenstein E, Hallowell P, Levine FH, Daggett WM, Austen G, Laver MB. Cardiovascular responses to large doses of intravenous morphine in man. N Engl J Med 1969;281:1389–93.
2. Stanley TH, Webster LR. Anesthetic requirements and cardiovascular effects of fentanyl-oxygen and fentanyl-diazepam-oxygen anesthesia in man. Anesth Analg (Cleve) 1978;57:411–6.
3. Sebel PS, Bovill JG, Boekhorst RAA, Rog N. Cardiovascular effects of high-dose fentanyl anaesthesia. Acta Anaesthesiol Scand 1982;26:308–15.
4. Lowenstein E. Morphine anesthesia—a perspective. Anesthesiology 1971;35:563–5.
5. Sebel PS, Bovill JG, Wauquier A, Rog P. Effects of high-dose fentanyl anesthesia on the electroencephalogram. Anesthesiology 1981;55:203–11.
6. Sebel PS, Bovill JG, Schellekens APM, Hawker CD. Hormonal responses to high-dose fentanyl anesthesia. Br J Anaesth 1981; 53:941–7.
7. James TN, Isobe JH, Urthaler F. Analysis of components in a cardiogenic hypertensive reflex. Circulation 1975;52:179.
8. Sonntag H, Larsen R, Hilfiker O, Kettler D, Brockschnieder B. Myocardial blood flow and oxygen consumption during high-dose fentanyl anesthesia in patients with coronary artery disease. Anesthesiology 1982; 56:417–22.

9. Bovill JG, Sebel PS, Wauquier A, Rog P, Schuyt HC. The influence of high-dose alfentanil anesthesia on the electroencephalogram: correlation with plasma levels. Br J Anaesth 1983;55:1995–2105.

10. Hall GM, Young C, Holdcroft A, Alaghband-Zadeh J. Substrate mobilization during surgery: a comparison between halothane and fentanyl anaesthesia. Anaesthesia 1978;33:924–30.

11. Bovill JG, Sebel PS, Fiolet JWT, Touber JL, Kok K, Philbin DM. The influence of sufentanil on endocrine and metabolic responses to cardiac surgery. Anesth Analg (Cleve) 1983;62:391–7.

12. Walsh ES, Paterson JL, O'Riordan JBA, Hall G. Effect of high-dose fentanyl anaesthesia on the metabolic and endocrine reponse to cardiac surgery. Br J Anaesth 1981;53:1155–64.

13. Kehlet H. The influence of epidural analgesia on the endocrine-metabolic response to surgery. Acta Anaesthesiol Scand [Suppl] 1978;70:39–42.

14. Hilgenberg JC. Intraoperative awareness during high-dose fentanyl oxygen anesthesia. Anesthesiology 1981;54:341–3.

15. Mummaneni N, Rao TLK, Montoya A. Awareness and recall with high-dose fentanyl oxygen anesthesia. Anesth Analg (Cleve) 1980;59:948–9.

16. Bovill JG, Sebel PS, Wauquier A, Rog P. Electroencephalographic effects of sufentanil anaesthesia in man. Br J Anaesth 1982;54:45–52.

17. Rao TLK, Mummaneni N. El-Etr AA. Convulsions: an unusual response to intravenous fentanyl administration. Anesth Analg (Cleve) 1982;61:1020–1.

9 PHARMACOKINETICS OF NEW SYNTHETIC NARCOTIC ANALGESICS

Carl C. Hug, Jr.

New narcotic analgesics of interest to American anesthesiologists include the agonists alfentanil (Alfenta, Rapifen) and sufentanil (Sufenta), and the antagonist analgesics butorphanol (Stadol) and nalbuphine (Nubain) [1].

Relatively little is known about the pharmacokinetics of butorphanol [2] and nalbuphine [3], especially in relation to the onset and duration of their effects (i.e., analgesia, ventilatory depression, antagonism of morphine-like agonists). Because of the ceiling to their agonistic actions, they cannot be used as primary anesthetic agents [4–6]. Current applications of antagonist analgesics include preanesthetic medication, supplementation of general and regional agents, and postoperative analgesia [1]. Investigation is under way regarding the use of nalbuphine to maintain postoperative analgesia while antagonizing the residual ventilatory depression effects of high-dose narcotic anesthesia [7,8]. In the latter context, pharmacokinetic information may be especially useful in predicting the duration of nalbuphine's antagonistic actions relative to the persistence of residual narcotic analgesic agonists in the body. Recurrence of ventilatory depression

as well as the initially excessive antagonism of analgesia and other narcotic effects after intravenous bolus doses of naloxone are predictable on the basis of its pharmacokinetics [9].

Alfentanil and sufentanil are chemical analogs of fentanyl with a very similar, if not identical, spectrum of effects. Their advantages and disadvantages compared to fentanyl are largely attributable to differences in the kinetics of their distribution in and elimination from the body.

OVERVIEW OF THE DISPOSITION OF NARCOTIC ANALGESICS

The narcotic analgesics can be compared in terms of their duration of action, pharmacokinetics (Table 9.1), receptor dissociation rates (Table 9.2), lipid solubility and other factors influencing their ability to penetrate the central nervous system (CNS) (Table 9.3).

Morphine has a short elimination half-life but is long acting due to its retention within the CNS [13]. The exit rate of narcotic an-

TABLE 9.1. Pharmacokinetics and duration of action*

Agent	$t_{1/2}\beta$ (hr)	Vd (L/kg)	Cl (ml/kg/min)
Long-acting (>4 hr)			
Morphine	2–3	2–6	10–23
Methadone (Dolophine)	9–87	2–12	1–8
Intermediate (1–4 hr)			
Fentanyl (Sublimaze)	2–4	3–5	10–22
Sufentanil (Sufenta)	2–4	2–3	9–14
Meperidine (Demerol)	3–5	3–6	8–18
Short-acting (<1 hr)			
Alfentanil (Alfenta)	1.4–1.6	0.4–1.0	3–8

*Modified from Hug [10].

$t_{1/2}\beta$ = elimination half-time; Vd = volume of distribution; Cl = plasma clearance.

algesics from the CNS is inversely related to their lipid solubility [14].

Alfentanil has a short duration of action that reflects its rapid dissociation from receptors, its facility to penetrate membranes, and its short elimination half-life. Fentanyl also dissociates rapidly from receptors and penetrates membranes rapidly; its duration of action varies with dose because of its pharmacokinetic characteristics. A small dose has a short duration due to its rapid redistribution from brain to other tissues; large doses are long acting because of their slow elimination from the body [15–19].

Sufentanil has a shorter elimination half-life than fentanyl but its dissociation from narcotic receptors is slower. At present, the data for sufentanil are too limited to explain fully the relationships among dose, duration of action, and pharmacokinetics.

Lofentanil is long acting because of its slow dissociation from narcotic analgesic receptors and in spite of its high degree of lipid solubility [11]. Methadone is long acting because of its slow elimination from the body [20].

PHARMACOKINETICS AND PHARMACODYNAMICS

The relationship between dose and concentration is determined by pharmaco*kinetic*

TABLE 9.2. Narcotic analgesic receptor interactions*

Agent	Dissociation Time		% Specific Binding	Kd (nmol)
	$t_{1/2}\alpha$ (sec)	$t_{1/2}\beta$ (min)		
Alfentanil	Too rapid to measure		50	<0.05
Fentanyl	5	1.2	75	1
Naloxone	11	1.7	50	6
Dihydro-morphine	7	5	60	2.6
Sufentanil	126	25	90	0.13
Lofentanil	—	208	80	0.06

*With permission of J. Leysen, Ph.D., Janssen Pharmaceutica, Beerse, Belgium [11].

$t_{1/2}\alpha$ = rapid dissociation half-time; $t_{1/2}\beta$ = slow dissociation half-time; KD = dissociation constant.

TABLE 9.3. Physiochemical factors affecting the disposition of narcotic analgesics*

Factor	Morphine	Alfentanil	Meperidine	Sufentanil	Fentanyl	Lofentanil
Ionization (pKa) constant	7.9	6.5	8.5	8.0	8.4	7.8
Percent un-ionized at pH 7.4	23	89	7.4	20	8.5	28
Octanol-water partition coefficients						
Un-ionized base	6	145	525	8,913	9,550	16,596
Ionized form	. . .	0.07	. . .	1.0	0.5	0.26
Apparent at pH 7.4	1.4	129	39	1,727	816	4,571
Ratio to morphine	1	89	28	1,241	676	3,265
Free fraction in human plasma (%) at pH 7.4	70	7.9	30	7.5	16	6.4
Relative potential for entering CNS†	1	10	12	133	155	299

*Modified from Meuldermans et al [12].

†Apparent partition coefficient at pH 7.4 multiplied by the free fraction of drug in plasma and divided by the value for morphine.

factors, and the relationship between concentration and effect is determined by pharmaco*dynamic* factors; together they determine the dose versus intensity of effect relationship (Figure 9.1). A proportional relationship between drug concentration in plasma and receptors exists in almost all cases of anesthetic drugs during steady state (e.g., long-term administration at a constant rate). During periods of rising and declining drug concentrations in plasma, the relationship of levels in plasma to concentrations at receptors and to the intensity of drug effects will be close only to the degree that the rate of change in plasma concentration is slow relative to the rate of drug equilibration between plasma and tissue receptors. Drugs that are limited in their ability to penetrate membranes—e.g., less lipophilic agents such as morphine [14]—or dissociate from receptors slowly—e.g., lofentanil [11]—exhibit poor correlations between their plasma levels and the intensity of their actions under nonsteady conditions. Even the most lipid-soluble drugs able to penetrate membranes rapidly—e.g., fentanyl [14,19]—do so at a finite rate, and when their concentrations in plasma are changing at a very rapid rate (e.g., immediately after an intravenous bolus dose), the relationships between concentrations and effects will not be close. A correlation between plasma concentration and intensity of effect can be expected for lipid-soluble narcotic analgesics such as fentanyl under relatively constant conditions (i.e., slowly changing concentrations and stability of factors affecting pharmacodynamics) [16,19,21].

CLINICAL IMPLICATIONS AND APPLICATIONS OF PHARMACOKINETICS: FENTANYL AND ALFENTANIL

As implied above, the most direct and significant relationship between plasma concentration and intensity of effect is evident for drugs equilibrating rapidly between plasma and their sites of action. This equilibration is rapid for fentanyl, alfentanil, and meperidine (Demerol). Observations published to date allow us to make estimates of the average plasma concentrations that are needed to produce certain effects (Table 9.4). One must remember that these are average concentrations estimated from observations during gradually changing plasma concentrations in selected groups of patients. Much work needs to be done (a) to identify and quantify pharmacodynamic factors that influence the patient's sensitivity to the drug (e.g., age, premedication, intensity of stimulation) and (b) to determine the intrinsic variability among patients even when all the recognized factors are controlled. By facilitating the rapid achievement of stable drug levels (not necessarily steady-state, but changing slowly), pharmacokinetics can be useful in determining pharmaco*dynamic* variability [21–25].

The anesthesiologist in the operating room faces a particularly challenging task, which is, to adjust anesthetic levels according to the varying intensity of stimulation. The objective is to provide satisfactory anesthetic conditions (analgesia, unconsciousness, relaxation, and suppression of somatic, autonomic, and endocrine reflexes) and at the same time avoid overdosage and toxicity (e.g., cardiovascular depression by excessive halothane, prolonged postoperative ventila-

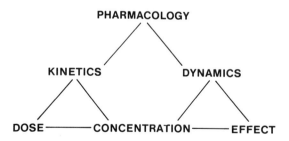

FIGURE 9.1. Relationships basic to pharmacology. Pharmaco*kinetic* variables determine the drug concentrations in plasma and tissues (receptors) that result from a given dose. Pharmaco*dynamic* factors influence the intensity of response produced by the concentration of drug achieved at receptor sites.

TABLE 9.4. Relationships of plasma concentrations
to the effects of narcotic analgesics*

Effects	Plasma Concentration (ng/ml)		
	Fentanyl	Alfentanil[†]	Meperidine
Mild analgesia, sedation, and ventilatory depression	1–2	50–150	100–200
Moderate analgesia, euphoria, and ventilatory depression; 33% decrease in MAC	2–5	150–350	200–500
Strong analgesia and marked ventilatory depression (apnea); 50% decrease in MAC	10–20	300–600	>500
Unconsciousness[†]	10–30	500–1500	. . . (seizures)

*Modified from Hug [10].
†Precise values not determined.

tory depression by excessive fentanyl). In the case of inhalational anesthetics, he is able to facilitate their elimination by way of the lungs by hyperventilating the patient. The decline of intravenous drug concentrations and effects depends entirely on the patient's ability to redistribute the drug away from sites of action and to eliminate it from the body. At least until drug concentrations in plasma have equilibrated with all body tissues, the decline of plasma levels (and drug effects) is dependent on both distributive and elimination processes.

To date, anesthesiologists have used three approaches to producing anesthesia by intravenous drugs, including narcotic analgesics: intermittent bolus doses, constant infusions, and variable-rate infusions.

Intermittent bolus doses are most often used to supplement nitrous oxide or other background anesthetic (including a large initial dose of the same intravenous drug). Intermittent doses produce rapidly fluctuating levels of drug in plasma and make it difficult to relate concentrations to effects (Figure 9.2). Although experienced anesthesiologists can become skillful in these techniques, some anesthetists regularly depend on the use of muscle relaxants to cover inadequate anesthesia and on the use of antagonists at the end of the operation to reverse the residual effects of excessive doses.

Some anesthetists attempt to avoid or to minimize the need for several intravenous doses by giving a single dose at the induction of anesthesia ("front end" or "up-front loading") (Figure 9.3). Their objective is to provide very high drug concentrations at the start of anesthesia and surgery when stimulation is usually most intense (e.g., laryngoscopy, skin incision, sternotomy, intraperitoneal dissection). Subsequently, they coast down the drug elimination curve as the operation is continued to completion. Of course some problems can be anticipated in at least some patients: (a) The patient becomes aware of intraoperative events when drug concentrations decline to ineffective levels before the completion of surgery. This situation may not be apparent to the anesthetist if the patient is paralyzed by muscle relaxants. (b) The operation is completed before the drug concentrations have declined to levels compatible with awakening and maintenance of satisfactory ventilation. Hence the recovery time is lengthy or the risks of antagonists are incurred. (c) The large initial dose produces acute side effects and toxicity (e.g., bradycardia, hypotension, rigidity). (d) The initial dose is inadequate and more of the

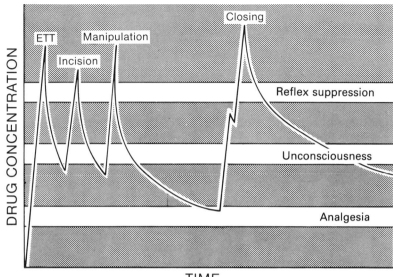

FIGURE 9.2.   Simulation of drug concentrations in plasma or tissues that result from intermittent intravenous bolus doses. Awareness may occur intermittently as the concentrations fall below those required for unconsciousness. Responses to noxious stimulation near the end of the operation may lead the anesthetist to administer a larger supplemental dose, with effects outlasting the duration of surgery.

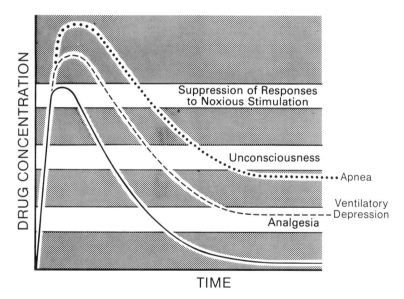

FIGURE 9.3.   Simulation of the consequences of administering a single large intravenous dose (three different sizes) at the induction of anesthesia. If the operation is short in relation to the time required for drug concentrations to decline, prolonged recovery may result. Inadequate anesthesia will result from drug doses that are small relative to the duration of the operation.

same drug or other drugs is administered, leading to prolonged recovery.

Constant intravenous infusions of narcotic analgesics have been used to produce anesthesia [24,25], to supplement nitrous oxide [26,27], and to provide postoperative analgesia [28]. Generally, the objective is to produce (priming dose) and to maintain (constant infusion) a stable drug level adequate to produce the desired degree of effect in 99% plus of patients (EC_{99} = effective concentration of 99%). Of course, this represents the equivalent of an overdose for the majority of patients. This is of little concern intraoperatively or postoperatively when ventilatory support is planned and provided. Ventilatory depression is of vital concern postoperatively when the patient is expected to maintain satisfactory spontaneous ventilation. If the infusion has been maintained

for a long time, steady state will have been approached, and the rate of recovery will depend on the rate of drug elimination (Figure 9.4). Before a steady state is reached and to the extent that redistribution of the drug from the central nervous system to other tissues can still occur, recovery time will be shortened (Figure 9.5).

Varying the rate of infusion of intravenous drugs is analogous to varying the inspired concentration of an inhalational anesthetic. Success with this technique requires constant feedback of signs of adequate or inadequate anesthesia. The technique begins with a loading dose (priming infusion, "overpressure") to induce anesthesia; subsequently, an attempt is made to use the least inspired concentration of intravenous infusion rate required to maintain the anesthetic objectives while avoiding unnecessary accu-

FIGURE 9.4. Elimination half-life predicts the rate of decline of drug concentrations after a steady state has been achieved during continuous administration of a drug at a constant rate. The concentrations will decline more rapidly (and presumably recovery will also occur more quickly) in the case of alfentanil than after fentanyl. *From Stanski and Hug [29]. By permission.*

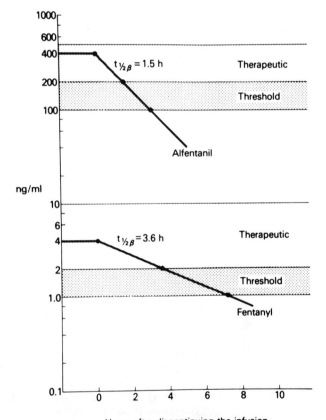

Hours after discontinuing the infusion

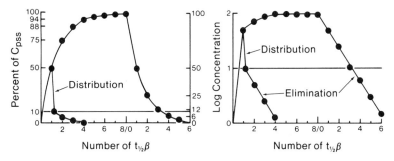

FIGURE 9.5. Both redistribution from brain to other tissues (rapid decline) and elimination (slower terminal phase) of the drug from the body are responsible for the decline of drug concentrations and recovery from its effects when administration is stopped prior to achievement of a steady state. Once steady state is achieved (i.e., complete equilibration between plasma and tissue levels; clearance rate equals the constant infusion rate), the decline of drug levels after discontinuing the infusion will depend solely on elimination processes.

mulation of the drug and the consequent prolongation of recovery. It is also important to anticipate the end of the operation and to discontinue drug inhalation or infusion at a time that will allow its concentration to fall to levels commensurate with recovery of consciousness and spontaneous maintenance of ventilation and other vital functions. In the case of a narcotic analgesic, preservation of analgesia in the postoperative period is desirable (Figure 9.6).

Using alfentanil in this manner to supplement nitrous oxide, Ausems et al were able to provide satisfactory anesthesia for lower abdominal gynecologic surgery lasting more than three hours in healthy young women and still have them awaken and breathe satisfactorily within ten minutes after completion of the operation [30]. Muscle relaxation was minimized to preserve somatic signs of anesthetic depth. None of the patients recalled any intraoperative event, although they all remembered their condition immediately before the induction of anesthesia (e.g., blurred vision after 1 mg pancuronium) and again 4 minutes after discontinuation of nitrous oxide at the end of surgery (16 minutes after stopping the alfentanil infusion) [30]. White has used intravenous infusions of fen-

tanyl or ketamine similarly to supplement nitrous oxide and thiopental for brief outpatient procedures [31].

COMPUTER-ASSISTED TITRATION OF INTRAVENOUS ANESTHESIA

With adequate knowledge of pharmacokinetics, pharmacodynamics, and their individual variation among patients, it is conceivable that computers can be useful in the rapid induction and maintenance of anesthesia with intravenous drugs [32,33]. It should be possible to categorize patients sufficiently well in terms of pharmacodynamics (i.e., useful range of drug concentrations in plasma) and pharmacokinetics (i.e., likely range of priming and maintenance infusions) to induce anesthesia rapidly without giving an excessive dose. With the ability to determine plasma levels rapidly in the operating room laboratory (to detect unexpected pharmacokinetic variability) and with reliable monitoring of anesthetic depth, especially in the patient given muscle relaxants, it should then be possible to vary the infusion rate appropriately to meet the challenge of stable anesthesia (i.e., varying anesthetic concen-

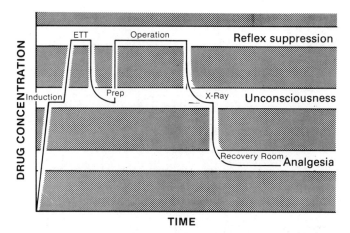

FIGURE 9.6. Simulation of the production of stable drug concentrations by a computer-assisted, variable-rate infusion. To lower the drug level, the infusion is stopped and distribution-elimination processes determine the rate of decline of drug concentrations to the lower level, which is then maintained by resumption of the infusion at a rate equivalent to the rate of drug clearance at that particular concentration in plasma.

The drug concentration should be sufficient to suppress autonomic and somatic reflexes to noxious stimulation (e.g., laryngoscopy for insertion of an endotracheal tube—ETT). Lower drug levels would be sufficient to induce and to maintain unconsciousness during periods of minimal stimulation (e.g., skin preparation, x-ray verification of missing surgical needle). An analgesic effect could be maintained postoperatively by a constant infusion.

trations in anticipation of changes in stimulus intensity) in the face of varying stimulus intensity and still provide for rapid recovery (Figure 9.6).

Such futuristic approaches to the efficient use of intravenous anesthetics will require that the anesthesiologist be as well versed in the dynamics and kinetics of intravenous drugs as he now is (or should be) in those features of inhalational anesthetics [22,34].

REFERENCES

1. Hug CC Jr. New narcotic analgesics and antagonists in anesthesia. Semin Anesth 1982;1:14–20.
2. Smyth RD, Pittman KA, Gaver RC. Human pharmacokinetics and metabolism of butorphanol. Clin Pharmacol Ther 1979; 25:250.
3. Nubain; Physicians's Monograph. Garden City, NY: Endo Laboratories, 1979:7.
4. Murphy MR, Hug CC Jr. The enflurane-sparing effect of morphine, butorphanol and nalbuphine. Anesthesiology 1982;57:489–92.
5. Lake CL, Duckworth EN, DiFazio CA, Durbin CG, Magruder MR. Cardiovascular effects of nalbuphine in patients with coronary or valvular heart disease. Anesthesiology 1982;57:498–503.
6. Moldenhauer CC, Hug CC Jr, Nagle DM, Youngberg JA. High-dose butorphanol (Stadol) in anesthesia for aortocoronary bypass surgery (ABS). Abstracts of the Third Annual Meeting of the Society of Cardiovascular Anesthesiologists, San Francisco, May 10–13, 1981:59–60.

7. Magruder MR, Delaney RD, Di Fazio CA. Reversal of narcotic-induced respiratory depression with nalbuphine hydrochloride. Anesthesiol Rev 1982;9:34–37.

8. Roach GW, Moldenhauer CC, Finalyson DC, et al. Nalbuphine reversal of respiratory depression following high-dose fentanyl anesthesia. Abstracts of the Fifth Annual Meeting of the Society of Cardiovascular Anesthesiologists, San Diego, April 24–27, 1983:140–1.

9. Ngai SH, Berkowitz BA, Yang JC, Hempstead J, Spector S. Pharmacokinetics of naloxone in rats and in man: basis for its potency and short duration of action. Anesthesiology 1976;44:398–401.

10. Hug CC Jr. Pharmacokinetics and dynamics of narcotic analgesics. In: Prys-Roberts C, Hug CC Jr, eds. Pharmacokinetics of anaesthesia. London: Blackwell Scientific, 1984:187–234.

11. Leysen J. Janssen Pharmaceutica, Beerse, Belgium (personal communication).

12. Meuldermans WEG, Hurkmans RMA, Heykants JJP. Plasma protein binding and distribution of fentanyl, sufentanil, alfentanil and lofentanil in blood. Arch Int Pharmacodyn Ther 1982;257:4–19.

13. Hug CC Jr, Murphy MR, Rigel EP, Olson WA. Pharmacokinetics of morphine injected intravenously into the anesthetized dog. Anesthesiology 1981;54:38–47.

14. von Cube B, Teschemacher H, Herz A. Permeation morphinartic wirksamer Substanzen an den Ord der antinociceptiven Wirkung in Gehirn in Abhängigkeit von ihrer Lipoidlöslichkcit nach intraventricularer Applikation. Naunyn Schmiedebergs Arch Pharmacol 1970;265:455–73.

15. Murphy MR, Olson WA, Hug CC Jr. Pharmacokinetics of ^{3}H-fentanyl in the dog anesthetized with enflurane. Anesthesiology 1979;50:13–19.

16. McClain DA, Hug CC Jr. Intravenous fentanyl kinetics. Clin Pharmacol Ther 1980;28:106–17.

17. Hug CC Jr, Murphy MR. Tissue redistribution of fentanyl and termination of its effects in rats. Anesthesiology 1981;55:369–75.

18. Hug CC Jr, McClain DA. Ventilatory depression by fentanyl in anesthetized patients. Anesthesiology 1980;53:S56.

19. Hug CC Jr, Murphy MR. Fentanyl disposition in cerebrospinal fluid and plasma and its relationship to ventilatory depression in the dog. Anesthesiology 1979;50:342–9.

20. Gorulay GK, Wilson PR, Glynn CJ. Pharmacodynamics and pharmacokinetics of methadone during the perioperative period. Anesthesiology 1982;57:458–67.

21. Murphy MR, Hug CC Jr. The anesthetic potency of fentanyl in terms of its reduction of enflurane MAC. Anesthesiology 1982; 57:485–8.

22. Quasha AL, Eger EI, Tinker JH. Determination and applications of MAC. Anesthesiology 1980;53:315–34.

23. Austin KL, Stapleton JV, Mather LE. Relationship between blood meperidine concentrations and analgesic response. Anesthesiology 1980;53:460–6.

24. Hug CC Jr, Moldenhauer CC. Pharmacokinetics and dynamics of fentanyl infusions in cardiac surgical patients. Anesthesiology 1982;57:A45.

25. Sprigge JS, Wynands JE, Whalley DG et al. Fentanyl infusion anesthesia for aortocoronary bypass surgery: plasma levels and hemodynamic response. Anesth Analg (Cleve) 1982;61:972–8.

26. Hengstmann JH, Stoeckel H, Schutter J. Infusion model for fentanyl based on pharmacokinetic analysis. Br J Anaesth 1980; 52:1021–5.

27. McQuay HJ, Moore RA, Paterson GMC, Adams AP. Plasma fentanyl concentrations and clinical observations during and after operation. Br J Anaesth 1979;51:543–50.

28. Stanski DR, Hug CC Jr. Alfentanil—a kinetically predictable narcotic analgesic. Anesthesiology 1982;57:435–8.

29. Ausems ME, Hug CC Jr, de Lange S. Variable rate infusion of alfentanil as a supplement to nitrous oxide anesthesia for general surgery. Anesth Analg (NY) 1983;62: 982–6.

30. White PF. Use of continuous infusion versus intermittent bolus administration of fentanyl or ketamine during outpatient anesthesia. Anesthesiology 1983;59:294–300.

31. Schwilden H. A general method for calculating the dosage scheme in linear pharmacokinetics. Eur J Clin Pharmacol 1981; 20:379–86.

32. Schwilden H, Stoeckel H, Lauven PM, Schuttler J. Pharmacokinetic data of fentanyl, midazolam and enflurane obtained by a new method for arbitrary application schemes. Br J Anaesth 1982;54:237P.

33. Eger EI II. Anesthetic uptake and action. Baltimore: Williams & Wilkins, 1974.

10 CHANGES IN THE ELECTROENCEPHALOGRAM DURING HIGH-DOSE NARCOTIC ANESTHESIA

N. Ty Smith, Holly Dec-Silver, Theodore J. Sanford, Jr., Charles J. Westover, Jr., Michael L. Quinn, Fritz Klein, and David A. Davis

It can be difficult clinically to estimate the depth of anesthesia during high-dose narcotic-oxygen anesthesia. Perhaps the electroencephalogram (EEG) could provide an indicator of anesthetic depth. Compared with inhalation agents, however, there are few data available about EEG effects of high-dose narcotic anesthesia [1]. This deficiency is compounded by the difficulty of interpreting raw EEG data in the operating room [2]. We therefore used two computerized analytical techniques quantitatively to analyze and compare the EEG patterns produced by high-dose morphine-oxygen, fentanyl-oxygen, or sufentanil-oxygen anesthesia.

INVESTIGATION OF EEG PATTERNS OF VARIOUS NARCOTICS

We compared the effects on EEG of morphine, fentanyl, or sufentanil in 49 male patients undergoing open heart surgery and receiving comparable preanesthetic medication consisting of morphine and scopolamine. To achieve comparable induction rates, we diluted morphine to 3 mg/ml and sufentanil to 10 μg/ml, concentrations approximately equivalent to fentanyl 50 μg/ml. We induced anesthesia slowly, injecting 1 ml/min for the first four minutes, 2 ml/min for the next three minutes, and 5 to 10 ml/min thereafter. After loss of response to verbal stimulation, we administered metocurine plus pancuronium.

We placed six gold-cup EEG electrodes in the FP1-O1 and FP2-O2 positions after abrading the skin and placing electrode jelly, collodion, and gauze. The high- and low-pass filters of our recorder were set at 0.5 Hz and 1000 Hz respectively. We calibrated the EEG, the EEG signals going into a tape recorder, and the signals from the recorder into the analyzers with 10-Hz, 100-μV wave forms. A continuous section of tape from preinduction to five minutes after sternal spread was played back into two EEG analyzers, the Klein and the Neurometrics analyzers.

The Klein analyzer is a period analyzer [3,4]. It uses a zero-crossing method [3,4] to obtain the amplitude (A0) and the averaged zero-axis crossing frequency (F0) of the fundamental wave. The raw signal is differentiated twice, and the resulting first- and second-derivative signals are used to generate two additional amplitudes (A1 and A2) and frequencies (F1 and F2). The raw EEG plus the seven outputs from the Klein analyzer— the six described above plus the electromyogram [3,4]—were recorded onto the strip-chart recorder with a slow (20-second time constant) filter. From the resulting strip-chart records, we measured each Klein variable during the control period, as well as just before and after each of seven events: oral airway insertion, Foley catheter insertion, laryngoscopy and 4% lidocaine spray, laryngoscopy and intubation, leg incision, chest incision, sternotomy, and sternal spread.

The Neurometrics analyzer uses aperiodic analysis [5,6], that is, instead of averaging wave forms over a given time period, an individual wave form is mapped in relation to its frequency, amplitude, and time of occurrence. We used a prototype Neurometrics EEG analyzer. For display, it uses a thinning process that preserves about 25% of the wave forms, combining some and eliminating others. Each recorded disk was examined visually on the Neurometrics display, and for each appropriate time period (before and after the previously mentioned events) the section most nearly artifact free was selected. From these selected segments, we analyzed one-minute epochs and printed out the numerical analysis for the display. Each printout included 153 data points: number of waves, total power, mean power per wave, percentage of power, and cumulative percentage of power for each of 30 1-Hz intervals (0.5–1.5, 1.5–2.5, etc.) and the total number of waves, total power, and mean power per wave for all frequencies. From these printouts we selected five variables

representative of some of the different types of information available from the Neurometrics: total number of waves, total power at 1 Hz (TP1), total power at 4 Hz (TP4), cumulative power at 3 Hz (CP3), and the frequency at a cumulative power of 90% (F90). Since the peak changes seemed to occur early with TP4, we measured the maximum TP4 between induction of anesthesia and insertion of the Foley catheter. Otherwise, the Neurometrics values were measured at the same intervals as the Klein values.

To eliminate muscle artifact from the control values for both analytic methods, we subtracted values obtained after the onset of neuromuscular blockade from those obtained just before administration of the agent, and in turn subtracted those values from control values. With the fentanyl and sufentanil records, we also compensated for the change in anesthetic depth that occurred during establishment of neuromuscular block (a time interval of about one minute) by subtracting that change from the correction factor.

RESULTS OF THE STUDY

Figure 10.1 shows EEG changes during the three anesthetics as demonstrated by the low-frequency amplitude (A0) from the Klein analyzer. With fentanyl and sufentanil, A0 increased, while the remaining variables decreased slightly to moderately. Although all variables changed significantly (except F2-sufentanil), many changes were relatively small. Steady states were reached with each variable except A0, which returned to control during incision, and A2, which tended to decrease during the relatively long interval between intubation and incision.

The results were somewhat different with morphine. The only change was with A1, which decreased. Amplitude A2 did not show any significant decreases until the time of laryngoscopy and F0 until the time of incision.

FIGURE 10.1. Mean amplitude of the raw EEG (A0) as determined by the Klein method. There are two controls: uncorrected control *(left)* and control corrected for noise *(next set of three points)*. See text for explanation of the events.

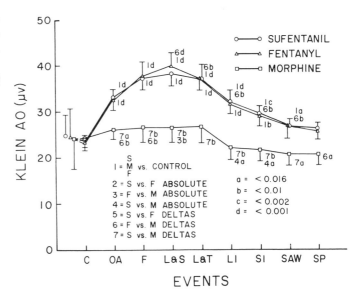

There were no significant differences between the absolute values, as well as the changes from control, with fentanyl and sufentanil. Significant differences between morphine and fentanyl occurred with A0, F0, and F1, while differences between morphine and sufentanil occurred with A0 and F0.

Four out of the five variables selected from the Neurometrics matrix changed during most of anesthesia. The total number of waves significantly decreased with fentanyl and sufentanil, but not with morphine. The values returned toward control by the time of incision. The TP4 did not change significantly with any agent, except for the very early changes with fentanyl and sufentanil, reflected by $TP4_{max}$, and just before laryngoscopy and spray with morphine. The TP4 did tend to be greater than control just before insertion of an oral airway with fentanyl and sufentanil anesthesia and until the incision with morphine, although the differences were not significant. Frequency F90 decreased significantly by over 50%, but returned toward control with fentanyl and sufentanil. The remaining two variables, TP1 and CP3, as well as F90, revealed considerable differences between fentanyl and sufentanil on the one hand and morphine on the

other. With fentanul and sufentanil, TP1 increased and then returned toward control at incision, while during morphine anesthesia it drifted slightly upward. The changes were highly significant with fentanyl and sufentanil, but not so with morphine. There was a marked increase in CP3 (Figure 10.2) with fentanyl and sufentanil and a somewhat smaller increase with morphine. The differences between fentanyl and sufentanil on the one hand and morphine on the other were highly significant with both TP1 and CP3.

CHARACTERISTICS OF EEG PATTERNS

Changes in the EEG have been studied during general anesthesia with a variety of agents [1]. These changes differ from agent to agent, but are consistent for any one drug. With the exception of ketamine, onset and deepening of general anesthesia from light stages are accompanied by a progressive slowing of EEG activity, that is, shift to the left of EEG frequency. This can consist of a decrease in the amplitude of high-frequency activity and an increase in low-frequency amplitude. With some agents, such as halothane, a distinct

FIGURE 10.2. The cumulative percent power at 3 Hz over a one-minute epoch as determined by the Neurometrics method. There are two controls: uncorrected control *(left)* and control corrected for noise *(next set of three points).* See text for explanation of the events and Figure 10.1 for the key to the significant differences.

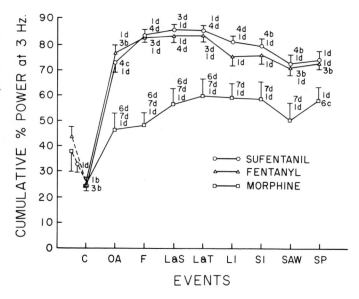

band is formed. This band shifts to the left with increasing concentrations.

The basic information from both methods of analysis suggests that with high-dose narcotic anesthesia there is also a considerable shift to the left of both frequency and amplitude. The aperiodic analysis, which retains more quantitative detail, reveals a sharp and marked increase in delta waves. During induction, we also observed with the Neurometrics a shift through the theta region at relatively light levels of fentanyl and sufentanil. This shift occurred within a very few minutes and was reflected by the significant difference between TP_{max} and control. With alfentanil the shift occurred in a matter of seconds (Smith NT et al, unpublished data, 1983).

We observed in the EEG a much more rapid onset of anesthesia with fentanyl and sufentanil than we did with morphine. This corroborates our clinically oriented data on the comparative rapidity of induction with these agents [7].

The fact that many of the EEG variables showed significant changes indicative of anesthetic lightening during the relatively long interval between laryngoscopy and incision suggests that the EEG reflects if not depth of anesthesia, then at least changes in brain concentrations of the agents. This speculation could be validated by measuring serum levels of the agents and correlating them with EEG values. Alternatively, clinical depth of anesthesia can be estimated and correlated with EEG levels. Preliminary evidence suggests that with fentanyl, aperiodic analysis can reliably estimate depth of anesthesia [8].

There were marked differences between the EEG effects of fentanyl and sufentanil on the one hand and morphine on the other. These differences were most apparent in the pattern on the Neurometrics screen, but were also reflected in the quantitative data and consisted of a greater concentration of EEG activity in the lower-frequency area during fentanyl and sufentanil. Thus either morphine produces a different EEG pattern, or patients anesthetized with morphine were in a lighter plane of anesthesia than those anesthetized with either fentanyl or sufentanil. The former is consistent with morphine's structural difference from fentanyl and its congeners. The latter is consistent with data which indicate that the cardiovascular system is more labile during morphine anesthesia and is also more subject to changes during stimulating events, such as laryngoscopy or incision (Smith NT et al, unpublished data, 1982).

Although great care was taken in recording the EEG, at least two considerations should be noted regarding the control values. First, preanesthetic medication with morphine and scopolamine could affect the baseline EEG. Second, and more important, was the unavoidable muscle noise occurring partly because of our use of global EEG leads, which were used to detect episodes of cerebral ischemia. These leads were particularly susceptible to noise induced by muscle tremor in a conscious or unparalyzed patient. This noise can be partially attenuated by appropriate filtering before analysis. In our case, the low-pass filter was set at 30 Hz before analysis. The subtraction process outlined above was able to compensate for much of the rest of this noise. We had to assume that muscle noise was nonspecific whether the patient was awake or lightly anesthetized, and therefore that we were justified in using a correction factor obtained while the patient was lightly anesthetized, that is, just before neuromuscular block. With fentanyl and sufentanil, we did have to modify the correction factor to account for the change in depth of anesthesia that occurred while the neuromuscular block was being established, usually about one minute.

COMPARISON OF TWO STUDIES

One of the few studies to investigate the EEG effects of high-dose narcotics in a similar way was that of Sebel et al [9]. These investigators examined the EEG during high-dose fentanyl anesthesia in patients undergoing open heart surgery. Except for our failure to detect the sharp waves observed by Sebel, their results were qualitatively similar to ours. The difference was in degree. Both studies demonstrated a marked shift to the left with fentanyl, although our relative changes were somewhat greater in the lower frequency ranges.

Several factors could have contributed to the quantitative differences between our studies: different preanesthetic medications, more fentanyl in our study, different EEG leads, the use of noise-canceling techniques in our study, different epochs, different frequency bins (1 Hz vs 3 to 15 Hz), and different analytic techniques. Sebel used Fourier analytic techniques, while we used zero-crossing and aperiodic techniques. Period analysis is somewhat similar to Fourier analysis in that both are averaging techniques. Aperiodic analysis examines individual wave forms, and as such retains considerably more detail for use.

Although the quantitative data were obtained off line after surgery, both the Klein and the Neurometrics can be used on line, and we observed the latter continually during all cases. The detail available with the Neurometrics is excellent for visual interpretation, and the shift to higher amplitudes at lower frequencies is readily seen; however, it gives too much detail to grasp quantitatively. Therefore we can still determine depth of anesthesia better with visual interpretation of the patterns on the Neurometrics screen than with any combination of numbers that we have been able to develop thus far.

The variables that we selected appear to give different information about these agents at different depths of anesthesia. At one extreme, CP3 seems to be very sensitive to small concentrations or light levels of anesthesia, as indicated by the fact that maximum changes were seen before insertion of the oral airway. Thus CP3, TP4, and F90 should be useful for low- to moderate-dose fentanyl or sufentanil, while TP1 should be more useful for moderate- to high-dose fentanyl or sufentanil anesthesia. Again, it would be useful to correlate quantitative EEG analyses with blood levels of the narcotic in question.

CONCLUSION

We recorded the EEG in 49 patients during morphine-oxygen, fentanyl-oxygen, or sufentanil-oxygen anesthesia, from induction through the period of the incisions. Marked and characteristic changes were seen, and these tended to return toward control with time. Although fentanyl and sufentanil produced similar changes in the EEG, these changes differed from those produced by morphine. Finally, we can speculate that these EEG changes probably reflect anesthetic depth and should be useful for monitoring this factor.

REFERENCES

1. Stockard JJ, Bickford RG. The neurophysiology of anesthesia. In: Gordon E., ed. A basis and practice of neuroanesthesia. New York: Excerpta Medica, 1981:1–49.
2. Levy WJ, Shapiro HM, Marvchale G, Meathe E. Automated EEG processing for intraoperative monitoring: a comparison of techniques. Anesthesiology 1980;53:223–36.
3. Klein FF. A waveform analyzer applied to the human EEG. IEEE Trans Biomed Eng 1976;23:246–52.
4. Klein FF, Davis DA. The use of the time domain-analyzed EEG in conjunction with cardiovascular parameters for monitoring anesthetic levels. IEEE Trans Biomed Eng 1981;28:36–40.
5. Demetrescu M. The aperiodic character of the electroencephalogram: a new approach to data analysis and condensation. Physiologist 1975;18:189.
6. Demetrescu M, Kavan E, Smith NT. Monitoring the brain condition by advanced EEG (abstract). Anesthesiology 1981;55:130.
7. Smith NT, Dec-Silver H, Harrison WK, Sanford TJ Jr, Gillig J. A comparison among morphine, fentanyl, and sufentanil anesthesia for open-heart surgery. Induction, emergence, and extubation. Anesthesiology 1982;57:A291.
8. Smith NT, Demetrescu M. The EEG during high-dose fentanyl anesthesia (abstract). Anesthesiology 1980;53:S7.
9. Sebel PS, Bovill JG, Wauquier A, Rog P. Effects of high-dose fentanyl anesthesia on the electroencephalogram. Anesthesiology 1981;55:203–11.

11 ELECTROENCEPHALOGRAPHY DURING HIGH-DOSE NARCOTIC ANESTHESIA: DISCUSSION

Michael G. Bazaral

Chapter 10 examined the electroencephalographic (EEG) changes associated with morphine, fentanyl, and sufentanil during induction of anesthesia and the beginning of surgery. The authors compared two techniques of EEG analysis: zero-crossing and Neurometrics spectral analysis. Relatively little was said about zero-crossing techniques. With respect to the hardware and software required, zero-crossing analysis is not difficult to implement, but the information it provides is not readily understandable in terms of a power spectrum. The method is empiric but apparently contains enough information to permit observation of the effects of fentanyl. Dr. Smith and his colleagues have demonstrated that it may be of some use.

Details on how the Neurometrics analysis is performed are not available to us, but the device is said to display each wave of the EEG decomposed according to its duration and amplitude. Dr. Smith's group developed important information that has been lacking: some quantitative results from the Neurometrics analysis. Unfortunately, the work is based on idiosyncratic techniques.

Neurometrics analysis and zero-crossing methods appear to have little future now that relatively inexpensive Fourier analysis devices are commercially available. The Fourier power spectrum provides the best-documented method for EEG analysis and is classic in this kind of work. Not commonly discussed is the fact that the results of Fourier analysis depend to an extent on the type of machinery being used and the algorithm by which the analysis is conducted. Therefore direct comparisons from one study to another cannot be made unless the machinery is at least similar.

The major finding reported by Smith et al is that the very lowest EEG frequencies are the most sensitive indicators of deep narcotic anesthesia. In light of the differences in technology used, it is not entirely clear that the findings of Smith's group are different from the power spectrum analysis of Sebel et al [1]. I suspect that the observation of changes at the very lowest frequencies reflects a new phenomenon, but confirmation by more broadly available methods is needed.

Dr. Smith raises the possibility of using an automated EEG analysis technique for gauging anesthetic levels. Questions must be addressed in this regard. For example, it is not immediately evident that automated titration could offer much to improve our use of fentanyl, which has a very flat dose-response curve. Abi-Nader, Wagner, Estafanous, and I have investigated the effects of high- and low-dose fentanyl and evaluated the EEG records obtained with the Neurometrics monitor. A brief description of the results follows.

EEG ANALYSIS IN FENTANYL ANESTHESIA

We studied induction of anesthesia with fixed doses of fentanyl in 40 patients who had at least good myocardial function. All were premedicated with morphine and scopolamine, and anesthesia was induced with muscle relaxant given concurrently with a fixed dose of fentanyl, either 15 or 60 μg per kilogram of body weight. The fentanyl was administered over 12 or 45 seconds depending on which dose was used. We worked by the clock and paid no attention to whether or not the patients appeared to be asleep.

Compared with controls, our patients showed a modest increase in heart rate with fentanyl, slightly greater with the higher than with the lower dose. Blood pressure decreased perhaps 10%. The average cardiac index remained similar to control values throughout induction, as did systemic vascular resistance and wedge pressure. Three minutes after the start of fentanyl, we intubated the patients and saw very minor hemodynamic effects. Wedge pressure increased by several torr, a change probably contingent upon the use of positive-pressure ventilation. Negligible differences were found between the 15- and 60-μg/kg doses overall.

If we succeeded in achieving anesthesia—and none of the patients remembered intubation or the early part of surgery—our results show that the amount of fentanyl makes little difference provided that some minimal level is achieved. Giving more of the agent produced no greater occurrence of hypotension, nor did giving less cause greater frequency of hypertension. There was variability in the course for individual patients in both groups. We are still analyzing these data.

When the Neurometrics EEG was used in these patients, all showed patterns characteristic of deep narcotic anesthesia within 110 seconds after either dose was given. The EEG was recorded for another nine minutes until we introduced halothane to maintain anesthesia. Low-frequency EEG activity remained and appeared to be unchanged for 13 minutes in both groups. It was not possible to make finer distinctions by eye using the Neurometrics cathode-ray display. I regret that we did not use some technique other than Neurometrics monitoring, as we do not have Smith's nice quantitative analysis programs.

EEG ANALYSIS DURING SURGERY

The other point I wish to make about narcotic anesthesia is that clinically, hypertension occurs in a fraction of patients upon manipulation of the aorta and during some other cardiac-related maneuvers. We certainly see hypertension during fentanyl anesthesia and thoracic aneurysm surgery. Reflexes that go from the thoracic aorta to the spinal cord or from the heart and other mediastinal structures to the spinal cord and back to sympathetic effector organs have been fairly well described [2]. No one has studied the effects that anesthetic agents—much less narcotic agents—exert on such reflexes under clinical circumstances. An EEG analysis, which examines the brain effects of narcotics, may be of little help when we try to achieve anesthesia as defined by hemodynamic stability while mediastinal structures are being manipulated. This remains to be seen. I look forward to what Dr. Smith will tell us as he continues to examine the relationship of the EEG to narcotic anesthesia.

REFERENCES

1. Sebel PS, Bovill JG, Wauquier A, Rog P. Effects of high-dose fentanyl anesthesia on the electroencephalogram. Anesthesiology 1981;55:203–11.

2. Malliani A. Cardiovascular sympathetic afferent fibers. Rev Physiol Biochem Pharmacol 1982;94:11–74.

12 HORMONAL CHANGES DURING NARCOTIC ANESTHESIA AND OPERATION

Daniel M. Philbin, Carl E. Rosow, Michael D'Ambra,
Edmond S. Freis, and Robert C. Schneider

Narcotics have been used to varying degrees from the very beginnings of anesthesia. Since the late 1960s, with the introduction of morphine in doses large enough to be the primary agent, narcotics as anesthetics have assumed a role of increasing importance [1]. This has been particularly true in the field of cardiac surgery where it became necessary to provide anesthesia in desperately ill patients with a severely compromised cardiovascular system without producing cardiovascular collapse. During this same period, rapid developments in the field of radioimmunoassays and radioenzymatic assays spilled over into the clinical field and for the first time, allowed accurate measurement of a variety of hormones during periods of stress such as anesthesia and surgery.

MORPHINE

The rapid development of cardiac surgery led gradually to the concept that large doses of morphine could be administered as the primary anesthetic agent [1]. This regimen met with widespread success and acceptance, particularly in the management of patients with valvular heart disease, primarily because of the minimal circulatory effects noted.

Subsequent studies investigated the effect of high-dose morphine on the various hormonal response that occurred after surgical stimulation. Evidence appeared that, in doses of 1 to 3 mg per kilogram of body weight, morphine was capable of blocking the cortisol and growth hormone response [2]. Shortly thereafter, data were published that investigated the relationships between morphine and antidiuretic hormone (ADH) in humans. It had generally been believed that morphine stimulates ADH release, but evidence now confirmed the clinical impression that ADH levels do not increase with morphine administration alone [3]. Significant increase in ADH could occur, however, with surgical stimulation, resulting in concentrations capable of producing a pressor effect. Larger doses of morphine were able to blunt but not eliminate this response [4].

The development of coronary artery bypass surgery, which changed the field of cardiac anesthesia considerably, paralleled the increasing problems with morphine anesthesia. Reports began to appear which suggested that morphine as the sole anesthetic agent was not adequately blunting the hormonal stress responses, particularly in patients with good left ventricular function. Other problems added to the situation, such as bradycardia (especially in patients with right coronary artery disease) [5], increased muscle tone [6], hypotension, probably due to histamine release [7], and patient recall. The use of increasingly larger doses of morphine was attempted in an effort to block many of those responses adequately, and it met with some success [8]. Although these enormous doses (up to 10 mg/kg) were reliably capable of blocking the hemodynamic (and presumably hormonal) responses to surgical stimulation, the clinical price was too high [9,10].

FENTANYL

This led to the introduction of a synthetic narcotic, fentanyl, a compound that is considerably more potent than morphine. It has the added advantage that in a single dose it has a relatively short duration of action because of rapid uptake by all tissues [11]. In addition, it provides relatively stable hemodynamics even when administered in moderately large doses, due in part to the fact that it does not release histamine in humans [12].

The majority of the early studies with fentanyl using doses in the range of 50 μg/kg demonstrated that it was indeed capable of blocking many, if not all, of the hormonal and hemodynamic responses to surgical stimulation. Hall et al reported in 1978 that the responses of cortisol and growth hormone during pelvic surgery could be prevented [13]. Subsequent studies using slightly larger doses (75 μg/kg) reported the same blunting effect on cortisol and growth hormone responses in patients undergoing cardiac surgery, but only in the period before bypass [14,15]. At these higher doses fentanyl had a similar effect on plasma ADH and cathecholamine levels [16,17]. As with morphine, however, significant increases in a variety of the stress hormones continued to occur during the period of cardiopulmonary bypass [16,18].

The relative hemodynamic stability seen even with very large doses of fentanyl and its ability to blunt many of the hormonal responses to surgical stimulation resulted in widespread acceptance of this technique. Within a short time, however, problems began to be reported in the literature. These included an alarmingly high frequency of hypertension and tachycardia [19] and metabolic evidence of myocardial ischemia [20] suggesting inadequate blunting of the stress response. Administration of these high doses significantly increased the frequency of patient rigidity as well as the occurrence of profound bradycardia. Finally, again as with morphine, there were disturbing reports of patient awareness during surgical procedures [21,22]. Increasingly larger doses of fentanyl were used in an effort to blunt hormonal responses totally and prevent some of these untoward results. These efforts to a large extent were only modestly successful and again, as with morphine, led to a reappraisal of the entire field of narcotic anesthesia [23,24].

SUFENTANIL AND ALFENTANIL

The increasing evidence of undesirable side effects and inadequate blunting of the hormonal stress response despite increasing dose of fentanyl spurred the search for newer and more potent narcotics. The hope was to find a drug that could be administered in amounts sufficient to blunt the hormonal responses and avoid side effects, or at least keep them to an acceptable level. One of the more promising of these is sufentanil, an analog of fentanyl, which is approximately five to seven times as potent and has a similarly short pharmacologic action [25,26]. As with fentanyl, it produces relatively stable hemodynamics during induction, which again may be related to lack of histamine release [27]. Preliminary data suggest that sufentanil in doses of 10 to 20 µg/kg is capable of blunting the hormonal stress responses to surgical stimulation except perhaps during the period of cardiopulmonary bypass [28]. Doses in the range of 30 µg/kg may prove more effective, but the data are incomplete [29]. It remains to be seen if sufentanil will be the answer to the problems encountered with high-dose morphine or fentanyl anesthesia.

Another synthetic narcotic undergoing investigation at present is alfentanil, which has the advantage of being short acting and thus is suitable for use in relatively short surgical procedures [30,31]. It is less potent than fentanyl, but early reports suggest that large doses produce relatively stable hemodynamics and can block the responses of cortisol, growth hormone, and ADH to surgical manipulation up to but not including the period of bypass [32,33]. Further studies are presently under way and more data are needed before alfentanil's position in clinical anesthesia is established.

CONCLUSION

Efforts to achieve an anesthetic environment that totally ablates the hormonal stress response to surgical stimulation have concentrated on high-dose narcotic anesthesia, particularly the new synthetic narcotics. This is because the high concentrations of drugs required can be administered with relative ease and side effects are either easily treatable or within acceptable range. High concentrations of potent inhalation agents could also blunt these hormonal responses but at a price unacceptable in the clinical situation. The basic question that remains is whether, in striving for this stress-free state, we are helping the patient. It seems clear from the variety of actions the various hormones have (Table 12.1) that a huge outpouring during the period of anesthesia and operation can and does contribute to patients' negative metabolic state. If, as some studies suggest [34,35], we are merely delaying this hormonal response and allowing it to occur in the postoperative period, then the benefit must be minimal and we should look to a different approach [36]. If this hormonal response, while being delayed, is also at least attenuated, however, perhaps this approach should be pursued.

The answer is not yet clear. The last two decades have convincingly demonstrated that narcotics can and do produce profound analgesia for surgical procedures and are capable of preventing, or at least attenuating, the hormonal stress response to operation, but not universally. High-dose narcotic anesthesia as presently practiced is far from perfect, and indeed, at times is totally inadequate. If preventing the hormonal stress response to anesthesia and operation is a

TABLE 12.1. Hormonal effects

Hormone	Effect
Antidiuretic hormone (vasopressin)	Water retention: vasoconstriction
Adrenocorticotropic hormone	Increased cortisol and aldosterone
Cortisol	Hyperglycemia, protein breakdown
Aldosterone	Sodium retention
Growth hormone	Hyperglycemia, ketogenesis
Catecholamines	Lipolysis, ketogenesis, hyperglycemia
Thyroxine	Increased catabolism
Renin	Vasoconstriction, increased aldosterone and angiotensin
Glucagon	Hyperglycemia, ketogenesis

worthwhile goal, it remains to be seen if the synthesis of narcotics with greater analgesic potency and/or shorter duration of action will provide the answer.

REFERENCES

1. Lowenstein E, Hallowell P, Levine FH, Daggett WM, Austen WG, Laver MD. Cardiovascular responses to large doses of intravenous morphine in man. N Engl J Med 1969;281:1389–93.

2. George JM, Reier CE, Lanese RR, Rower JM. Morphine anaesthesia blocks cortisol and growth hormone response to surgical stress in humans. J Clin Endocrinol Metab 1974;38:736–41.

3. Philbin DM, Wilson N, Sokoloski J, Coggins CH. Radioimmunoassay of antidiuretic hormone during morphine anaesthesia. Can Anaesth Soc J 1976;23:290–5.

4. Philbin DM, Coggins CH. Plasma antidiuretic hormone level in cardiac surgical patients during morphine and halothane anesthesia. Anesthesiology 1978;49:95–8.

5. Thomas M, Malcrona R, Fillmore S, et al. Haemodynamic effects of morphine in patients with acute myocardial infarction. Br Heart J 1965;27:863–75.

6. Freund FG, Martin WE, Wong KC, Hornbein TF. Abdominal muscle rigidity induced by morphine and nitrous oxide. Anesthesiology 1973;38:358–62.

7. Philbin DM, Moss J, Akins CW, et al. The use of H_1 and H_2 histamine antagonists with morphine anesthesia: a double-blind study. Anesthesiology 1981;55:292–6.

8. Hasbrouk JD. Morphine anesthesia for open heart surgery. Ann Thorac Surg 1970; 10:364–9.

9. Stanley TH, Gray NH, Stanford DW, et al. The effects of high-dose morphine on fluid and blood requirements in open-heart operation. Anesthesiology 1973;38:536–41.

10. Lowenstein E. Morphine "anesthesia"—a perspective. Anesthesiology 1971;35:563–5.

11. Hug CC Jr. Pharmacokinetics of drugs adminstered intravenously. Anesth Analg (Cleve) 1978;57:704–32.

12. Rosow CE, Moss J, Philbin DM, Savarese JJ. Histamine release during morphine and fentanyl anesthesia. Anesthesiology 1982; 56:93–6.

13. Hall GM, Young C, Holdcroft A, Alaghband-Zadeh J. Substrate mobilization during surgery. A comparison between halothane and fentanyl anesthesia. Anaesthesia 1978;33:924–30.

14. Sebel PS, Bovill JG, Schellekens APM, Hawker CD. Hormonal responses to high-dose fentanyl anaesthesia. Br J Anaesth 1981;53:941–7.

15. Kono K, Philbin DM, Coggins CH, et al. Renal function and stress response during halothane or fentanyl anesthesia. Anesth Analg (Cleve) 1981;60:552–6.

16. Stanley TH, Philbin DM, Coggins CH. Fentanyl-oxygen anaesthesia for coronary artery surgery: cardiovascular and antidiuretic hormone responses. Can Anaesth Soc J 1979;26:168–72.

17. Stanley TH, Berman L, Green O. Plasma cathecholamine and cortisol responses to fentanyl-oxygen anesthesia for coronary artery operations. Anesthesiology 1980; 53:250–3.

18. Philbin DM, Coggins CH, Emerson CW, Levine FH, Buckley MJ. Plasma vasopressin levels and urinary excretion during cardiopulmonary bypass: a comparison of halothane and morphine anesthesia. J Thorac Cardiovasc Surg 1979;77:582–5.

19. Waller JL, Hug CC Jr, Nagle DM, Craver JM. Fentanyl-oxygen "anesthesia" and coronary bypass surgery. Anesth Analg (Cleve) 1980;59:562–3.

20. Sonntag H, Larsen R, Hilfiker D, Kettler D, Buckschneider B. Myocardial blood flow and oxygen consumption during high-dose fentanyl anesthesia in patients with coronary artery disease. Anesthesiology 1982; 56:417–22.

21. Mummaneni N, Rao TL, Montoya A. Awareness and recall with high-dose fentanyl oxygen anesthesia. Anesth Analg (Cleve) 1980;59:948–9.

22. Hilgenberg JC. Intra-operative awareness during high-dose fentanyl-oxygen anesthesia. Anesthesiology 1981;54:341–3.

23. Lowenstein E, Philbin DM. Narcotic "anesthesia" in the eighties. Anesthesiology 1981;55:195–7.

24. Sebel PS, Bovill JG. Opioid anaesthesia—fact or fallacy? Br J Anaesth 1982;54:1149–50.

25. Rolly G, Kay B, Cockx F. A double-blind comparison of high doses of fentanyl and sufentanil in man. Acta Anesthesiol Belg 1979;30:247–54.

26. de Lange S, Boscoe MJ, Stanley TH, Pace N. Comparison of sufentanil-O_2 and fentanyl-O_2 for coronary artery surgery. Anesthesiology 1982;56:112–18.

27. Philbin DM, Rosow CE, Moss J, Tomichek RC, Schneider RC. Histamine release during induction with high-dose fentanyl. Abstract of the Sixth European Congress of Anesthesiology. London: Academic Press, 1982:322–3.

28. Bovill JG, Sebel PS, Fiolet JWT, Touber JL, Kosk K, Philbin DM. The influence of sufentanil on the endocrine metabolic responses to cardiac surgery. Anesth Analg (NY) 1983;62:391–7.

29. Rosow CE, Philbin DM, Moss J, Keegan CR, Schneider RL. Sufentanil vs. fentanil. I. Suppression of hemodynamic responses. Anesthesiology 1983;59:A323.

30. Bovill JG, Sebel PS, Blackburn CL, Heykants J. The pharmacokinetics of alfentanil (R 39209): a new opioid analgesic. Anesthesiology 1972;57:439–43.

31. Stanski DR, Hug CC Jr. Alfentanil—a kinetically predictable narcotic analgesic. Anesthesiology 1982;57:435–8.

32. de Lange S, Boscoe MJ, Stanley TH, de Bruijin N, Philbin DM, Coggins CH. Antidiuretic and growth hormone responses during coronary artery surgery with sufentanil-oxygen and alfentanil-oxygen anesthesia in man. Anesth Analg (Cleve) 1982;61:434–8.

33. de Lange S, Stanley TH, Boscoe MJ, et al. Cathecholamine and cortisol responses to sufentanil-oxygen and alfentanil-oxygen anesthesia during coronary artery surgery. Anesth Analg (Cleve) 1982;61:177–8.

34. Walsh ES, Paterson JL, O'Riordan JBA, Hall GM. Effect on high-dose fentanyl anaesthesia on the metabolic and endocrine response to cardiac surgery. Br J Anaesth 1981;53:1155–65.

35. Cooper GM, Paterson JL, Ward ID, Hall GM. Fentanyl and the metabolic response to gastric surgery. Anaesthesia 1981;36:667–71.

36. Philbin DM, Levine EH, Kono K, et al. Attenuation of the stress response to cardiopulmonary bypass by the addition of pulsatile flow. Circulation 1981;34:808–12.

13 EFFECTS OF INTRATHECAL AND EPIDURAL MORPHINE ON ENDOCRINE FUNCTION

Tsutomu Oyama

In Chapter 12 Dr. Philbin nicely summarized the attempts that have been made to suppress the hormonal stress response during surgery with high-dose narcotic anesthesia. The discussion centered mostly on cardiovascular procedures. We have investigated the effects of morphine on endocrine function when the agent was administered intrathecally or epidurally to patients undergoing gynecologic surgery. This chapter briefly describes the protocols and presents our results.

EFFECTS OF INTRATHECAL MORPHINE ON PAIN AND STRESS

Twenty patients who underwent gynecologic abdominal surgery were divided into three groups at random. Four patients served as controls and were anesthetized with halothane–nitrous oxide. Eight patients comprising a β-endorphin group were given 2 mg of that synthetic human opiate peptide intrathecally. The remaining eight patients, the

morphine group, received morphine hydrochloride, 0.2 mg intrathecally, before anesthesia and surgery. To avoid diurnal variations in plasma concentrations of the various hormones, anesthesia was started at around 8:30 AM in all cases.

In the β-endorphin and morphine groups, administration of 0.5% inspired halothane was sufficient to maintain an adequate depth of anesthesia during surgery. Inhalation of more than 1.5% halothane was necessary in the control group, however. Mean duration of analgesia after the initial postoperative injection was 5.5 hours in the control group, 14.3 hours in the β-endorphin group, and 24.7 hours in the morphine group. No major complications such as respiratory or circulatory depression were found in any of the patients [1].

Levels of plasma growth hormone increased significantly during halothane anesthesia and surgery in the control group. In the patients who received β-endorphin or morphine, levels rose slightly during surgery and continued to increase postoperatively.

Plasma adrenocorticotropic hormone (ACTH) increased much less in the β-endorphin and control groups than in the morphine group during halothane anesthesia and surgery [2].

Levels of plasma cortisol rose during surgery and the postoperative period in all patients. The increase was much less marked in the β-endorphin and morphine groups compared with controls. Plasma prolactin levels increased about threefold above preanesthetic levels during halothane anesthesia and surgery in all patients, and there was no significant difference among the groups [2].

Thus intrathecal morphine was effective in relieving pain and generally provided some degree of control over the stress hormones.

EFFECTS OF EPIDURAL MORPHINE ON PAIN AND STRESS

The effects of epidural morphine on postoperative pain relief and endocrine function were investigated in 25 patients undergoing transabdominal gynecologic operations. In 15 patients, 2 mg of morphine hydrochloride in 10 ml of physiologic saline was injected epidurally through the second and third lumbar intervertebral space prior to halothane–nitrous oxide anesthesia. The remaining 10 patients received 10 ml of physiologic saline as controls.

Profound relief of pain was achieved in the morphine group postoperatively and lasted 19.7 hours, versus 11.8 hours for the control group. Nausea, vomiting, respiratory depression, and prolonged postoperative flatus were observed in several patients who had received morphine, however [3].

The increase in plasma ACTH and cortisol levels was not so high in the morphine group as it was in the control group two hours after the start of operation and when the patients recovered from anesthesia. Levels of plasma antidiuretic hormone and aldosterone decreased and plasma renin activity increased after epidural administration of mor-

phine as compared with the control group. Urine osmolality and volume decreased and the sodium-potassium ratio rose in the morphine group compared with control values [4].

Plasma growth hormone levels decreased during surgery, but they increased significantly on the first postoperative day in patients who received morphine compared with controls. Compared with the preinduction level, plasma insulin levels in the morphine group decreased slightly two hours after the start of operation and in the recovery room when the patients awoke adequately from anesthesia. Thereafter they increased gradually, as in the control group. Plasma glucose levels decreased significantly two hours after the start of operation in the morphine group as compared with controls. Significant increases in plasma prolactin occurred in both groups after anesthesia and surgery; no significant difference in prolactin levels was found between the groups [5].

Plasma concentrations of β-endorphin increased significantly during and after anesthesia and surgery. In the morphine group, a marked increase was not detected in the recovery room when the patients had completely recovered from anesthesia (Figure 13.1). Changes in plasma β-endorphin and ACTH levels paralleled each other during the surgical procedure [6]. Plasma concentrations of β-lipotropic hormone increased after halothane–nitrous oxide anesthesia and surgery in both groups. Plasma norepinephrinc levels increased significantly during surgery and in the recovery room, but no significant difference was detected between the groups. Plasma epinephrine levels in the patients who received morphine were significantly depressed compared with controls.

CONCLUSION

To summarize our results with epidural morphine (Table 13.1), our findings suggest that

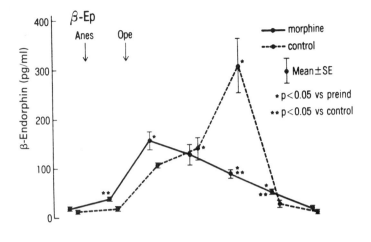

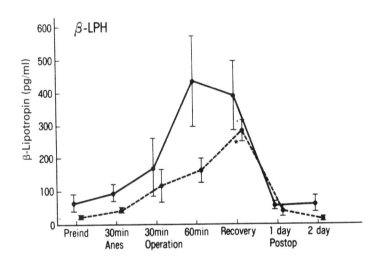

FIGURE 13.1. Plasma β-endorphin and β-lipotropin levels after anesthesia and surgery.

it can suppress the elevation of plasma ACTH and cortisol levels after halothane–nitrous oxide anesthesia and surgery. Concentrations of plasma growth hormone and glucose are also maintained near baseline values, while morphine helps to increase plasma growth hormone levels on the first postoperative day. Finally, epidural morphine prevents an increase in plasma β-endorphin and epinephrine levels after halothane–nitrous oxide anesthesia and surgery. Thus our results suggest that epidural morphine attenuates the endocrine nociceptive response to surgical stress.

TABLE 13.1. Plasma hormones after anesthesia and surgery

Anesthesia	ACTH	Cortisol	ADH	Aldosterone	PRA	PRL	HGH	β-Ep	β-LPH
Halothane–N₂O	↑↑	↑↑	↑↑	↑↑	↑↑↑	↑↑	↑↑	↑↑	↑↑
Morphine–N₂O	↑	↑↑	↑	↑↑	↑↑↑	↑↑	↑↑	↑↑	↑ or→
Epidural	↑	↑	↑	↑	↑	↑	↑	↑ or→	↑ or→
Halothane–N₂O		↑↑	↑↑	↑↑	↑↑	↑↑	↑	↑	↑↑
Epidural morphine	↑								

REFERENCES

1. Taniguchi K, Yamashita M, Ishida K, Matsuki A, Oyama T. Effects of intrathecal β-endorphin and morphine on postoperative pain. Jpn J Anesthesiol 1981;30:1105–11.
2. Taniguchi K, Yamashita M, Kudoh T, Matsuki A, Oyama T. Effects of intrathecal β-endorphin and morphine on endocrine response during halothane anesthesia and surgery in man. Jpn J Anesthesiol 1981;30:1175–82.
3. Yao M, Yamaya R, Ishihara H, Kudo T, Matsuki A, Oyama T. Endocrine function following epidural morphine in man. I. Effects on postoperative pain and plasma ACTH and cortisol levels. Jpn J Anesthesiol 1981;30:1168–74.
4. Yao M, Tanioka F, Ishihara H, Kudo T, Matsuki A, Oyama T. Endocrine functions following epidural morphine in man. II. Effects on renal function and plasma ADH and aldosterone levels and plasma. Jpn J Anesthesiol 1981;30:1353–63.
5. Yao M, Miyahara T, Ishihara H, Kudo T, Matsuki A, Oyama T. Endocrine function following epidural morphine in man. III. Effects on plasma prolactin, growth hormone and insulin levels. Jpn J Anesthesiol 1982;31:1211–17.
6. Yao M, Kudoh T, Jin T, Fukushi S, Matsuki A, Oyama T. Endocrine function following epidural morphine in man. IV. Effects on plasma β-endorphin and β-lipotropin levels in man. Jpn J Anesthesiol 1983;32:1104–9.

Part II DISCUSSION

DR. M. M. GHONEIM: My first question is directed to Dr. Hug. I am trying to understand how the attachment of the various opioids to the opiate receptors relates to the duration of action of each drug. With alfentanil, for example, the correlation seems clear. Alfentanil is attached loosely to the receptor and it has a short duration of action. Fentanyl and sufentanil, however, have almost the same duration of action but the tightness with which they bind and remain attached to receptors is completely different.

DR. CARL C. HUG, JR.: We are just starting to investigate how tightly drugs are bound and how rapidly they dissociate from receptors, and we don't have the full explanation yet. I did speculate that perhaps sufentanil has a very tight interaction with the receptor that helps to sustain its effect, but we still need to look at different situations with various narcotics. Long-acting morphine, for example, has a kinetic profile comparable in many ways to that of fentanyl, and I think morphine is longer acting because of its rate of exit from the central nervous system. There are probably different reasons for the various durations of action of narcotic analgesics, and one might be the rate of dissociation of a drug from its receptors.

DR. MICHAEL F. ROIZEN: I have two questions, both for Dr. Smith. Does the theta activity or the very low frequency electroencephalographic (EEG) activity (delta) continue to decline as anesthesia is deepened, or does it reach a basement threshold and stop declining? Also, how can we relate the EEG changes you observed to actual clinical events?

DR. N. TY SMITH: Theta activity appears to be related to very light narcotic depth; it increases initially and then declines rapidly as more fentanyl or sufentanil is administered. We have seen it reappear only with alfentanil, whose course we can follow over 10 to 15 minutes. If one administers enough agent, almost all EEG activity above delta disappears; delta activity increases as more drug is given. We have not reached a peak delta effect, but we have not given the large amounts that Dr. Moldenhauer has. Delta wave activity appears to be a good marker for deep narcotic anesthesia, in contrast to theta activity.

In response to your second question, we have watched EEG readings return toward waking levels and can correlate this return with the patient's clinical state. In the course of fentanyl anesthesia during cardiovascular surgery, we can predict within 90% accuracy whether a patient is going to have a cardiovascular response to intubation, incision, sternal spread, or other surgical events.

DR. ROIZEN: Which of the EEG components or wave forms let you make these predictions?

DR. SMITH: The alpha, beta, theta, and delta waves all give us clues, and we look at them in combination. Until now, we have been using the changing patterns on the Neurometrics screen; however, we are just beginning to learn how to use the information from the large matrix that I showed earlier. By dividing the EEG information into 1-Hz bins, instead of four bands, we can achieve certainly more detailed and perhaps more useful information for estimating depth of anesthesia.

DR. THEODORE H. STANLEY: I have two conceptual questions, one for Dr. Janssen, and one for Dr. Hug or Dr. Stanski. Dr. Janssen, we have seen the narcotic anesthetics evolve from morphine through phenoperidine to fentanyl and now sufentanil, and you spoke about the quest for greater and greater potency. Do you think a drug with a potency of one million times morphine, or ten million times morphine, is going to provide any clinical advantages over the agents available to us now, or have we reached the limit?

DR. PAUL A. J. JANSSEN: My guess is that with greater potencies we will probably find more of the same types of effects. I was talking about morphinomimetic drugs, or compounds that mimic morphine. The differences between these drugs are almost entirely quantitative, not qualitative. Perhaps further progress will be achieved in anesthesia with drugs that have nothing to do with morphine. But these drugs are not known today, and I'm not a prophet so I can't say.

DR. STANLEY: Dr. Hug, my second question concerns pharmacokinetics. How much patient-to-patient variability exists in the amount of drug needed to produce analgesia or to alter respiration?

DR. HUG: I really can't answer that question. A tremendous number of variables influence a patient's response to a narcotic analgesic. I mentioned sleep as one example, and data described by the San Francisco group a few years ago show that stimulus level can also affect the extent to which respiration becomes depressed. So if the stimulus level or any of a number of other factors were to change, the dosage and concentration requirements would need to change along with them.

The issue of drug requirement with narcotic anesthetics is only vaguely defined at present, but we are starting to home in on it a bit. We have developed techniques for correlating respiration and analgesia with dosage, and now we must begin studying the effects of different variables. But at least we are gaining the techniques and procedures that will allow us to make these estimations.

DR. STANLEY: As a corollary to that thought, you suggested, Dr. Hug, that administering an agent by continuous intravenous infusion to regulate the level of anesthesia is a desirable goal. I agree, but obviously surgical stimulation changes during an operation, and therefore adjustments might be needed to maintain an appropriate infusion rate.

DR. HUG: Yes. In fact, we may begin using these agents in much the same way we've used inhalation agents over the years: we may vary drug concentrations throughout the surgical procedure according to fluctuations in the intensity of surgical stimulation. This has been done, in fact. Dr. Ausems, at the University of Leiden in the Netherlands, has been administering variable-rate alfentanil infusions, and he has maintained satisfactory anesthesia by manipulating the rate in anticipation of or in response to differences in stimulation.

DR. HARVEY SHAPIRO: It is well recognized that narcotics have a dose-related neuroexcitatory effect, which in animals culminates in seizures. We have seen this with fentanyl in our laboratory, and we've localized the sites of these seizures to subcortical areas of the hippocampus and other parts of the limbic system, which is well known to have a bimodal response to a dose: at very low doses it does not occur, and at very high levels it is suppressed. It seems that in humans this neuroexcitatory effect does not occur. Is it because of the doses we use? Has anyone seen this type of effect?

DR. SMITH: There are several possible explanations for the lack of seizure activity in human beings. First, the drug may produce different effects in different species. Second, the doses we have used may be too low to produce seizures.

Third, the agent may not have been injected rapidly enough to produce a high peak level. A fourth possibility is that we are not recording the right things in the right places. For example, an agent could be producing seizures in areas deep within the brain so that they cannot be detected with surface EEGs, which measure only a few millimeters below the surface of the skull.

DR. SHAPIRO: Let me elaborate on Dr. Smith's last comment. The brain areas in which we observe the metabolic activity associated with seizures are easy to measure by surface EEG in the rat. In humans, these areas are very difficult to record with surface EEGs, and we might not detect activity even if it were occurring. I'd like to ask our experts in EEG technology if they could help us to improve our means of recording, or to comment on whether this is indeed a problem.

DR. SMITH: Perhaps in your next patients undergoing brain surgery, Harvey, you can ask your neurosurgeon to place some EEG electrodes into subcortical areas in the limbic system. You could then observe the effect in these areas after administration of a narcotic such as fentanyl.

DR. JANSSEN: From a pharmacologic point of view, I would like to point out that only two narcotics are clear-cut convulsants. The best known, of course, is codeine, which in sufficient doses has produced convulsions in 100% of all animals tested. The second convulsant is meperidine. With many of the other narcotics, seizures are extremely rare. For instance, fentanyl, sufentanil, and similar compounds have been used in more than 200 species, and I'm not aware of a single one in which they produced convulsions.

DR. HUG: Dr. Moldenhauer and Dr. Merkin have completed studies using fentanyl with EEG monitoring, and they saw no signs of the grand mal seizure activity reported by Dr. Rao. The patients were paralyzed and 150 µg/kg of fentanyl was administered in 90 seconds, so the EEG was being recorded without interference from the outward manifestations of muscle rigidity.

Dr. Shapiro is talking about metabolic changes at the subcortical level. As I understand it, the implications of these changes in our patients are unclear, nor is it known for certain that they represent a stress on the brain due to imbalance between oxygen supply and demand. Is that correct?

DR. SMITH: This seizure activity is not a phenomenon unique to the opioid drugs. Most of the inhalation agents, particularly most of the inhalation ethers, will produce seizures when given in high enough doses. We see this with the barbiturates as well. It is interesting that excitation and depression can be produced by the same agent—sometimes at the same time.

DR. HUG: Some seizure activity, in fact, may stem from a drug-induced reduction in factors that inhibit neural firing. This, as we understand it, may be a distribution phenomenon of the drug.

DR. DAVID DAVIS: Let me attempt to prevent some misconceptions about the EEG effects of fentanyl. So far we have heard that a large dose, given rapidly, produces the large slow waves that are fairly typical of depression by an anesthetic. My experience with fentanyl has been with the low-dose technique, consisting of induction with a barbiturate, loading with fentanyl, and concomitant administration of nitrous oxide and muscle relaxants. In these situations, fentanyl does not produce the typical increase in amplitude that is associated with many other anesthetic agents. We do slow the frequency, but a great deal of very high-frequency EEG activity remains. I would like to know what your spectral analysis would show under these conditions, Dr. Smith.

DR. SMITH: I agree with your first point: the changes in amplitude and frequency we have been talking about don't occur except at moderate or higher doses. Also, as you stated, the frequency information may begin to change before we see alterations in amplitude. Perhaps more accurately, frequency and amplitude information should be combined. For example, we can describe light narcotic anesthesia partly by observing the amplitude and number of the theta waves. Yet if we look at only amplitude or only frequency, we will miss this information.

In response to your second point, we do see small slow waves accompanied by some high-fre-

quency waves when we administer fentanyl in the low-dose technique. But we don't interpret these as seizure waves. They are not at all like the so-called epileptiform activity or the frank seizures we see with enflurane, for example, and the small rapid waves disappear with higher drug concentrations.

DR. J. EARL WYNANDS: A remark for Dr. Philbin: I wonder if some of the cardiovascular effects that occur during cardiopulmonary bypass may be related to catecholamine release and the fentanyl dosage. We looked at two groups of patients. One group, with a mean plasma fentanyl concentration of 12 ng/ml, had a 100% incidence of hypertension after 60 minutes of extracorporeal perfusion. The other group, with a plasma fentanyl concentration of 25 ng/ml, had only a 20% incidence of pump hypertension at 60 minutes. The hypertension was not altered by saralasin infusion and was not associated with increased renin release, so we assume catecholamines were responsible. For that reason, we think we may be able to limit the rise in catecholamines during cardiopulmonary bypass in at least some patients by maintaining fairly high plasma fentanyl concentrations.

DR. DANIEL M. PHILBIN: I think you are probably largely correct that the higher the fentanyl concentration rises, the less cardiovascular response occurs. But I think it also depends on what happens after hypothermia, since catecholamines rise during rewarming. It is also important to keep in mind that the hormonal effects we see are not necessarily reflected in a patient's hemodynamic responses. Blood pressure and heart rate may not change very much despite significant increases in catecholamine levels. It bothers me that we concern ourselves so much with suppressing the catecholamine response, because clinically it may have no great effect on the patient.

III ULTRA-SHORT-ACTING OPIOIDS

14 ALFENTANIL: AN ULTRA-SHORT-ACTING NARCOTIC FOR THE INDUCTION OF ANESTHESIA

Richard R. Bartkowski and Thomas McDonnell

Opioids have been a part of anesthesia for many years. For much of this time, however, narcotics were used as analgesics to alleviate pain in the still conscious patient or as supplements to traditional anesthetics such as nitrous oxide. The use of a narcotic as a complete anesthetic to provide unconsciousness and obtundation of the responses to surgical stimulation is a more recent development. Until the advent of respiratory intensive care with reliable controlled ventilation, the profound respiratory depression of narcotics limited their use to a supplementary role. The problem of ventilatory depression was aggravated by the long-lasting qualities of the traditional opioids, such as morphine, whose action persisted for many hours. Studies by Lowenstein et al [1] opened the era of morphine anesthesia by exploring the properties of this drug. They confirmed the lack of cardiac depression by morphine, which separated it from other anesthetics whose action was associated with significant and sometimes profound depression of cardiac function. They found that morphine was suitable as an anesthetic in their patients who were undergoing cardiac surgery.

DEFICIENCIES OF MORPHINE

While the positive aspects of morphine led to a major expansion in its use, deficiencies were pointed out that were ultimately limiting. Among these was the histamine release long attributed to this particular narcotic; this was recently investigated in detail [2]. Histamine was clearly associated with the vasodilation and hypotension that often accompanied morphine use. It was also pointed out by Conahan et al [3] that morphine anesthesia had a higher prevalence of hypertensive episodes than inhalational anesthesia and that these had to be treated by another agent. Finally, many questioned whether morphine could be a complete anesthetic and produce unconsciousness in a healthy person not debilitated by end-stage cardiac disease [4]. Indeed, it was common practice to supplement morphine anesthesia with a variety of adjuvants to ensure unconsciousness.

REQUIREMENTS OF NARCOTICS

The positive aspects of narcotic anesthesia provided the impetus to find new narcotics that preserved the best features of morphine while being both shorter acting and free of histamine release. The introduction of the more potent and shorter-acting drug fentanyl further expanded the horizons. Fentanyl was free of histamine release, allowing a greater narcotic effect without histamine side effects. In general, fentanyl in anesthetic doses (usually about 25 μg/kg) was able to produce unconsciousness rapidly in sedated patients without producing cardiac depression [5]. It could be given in a high enough dose to block the hypertensive and tachycardic responses to laryngoscopy and intubation. Fentanyl, therefore, showed several qualities desirable in an anesthetic induction drug. Its limitation in this regard was in its duration of action. When given at dose levels required for anesthetic induction, it produced hours of respiratory depression.

To examine the suitability of narcotics as induction agents, it is worthwhile to list the properties that we are seeking.

1. An induction agent must provide rapid onset of anesthesia. Anesthesia in this context can be defined as loss of consciousness and freedom from response to stimulation.
2. An induction agent should be free of undesirable or uncontrollable side effects such as hypotension, tachycardia, seizures, or pain on injection.
3. An induction agent should be short acting. The difference between an induction agent and another anesthetic is that the former provides anesthesia rapidly and smoothly, allowing for maintenance by any technique.

Thiopental, our standard induction drug, generally fits these criteria. It can produce anesthesia and is ultra short acting; its clinical duration is measured in minutes. It meets the second criterion inconsistently, since it may cause hypotension in a debilitated or compromised patient.

Fentanyl, which was introduced as a short-acting narcotic, only partially fits these criteria. When given at the dose level needed to provide anesthesia, its duration of action is more prolonged, extending for several hours. Its advantage is in criterion number 2 in that it provides cardiovascular stability and lack of cardiac depression. Among its untoward side effects, muscle rigidity is common, as with other opioids, but this can be controlled by muscle relaxants.

More recently, an even shorter-acting narcotic has become available for study: alfentanil (N-[1-[2-(4-ethyl-4,5-dihydro-5-oxo-1H-tetrazol-1-yl)ethyl]-4-(methoxymethyl)-4-piperidinyl]-N-phenylpropanamide monohydrochloride). Because its duration of action was approximately one-third that of fentanyl, it showed promise as a narcotic anesthetic induction agent whose use would not be limited to major surgery or procedures requiring postoperative ventilator support.

Alfentanil is ultra short acting. This apparently reflects its rapid distribution to the brain and other central organs, followed by rapid redistribution to a more remote site. In small analgesic doses, its duration is measured in minutes. Early reports [6] found that alfentanil was significantly shorter in duration than fentanyl and that its effects were terminated in 5 to 20 minutes when analgesic doses were given. Since alfentanil is a structural analog of fentanyl, it is reasonable to expect that the drug has similar properties. Because alfentanil is significantly shorter acting that other opioids, it is worthwhile to test it against our induction criteria.

RESULTS WITH ALFENTANIL

De Lange et al [7] found that alfentanil could serve as the sole anesthetic for coronary surgery in patients with coronary disease who were premedicated with lorazepam. Nauta et al [8] induced anesthesia with alfentanil in patients premedicated only with atropine. Both groups infused alfentanil at 3 mg/min to produce unconsciousness and followed this with muscle relaxation and intubation. Both reported some muscle rigidity during induction, while the latter group found less frequency of this side effect in a subgroup of patients premedicated with lorazepam. The latter study also reported minimal changes in cardiovascular variables during induction of anesthesia, initiation of paralysis, and endotracheal intubation.

The authors [9] administered alfentanil as a bolus (0.10, 0.15, 0.20, or 0.25 mg/kg) to 28 unpremedicated young adults to evaluate its anesthetic induction capabilities. Except for two patients, all became unconscious at the lowest dose level. As a test of anesthetic adequacy, each patient was stimulated by the placement of a nasal airway 90 seconds after alfentanil administration. Patients were scored on the presence or absence of a withdrawal response and the results were analyzed by probit regression to determine a dose effective in 90% of the patients (ED_{90}) and a median effective dose (ED_{50}). This yielded an ED_{90} for unconsciousness of 0.11 mg/kg while the ED_{50} and ED_{90} for anesthesia were 0.11 and 0.17 mg/kg respectively. Observations at this time found a high degree of muscle activity. Seventy-five percent of the patients had chest rigidity, making ventilation difficult to impossible. At the same time, 54% showed spasmodic tightening of the arm muscles, leading to fist clenching together with wrist and forearm flexion. At this time, patients were intubated with the aid of succinylcholine relaxation while the blood pressure and heart rate were monitored. The hemodynamic responses to intubation were modest: a significant rise in mean heart rate from 81.4 to 98.3 per minute and a rise of mean blood pressures from 123/79 to 136/84 mm Hg. The hemodynamic response to alfentanil alone was unexpected in that the mean heart rate had risen from 81.4 to 91.8 per minute prior to any stimulation. This is in contrast to the bradycardia that has been reported [10] at lower doses.

The action of alfentanil appeared to be short lived. Patients were seen to open their eyes in as little as six minutes after drug administration. Anesthesia, therefore, was continued with inhalational agents. Emergence from anesthesia was affected minimally by this induction agent. Naloxone in 0.05-mg increments was given if spontaneous respiration had not returned by five minutes after all inhalational anesthetics were terminated and end-tidal arterial carbon dioxide partial pressure (PCO_2) exceeded 48 mm Hg. By this criterion, 35% of the patients received naloxone after procedures ranging in length from one to four hours. Further measurements of end-tidal PCO_2 over the next hour showed no increases, and no patient received additional naloxone.

These encouraging results led us to evaluate alfentanil as an induction agent in a more demanding clinical setting [11]. Sixteen patients with cardiovascular disease (American Society of Anesthesiologists physical status II or III) were randomly assigned to receive either alfentanil, 0.175 mg/kg, or thiopental, 3 to 4 mg/kg, plus lidocaine, 1.5 mg/kg, as the induction agent. Immediately after the induction drugs were administered, patients in both groups received succinylcholine to facilitate tracheal intubation, which was performed 90 seconds later. In these compromised patients, both drug regimens produced a drop of mean arterial pressure averaging 31 mm Hg. The heart rate did not change significantly in either group. The only difference up to this point was transient muscle activity in a majority of patients who received alfentanil. The most common manifestations were wrist and forearm flexion together with clenching of the fingers. Less frequent were facial movements and masseter tightness; these lasted only 20 to 40 seconds, at which time the muscles became flacid.

At the time of laryngoscopy and intubation, however, the behavior of the two groups diverged. Intubation produced a marked blood pressure rise from a mean control value of 171/69 to 193/105 mm Hg by 90 seconds after laryngoscopy in the thiopental-lidocaine group. This was accompanied by a rise in heart rate from a control of 76 per minute to 92 per minute over the same time interval. The arterial pressure of patients who received alfentanil rose to 148/73 mm Hg at this time, a value somewhat less than the control of 171/69 mm Hg. No patient in either group had recollection of the induction events and all were extubated normally at the end of their procedures. Five of the eight patients who received alfentanil required naloxone, 0.05 to 0.15 mg, when their end-tidal P_{CO_2} rose above 50 mm Hg at the termination of anesthesia.

CONCLUSION

Alfentanil can serve as an induction agent. Even unsupplemented, it is capable of producing unconsciousness and blocking both the withdrawal responses to stimulation and the cardiovascular responses to laryngoscopy and intubation. In practice, however, some shortcomings are evident. Muscle activity, both rigidity and flexor spasm, is a prominent feature when this drug is given rapidly unless it is blocked by muscle relaxants. Rapid drug administration was also associated with an elevated heart rate, possibly reflex, in the young healthy population. This same rapid administration produced a fall of blood pressure, sometimes to worrisome levels, in compromised patients. Alfentanil's major advantage over earlier opioids is its brief duration of action. This has been well documented in clinical and pharmacokinetic studies, and confirmed in the authors' studies. Patients awaken from the substantial narcotic effect of alfentanil in times as short as one hour after administration. So, while this drug is not the perfect induction agent, its unique properties challenge us to find ways to take advantage of its benefits while minimizing its side effects.

REFERENCES

1. Lowenstein E, Hallowell P, Levine FH, Daggett WM, Austen WG, Laver MD. Cardiovascular response to large doses of intravenous morphine in man. N Engl J Med 1969;281:1389–93.
2. Philbin DM, Moss J, Akins CW, et al. The use of H_1 and H_2 histamine antagonists with morphine anesthesia: a double-blind study. Anesthesiology 1981;55:292–6.
3. Conahan TJ, Ominsky AJ, Wollman H, et al. A prospective random comparison of halothane and morphine for open-heart anesthesia. Anesthesiology 1973;38:528–35. artery surgery. Br J Anaesth 1981;53: 1291–6.
4. Lowenstein E. Morphine "anesthesia"—a perspective. Anesthesiology 1971;35:563–5.
5. Stanley TH, Webster LR. Anesthetic requirements and cardiovascular effects of fentanyl-oxygen and fentanyl-diazepam-oxygen anesthesia in man. Anesth Analg (Cleve) 1978;57:411–16.
6. Kay B, Pleuvry B. Human volunteer studies of alfentanil (R 39209), a new short-acting narcotic analgesic. Anaesthesia 1980;35:952–6.
7. de Lange S, Stanley TH, Boscoe MJ, et al. Alfentanil-oxygen anaesthesia for coronary artery surgery. Br J Anaesth 1981;53:1291–6.
8. Nauta J, de Lange S, Koopman D, et al. Anesthetic induction with alfentanil: a new short-acting narcotic analgesic. Anesth Analg (Cleve) 1982;61:267–72.
9. McDonnell TE, Bartkowski RR, Williams JJ. ED_{50} of alfentanil for induction of anesthesia in unpremedicated young adults. Anesthesiology 1984;60:136–40.
10. Kay B, Stephenson DK. Alfentanil (R 39209): initial clinical experiences with a new narcotic analgesic. Anaesthesia 1980;35:1197–1201.
11. Bartkowski RR, McDonnell TE. Alfentanil as an anesthetic induction agent—a comparison with thiopental-lidocaine. Anesth Analg (Cleve) 1984;63:330–4.

15 HYPOTENSION DURING ANESTHETIC INDUCTION WITH ALFENTANIL

Michael R. Murphy

Because the rationale for the use of alfentanil for induction of anesthesia is not only its short duration of action but also its alleged cardiovascular stability, the production of hypotension by alfentanil during induction is noteworthy. Drs. Bartkowski and McDonnell have produced two very interesting and clinically relevant studies in this regard, one demonstrating significant hypotension, the other not [1,2]. The previous literature describes slight or clinically insignificant changes in heart rate and blood pressure when alfentanil was used for induction in combination with other anesthetic induction agents [3–5]. In other studies, alfentanil was employed as the primary induction agent for patients with severe cardiovascular disease [6–9]. In these patients, alfentanil was given at a rate of approximately 50 μg per kilogram of body weight per minute. Again, in general, the investigators found slight decreases in blood pressure and heart rate with loss of consciousness, which returned toward control with intubation.

At Emory University Hospital, several studies were performed which examined the potential of alfentanil for induction of anesthesia. The resulting blood pressure changes

and our interpretation of them are compared to the studies of Bartkowski and McDonnell in this chapter.

INVESTIGATION OF THE HYPOTENSIVE POTENTIAL OF ALFENTANIL

In one study (Murphy), alfentanil was used as the sole anesthetic induction agent in nine healthy patients (ASA class I or II) after diazepam, 0.15 mg/kg orally, and glycopyrrolate, 0.3 mg/70 kg intramuscularly, 90 minutes prior to induction of anesthesia. The patients were given d-tubocurarine, 3 mg, approximately two minutes before induction with alfentanil. Anesthesia was then induced in a manner similar to that used in the study by Bartkowski and McDonnell [1]. Alfentanil, 150 μg/kg, was administered intravenously as a rapid bolus (less than 30 seconds). After the patients lost consciousness, they were ventilated with 60% nitrous oxide in oxygen and were intubated within four to six minutes of the alfentanil dose, after being given succinylcholine.

Table 15.1 shows the hemodynamic changes in these patients (Murphy) compared to those of Bartkowski and McDon-

TABLE 15.1. Hemodynamic changes after induction of anesthesia with alfentanil*

Determination	Bartkowski and McDonnell (N = 8)	Murphy (N = 9)	Griesemer et al I (N = 8)	Griesemer et al II (N = 5)
CONTROL: BEFORE ALFENTANIL				
Blood pressure (mm Hg)				
Systolic	171 ± 41	117 ± 12	145 ± 19	166 ± 43
Mean	103 ± 16	88 ± 9	94 ± 8	104 ± 22
Heart rate (beats/min)	76 ± 11	79 ± 15	76 ± 14	84 ± 10
HEMODYNAMICS FOLLOWING ALFENTANIL (150–175 µg/kg)				
Before laryngoscopy				
Blood pressure (mm Hg)				
Systolic	113 ± 51 (−34)	99 ± 12 (−15)	110 ± 32 (−25)	144 ± 36 (−12)
Mean	71 ± 22 (−31)	75 ± 9 (−15)	71 ± 21 (−25)	89 ± 16 (−16)
Heart rate (beats/min)	78 ± 13 (+3)	71 ± 12 (−10)	75 ± 12 (−1)	73 ± 7 (−13)
After laryngoscopy				
Blood pressure (mm Hg)				
Systolic	148 ± 36 (−13)	113 ± 21 (−4)	140 ± 45 (−4)	160 ± 44 (−3)
Mean	92 ± 9 (−11)	82 ± 12 (−7)	91 ± 31 (−3)	100 ± 21 (−4)
Heart rate (beats/min)	77 ± 10 (+1)	68 ± 18 (−14)	79 ± 14 (+4)	69 ± 5 (−17)

*Values are mean ± SD with percent change from control in parentheses.

nell [1]. Control values for blood pressure and heart rate were taken in the operating room just prior to induction with alfentanil. The lowest values for blood pressure after alfentanil and before laryngoscopy are shown, as well as the highest values after laryngoscopy but before surgical stimulation. There was a decrease in blood pressure in each of our patients, with a mean decrease of 15% of control before laryngoscopy. Heart rate also decreased an average of 10% from control. After laryngoscopy, blood pressure returned toward control. To summarize the findings in the Murphy group: in healthy patients given large doses of alfentanil (150 µg/kg) as a rapid bolus, there were no *clinically* significant alterations in heart rate and blood pressure.

Also at Emory University, Drs. Griesemer, Moldenhauer, and Hug performed a similar study in eight patients, ASA class II to IV, scheduled for elective thoracotomy. These patients had more cardiovascular impairment than the Murphy group. Griesemer et al induced anesthesia with alfentanil, 150 µg/kg, given as a rapid intravenous bolus. They found a decrease in blood pressure in each case, with a mean decrease of 25% for the eight patients (Table 15.1, Griesemer et al, I). It is noteworthy, however, that two patients had severe drops in blood pressure (50%), similar to those seen in the study by Bartkowski and McDonnell.

Because of the hypotension produced by the rapid administration of alfentanil, Griesemer et al studied a second group of five patients (Table 15.1, Griesemer et al, II) with the same protocol except that the alfentanil dose, 150 µg/kg, was administered at a slower rate of 50 µg/kg/min. The average decrease in blood pressure for this group (14%) is very similar to values reported in the literature and to the declines noted in the healthy patients.

FACTORS RESPONSIBLE FOR ALFENTANIL-RELATED HYPOTENSION

These studies demonstrate that hypotension can result after administration of alfentanil, but why? Three points should be mentioned.

In Dr. Bartkowski's study of patients with impaired cardiac function, the systolic blood pressure averaged 171 mm Hg with a mean blood pressure of 103 mm Hg. These patients were hypertensive before they came to surgery, or at least on the day of surgery. Generally, when anesthesia is induced in hypertensive patients, blood pressure drops more severely than in normotensive patients. Other drugs these patients may have been taking could have affected their blood pressure. Furthermore, what is the actual normal blood pressure for a patient? If blood pressures are taken in the operating room, which is commonly done to obtain control values, the patient's anxiety about the surgical procedure may cause pressures to be higher than the actual normal for the patient. When anesthesia is induced, the blood pressure may simply return to more normal levels for that individual.

The second point concerns the patients' physical status. In general, healthy individuals withstand surgery relatively satisfactorily. In the studies cited, no healthy patients demonstrated clinically significant blood pressure changes, while in those with ASA class III and IV physical status, Bartkowski's hypertensive patients, and those subjected to thoracotomy by Griesemer et al, there was severe hypotenion in several instances.

The third point is the rate of administration. A rapid bolus of 150 to 175 µg/kg did not cause clinically significant blood pressure decreases in healthy patients in any of the studies. This rate of administration did, however, cause severe hypotension in several patients with poor cardiac function. When the rate was slowed to 50 µg/kg/min, the same dose of alfentanil (150 µg/kg) produced the slight decreases in blood pressure that were seen in healthy patients. This change again agrees with previous studies in the literature.

CONCLUSION

Clinically significant decreases in blood pressure are not seen in healthy patients when anesthesia is induced with large doses of alfentanil, even with rapid administration. Significant decreases are seen in patients with cardiovascular instability when an induction dose of alfentanil is given very rapidly. Finally, if administration of alfentanil is slowed to 50 μg/kg/min, clinically significant hypotension will not be produced even in the sick patient.

REFERENCES

1. Bartkowski RR, McDonnell TE. Alfentanil as an anesthetic induction agent—a comparison with thiopental-lidocaine. Anesth Analg (Cleve) 1984;63:330–4.
2. Bartkowski RR, McDonnell TE, Williams JJ. ED_{50} of alfentanil for induction of anesthesia in unpremedicated young adults. Anesthesiology 1982;57:A352.
3. van Leeuwen L, Deen L. Alfentanil, a new, potent and very short-acting morphinomimetic for minor operative procedures. Anaesthesist 1981;30:115–17.
4. Helmers JHJH, van Leeuwen L, Adam AA, et al. Double-blind comparison of the postoperative respiratory depressant effects of alfentanil and fentanyl. Acta Anaesthesiol Belg 1982;33:13–21.
5. McLeskey CH. Alfentanil-loading dose/continuous infusion for surgical anesthesia. Anesthesiology 1982;57:A68.
6. de Lange S, Boscoe MJ, Stanley TH, et al. Antidiuretic and growth hormone responses during coronary artery surgery with sufentanil-oxygen and alfentanil-oxygen anesthesia in man. Anesth Analg (Cleve) 1982; 61:434–8.
7. de Lange S, Stanley TH, Boscoe MJ. Alfentanil-oxygen anaesthesia for coronary artery surgery. Br J Anaesth 1981;53:1291–6.
8. Sebel PS, Bovill JG, van der Haven A. Cardiovascular effects of alfentanil anaesthesia. Br J Anaesth 1982;54:1185–9.
9. Nauta J, de Lange S, Koopman D, et al. Anesthetic induction with alfentanil: a new short-acting narcotic analgesic. Anesth Analg (Cleve) 1982;61:267–72.

16 ALFENTANIL FOR USE IN SHORT SURGICAL PROCEDURES

Carl E. Rosow, William B. Latta, Christine R. Keegan, and Daniel M. Philbin

The use of high doses of opioids to produce both analgesia and hypnosis is simply impractical for the majority of operations, and the opioids are restricted to a lower dosage range. This chapter deals with a study on the use of opioids in relatively low doses as the analgesic component of balanced anesthesia.

Alfentanil hydrochloride is a synthetic opioid with a significantly faster onset and shorter duration than its parent drug, fentanyl [1–3]. Alfentanil is one-third as potent an analgesic as fentanyl, but the differences otherwise are almost totally pharmacokinetic. The rapid elimination of this drug suggested to us and others that it would be particularly appropriate for use in short outpatient surgical procedures [4].

Our study was designed to compare the intensity and duration of opioid effect with alfentanil and fentanyl and to characterize the quality of the recovery. More specifically, we hypothesized that alfentanil could be used to produce a more intense analgesic effect without significant prolongation of recovery. We also included a group receiving barbiturate–nitrous oxide anesthesia without opioid. The data from this last group clearly show the rationale behind the use of opioids in this setting.

COMPARISON OF ANALGESIC EFFECTS OF ALFENTANIL AND FENTANYL

Fifty-two unpremedicated patients gave written informed consent to participate. All were in ASA class I or II, their ages ranged from 20 to 79 years, and their operations lasted from 2 to 59 minutes. Forty-four patients were admitted through our ambulatory surgical facility. All but five underwent urologic procedures. We felt that the wide range of patient ages and operative times would give this study broad clinical applicability.

Fentanyl was given in doses commonly used for outpatient surgery in this institution. The alfentanil doses selected for this study were determined by an open pilot study involving ten patients. Doses lower than 10 μg per kilogram of body weight were of such short duration that they were inconvenient to give by an intermittent bolus technique. On the basis of our experience we felt comfortable with doses of alfentanil in the 10- to 20-μg/kg range, which were previously shown to produce a very short period of respiratory depression [5].

Opioid or saline was prepared in coded vials ("study medication"), and each patient was randomly and blindly assigned to one of five experimental groups.

Fentanyl, low dose   (FL)   1 μg/kg
Fentanyl, high dose   (FH)   2 μg/kg
Alfentanil, low dose (AL)   10 μg/kg
Alfentanil, high dose (AH)   20 μg/kg
Saline   (S)

After administration of the initial dose of 0.04 ml/kg study medication (SM), anesthesia was induced and maintained with sodium thiamylal, 3 mg/kg, and 66% nitrous oxide in oxygen. Supplemental SM or thiamylal was given as needed, but muscle relaxants and potent inhalation anesthetics were not used unless necessary for the safe conduct of anesthesia. The elapsed times from discontinuation of nitrous oxide until responsiveness (recovery of response to verbal command) and alertness (orientation to person, place, and time) were measured. Intraoperative and postoperative side effects were recorded, and the occurrence of delayed side effects was ascertained by specific questionnaire.

FINDINGS OF THE STUDY

The five groups were demographically comparable. The total doses of SM and barbiturate administered are shown in Table 16.1. Total SM doses differed significantly between high- and low-dose groups, since total dose was primarily a reflection of initial dose. In fact, most patients in the opioid groups required two injections or less. The requirement for barbiturate was roughly equivalent in the four opioid groups, but significantly higher in the saline group.

At induction of anesthesia, both opioids produced small decreases in pulse and in-

TABLE 16.1. Drug requirements

| Regimen | Drug | |
	Study medication (μg)	Thiamylal (mg)
FL	118 ± 15	459 ± 62
FH	241 ± 22	548 ± 45
AL	1150 ± 177	540 ± 93
AH	2060 ± 193	450 ± 25
S	· · ·	720 ± 73
Significance	$p<0.001$*	$p<0.01$†

See text for explanation of abbreviations.
*Significant dose effect for each drug.
†S vs. all opioid groups.

consistent effects on blood pressure. Respiratory depression and frank apnea occurred in many patients in groups FL, FH, AL, and AH, although few required more than one or two minutes of controlled ventilation. Some clinically detectable loss of chest wall compliance was reported in 50% of patients in groups AH and FH (Figure 16.1), although only 3 out of 52 patients had sufficient rigidity to require treatment with succinylcholine. No patient in group S had chest wall rigidity. Supplemental SM was given to 44% of patients prior to the first surgical stimulus (insertion of cystoscope or incision)

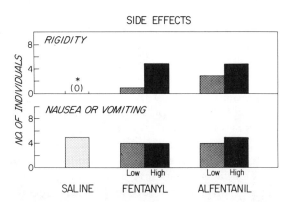

FIGURE 16.1. *(Top)* Number of patients in each group with loss of chest wall compliance. High-dose opioid groups were significantly different from saline ($p < 0.05$). *(Bottom)* Number of patients having postoperative nausea or vomiting. No significant differences between groups.

FIGURE 16.2. *(Top)* Number of patients in each group requiring supplemental study medication prior to the first surgical stimulus. The difference between saline and opioid groups was significant (*p* < 0.01); fewer patients required supplemental alfentanil than fentanyl (*p* < 0.06). *(Bottom)* Number of patients who moved one or more times intraoperatively. More patients moved in the saline group than in the opioid groups (*p* < 0.06).

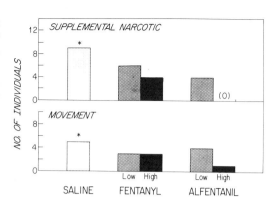

(Figure 16.2). No patient in group AH required supplemental medication at this time, while 82% in group S received supplemental doses. Movement occurred in 5 of 11 patients in group S, but only 1 in 10 in group AH.

The duration of opioid effect (measured indirectly as the time until the first supplemental dose) was dose related and similar for fentanyl and alfentanil at this 1:10 dose ratio. In patients given 20 μg/kg of alfentanil or 2 μg/kg of fentanyl, the first supplemental narcotic was needed after 15 to 18 minutes. The average number of opioid injections in the FH and AH groups was 2.1 and 1.5 respectively; that is, many patients needed only one injection of alfentanil for the entire procedure.

The times to responsiveness and alertness were significantly longer in the S group than in any of the opioid groups (Figure 16.3). This difference is almost totally accounted for by the differences in total thiamylal dose (*p* = 0.0008).

Postoperative side effects were relatively frequent, probably due to the omission of premedication, antiemetics, and the like. There was 40% prevalence of nausea and/or vomiting in all five groups (Figure 16.1). Sixteen patients complained of headache, and

FIGURE 16.3. *(Top)* Total doses of thiamylal for saline-, fentanyl-, and alfentanil-treated patients. Saline > opioid (*p* < 0.01). *(Bottom)* Elapsed time from discontinuation of nitrous oxide until alertness *(see text)*. Saline > opioid (*p* = 0.0015).

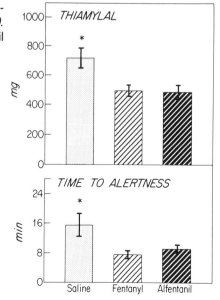

these were evenly divided among the groups. One patient in the FH group required naloxone for respiratory depression and chest wall rigidity. Eleven patients did not wish to have the same anesthetic again. Nausea was the apparent reason for dissatisfaction in 8 of the 11 patients; 5 of these 11 received saline.

CONCLUSIONS

Since there is no single valid measure of opioid agonist effect, we resorted to indirect measurements to compare the intensity and duration of opioid effect with alfentanil and fentanyl. Admittedly, these measurements are imprecise, but they gave us some indication that the intensity of narcotic effect was greatest with alfentanil (Table 16.2). Based upon analgesic potency estimates in animals, this was an expected result [6]. Of equal interest was the fact that these doses of alfentanil and fentanyl had similar durations. Patients receiving either agent in this study had extremely rapid return of consciousness and orientation.

Anesthesia with thiamylal and nitrous oxide alone was different in several respects from opioid-supplemented anesthesia. There was no chest wall rigidity, bradycardia, or respiratory depression; however, induction

TABLE 16.2. Intensity and duration of opioid effect

Measurement	Agents
Intensity	
↓ Supplemental study medication	A > F > S
↓ Supplemental barbiturate	A = F > S
↓ Movement	A > F > S
↑ Rigidity	A > F > S
Duration	
Time to second dose	A = F > S
Time to alertness	A = F > S

A = alfentanil; F = fentanyl; S = saline.

and maintenance were not smooth, there was more patient movement, and much more supplemental barbiturate was required. The time to alertness was nearly double that of opioid-treated patients.

Nausea with vomiting is clearly a multifactorial problem in this surgical setting, the presence or absence of an opioid being only one precipitating factor. In this study, postoperative nausea was the same in saline and opioid groups. On our postoperative questionnaire we found it was the single most important factor determining patient satisfaction with the anesthetic experience. The value of antiemetic premedicants is well established [7,8], and it seems prudent to use agents such as droperidol with a fentanyl or alfentanil technique.

In summary, the amount of movement and the requirement for supplemental drug suggest that our opioid doses were too low in these otherwise unmedicated patients. In retrospect, only the high dose of alfentanil was adequate for the purpose: 20 μg/kg of alfentanil produced good operating conditions and rapid recovery in this patient population. (Under more typical clinical conditions, patients may receive premedication, muscle relaxants, and other adjuvants, so lower doses of opioid may suffice.)

Although alfentanil may be particularly well suited to administration by infusion [9], clinician familiarity with the traditional bolus techniques makes it likely that this drug will be given by intermittent injection in most cases. Alfentanil was easily used in this manner, and one dose of 20 μg/kg was frequently sufficient for a 15- to 20-minute procedure. This dose produces a more intense narcotic effect than 2 μg/kg of fentanyl without prolonging recovery time or increasing the incidence of side effects.

REFERENCES

1. Camu F, Gepts E, Rucquoi M, Heykants J. Pharmacokinetics of alfentanil in man. Anesth Analg (Cleve) 1982;61:657–61.

2. Bovill JG, Sebel PS, Blackburn CL, Hey-
    kants J. The pharmacokinetics of alfentanil
    (R 39209): a new opioid analgesic. Anesthe-
    siology 1982;57:439–43.
3. Stanski D, Hug CC Jr. Alfentanil—kineti-
    cally predictable narcotic analgesic. Anesthe-
    siology 1982;57:435–8.
4. van Leeuwen L, Deen L, Helmers JH. A
    comparison of alfentanil and fentanyl in short
    operations with special reference to their du-
    ration of action and postoperative respiratory
    depression. Anaesthesist 1981;30:397–9.
5. Scamman FL, Ghoneim MM, Kortilla K.
    Ventilatory and mental effects of alfentanil
    and fentanyl. Anesthesiology 1982;
    57(3A):A364.

6. Niemegeers CJE, Janssen PAJ. Alfentanil (R
    39209)–a particularly short-acting intrave-
    nous narcotic analgesic in rats. Drug Dev Res
    1981;1:83–8.
7. Abramowitz MD, Epstein BS, Friendly DS,
    Oh T, Greenwald M. The effect of droperi-
    dol in reducing vomiting in pediatric strabis-
    mic outpatient surgery. Anesthesiology
    1981;55(3A):A329.
8. Chen LH, Watkins ML. Antiemetic premed-
    ication in outpatient anesthesia. Anesthe-
    siology 1981;55(3A):A280.
9. McLeskey CH. Alfentanil—loading dose/
    continuous infusion for surgical anesthesia.
    Anesthesiology 1982;57(3A):A68.

17 COMPARISON OF ALFENTANIL VERSUS FENTANYL FOR OUTPATIENT SURGERY

Eli M. Brown

In our institution, a balanced anesthesia technique is frequently employed for outpatient pelvic laparoscopy. It involves induction of anesthesia with thiopental, 4 to 5 mg/kg, pancuronium 60, µg/kg, to facilitate intubation, and nitrous oxide–oxygen–fentanyl for analgesia. In animal studies, alfentanil is purported to have a shorter duration of action than fentanyl [1]. Accordingly, it would appear that substitution of alfentanil for fentanyl in our technique would be advantageous for short surgical procedures in an ambulatory setting.

DETAILS OF THE STUDY

To test this hypothesis, we designed a double-blind study to compare the two narcotics in 80 patients scheduled for pelvic laparoscopy. The groups that received alfentanil and fentanyl respectively were comparable. The total dose of alfentanil administered averaged 2.06 mg (range 1.5 to 2.5 mg), whereas the dose of fentanyl averaged 0.21 mg (range 0.1 to 0.25 mg). There was little difference in the cardiovascular effects of the two narcotics. During induction of anesthesia, the heart rate and blood pressure were maintained within 20% of preanesthetic values. After intubation of the trachea, there was a significant rise in blood pressure in both groups, but the increase was noticeably greater in patients receiving fentanyl. There was no significant difference between the groups in duration of anesthesia, time to extubation, verbal response time, or time to orientation to person, place, and time (Table 17.1). Postoperatively, the respiratory rate was not below 12 breaths per minute for any patient in the study and was comparable for the two groups. The only significant untoward side effect that occurred in these patients was nausea and/or vomiting. Nausea occurred in over 40% of patients in each group, but in most instances it was characterized by the patient as mild. The frequency of nausea and vomiting was not significantly different between the groups.

TABLE 17.1. Time to reaction on emergence (minutes)

Measurement	Alfentanil	Fentanyl	Difference
Duration of anesthesia	31.5 ± 8.0	35.1 ± 13.4	NS
Time to extubation	3.3 ± 2.4	3.3 ± 2.2	NS
Verbal response time	3.6 ± 2.0	4.0 ± 2.0	NS
Time to orientation	4.9 ± 2.7	5.6 ± 3.9	NS

NS = not significant ($p > 0.05$).

COMPARISON OF THE DRUGS

Since both drugs were administered on the basis of clinical signs (movement, tearing, pupillary dilatation, rise in heart rate and/or blood pressure) the total dose of alfentanil was approximately twice the amount that would have been predicted on the basis of relative potency in animal studies. This may indicate a difference between relative potency of the drugs in animals and humans, or that narcotic requirement varies considerably among patients. Despite the apparently larger dose of alfentanil, the time to extubation, verbal response, and orientation were not significantly different. Failure to detect a difference in awakening time is not surprising because of the relatively small total dose of narcotic used. At these doses, redistribution mechanisms account for the termination of narcotic effect. Since the major pharmacokinetic difference between fentanyl and alfentanil is in the terminal elimination phase, one would expect to see a difference in awakening time only when larger total doses of the drugs are used. Respiratory depression was not a problem with either agent. All patients had a respiratory rate greater than 12 breaths per minute at the completion of the anesthetic. Consequently, it was not necessary to use naloxone in any of the 80 patients included in this study.

The frequency of nausea was quite high in both groups, however, in most instances it was not distressing. There are several factors (age, emotional state, type and duration of surgical procedure) other than the narcotic that could contribute to nausea and

vomiting [2–4]. In addition, the large quantity of carbon dioxide introduced into the peritoneal cavity during pelvic laparoscopy may have contributed to the high incidence of nausea.

All patients in both groups indicated that the anesthetic was satisfactory, except for the few who complained of severe nausea and/ or vomiting.

CONCLUSION

We conclude that alfentanil is a suitable narcotic drug for short surgical procedures on ambulatory patients. It has no marked advantage over fentanyl when relatively small total doses are administered. It appears that the best application of alfentanil, therefore, is for procedures in which larger doses of a narcotic drug are necessary because of longer duration or more intense surgical stimulation.

REFERENCES

1. Bovill JG, Sebel PS, Blackburn CL, Heykants J. The pharmacokinetics of alfentanil (R 39209): a new opioid analgesic. Anesthesiology 1982;57:439–43.
2. Bodman RI, Morton HJV, Thomas ET. Vomiting by outpatients after nitrous oxide anaesthesia. Br Med J 1960;1:1327–30.
3. Steward DJ. Experiences with an outpatient anesthesia service for children. Anesth Analg (Cleve) 1973;52:877–80.
4. Fahy A, Marshall M. Postanaesthetic morbidity in outpatients. Br J Anaesth 1969; 41:433–8.

18 THE USE OF SHORT-ACTING NARCOTICS IN OBSTETRIC ANESTHESIA AND THE EFFECTS ON THE NEWBORN

John H. Eisele, Jr.

Many elective and most emergent cesarean sections are performed under general anesthesia; however, narcotic drugs are very infrequently used. The usual technique employs thiopental and nitrous oxide with some muscle relaxants. Within the past ten years, small doses of ketamine and subanesthetic concentrations of halogenated inhalation agents have been used successfully. These latter techniques indicate a need for more profound analgesia/anesthesia during operative delivery, and thus a desire to reduce stress that has been shown to have the potential for harmful effects on fetal blood flow and oxygenation [1]. Narcotic transport studies are limited but indicate substantial differences between the older and newer compounds.

MEPERIDINE

Meperidine rapidly crosses the placenta and is detected in the fetal cord blood less than two minutes after intravenous administration to the mother. Fetal meperidine concentrations approach maternal concentrations over 5 to 10 minutes and have a decay course similar to that of the drug in the mother [2]. The newborn infant excretes meperidine preferentially in the unchanged form rather than the demethylated form. The above investigation also noted differences in fetal drug excretion depending on the route of administration to the mother.

A classic study by Shnider and Moya [3] pointed out that small doses (50 mg) of meperidine given intravenously to the mother can significantly depress the newborn and that the time interval between administration and delivery is important. In this investigation there was a significant increase in neonatal depression as measured by Apgar scores and time to spontaneous respiration during the second hour after drug administration. The time of maximum depression was seen when meperidine was given during the fourth hour before birth. This suggests delayed clearance of meperidine in fetal/newborn brain tissue. Such a time lag in plasma-brain equilibration after intramuscular injection of meperidine has been documented in pregnant ewes [4]. The data suggested that the fetal brain should be considered as a peripheral rather than central compartment, and that the respiratory effects of meperidine may correspond more closely to the time course of meperidine in the peripheral compartment.

ALPHAPRODINE

Alphaprodine (Nisentil) is a synthetic narcotic that, like meperidine, is derived from piperidine. Its time of onset is similar to meperidine's, as is its metabolite (nor-alphaprodine). Its elimination half-life is two hours compared to four hours for meperidine. In addition, the respiratory depression is slightly less with alphaprodine given in equianalgesic concentrations, at least in healthy volunteers [5].

MORPHINE

Morphine has long been known to produce neonatal depression, as Shute and Davis [6] noted that babies delivered less than one hour or more than six hours after drug was administered to the mothers seldom showed signs of narcosis. Kupferberg and Way [7] observed an increased sensitivity to morphine in newborn rats compared to adults, and they related this to increased permeability of the newborn's brain. Morphine has been shown to have a clinically significant effect on fetal heart rate [8] and on fetal heart rate variability [9]; consequently, it is not used much today in obstetrics.

METHADONE

Studies have been performed in sheep to examine placental transfer of methadone [10], which readily crosses after maternal intra-

venous infusion, but the fetal concentration remained substantially lower than maternal concentration at all times. One explanation the authors offered for this difference was that methadone is bound to plasma proteins in the mother considerably more than in the fetus. Similar infusion studies of meperidine in sheep show the steady-state distribution ratio between fetal and maternal plasma to be 0.30 for both methadone and meperidine [11].

FENTANYL

A study in humans examined the fetal and neonatal effects of fentanyl (1 μg/kg) given intravenously just prior to cesarean section [12]. At delivery, blood was sampled from maternal vein and from both artery and vein of the umbilical cord for fentanyl and blood gas analysis. The newborns were handled in the usual way by a pediatrician who assigned Apgar scores at one and five minutes. One investigator examined the newborns at 4 and 24 hours of age using a modification of the neurobehavioral test described by Scanlon [13], which scores muscle tone, reflexes, state of alertness, and overall condition. Eleven of the 15 patients received general anesthesia with pentothal and nitrous oxide. In this group, one infant had a low one-minute Apgar score of 3. In this case the mother had received 11 minutes of general anesthesia prior to delivery. Among the control patients not receiving fentanyl, 6 of 13 had general anesthesia and one newborn had a low one-minute Apgar score of 6; again, the mother had nine minutes of general anesthesia before delivery.

There were minimal neurobehavioral differences between the fentanyl and control groups. Figure 18.1 shows the percentage of normal scores at four hours in the fentanyl compared to the control group. At 24 hours the scores for the fentanyl group were slightly higher for awakeness, muscle tone, and reflex quality, but these differences were not significant. Another way of looking at neu-

FIGURE 18.1. Neurobehavioral examination at 4 hours *(top)* and 24 hours *(bottom)* comparing newborns of mothers receiving fentanyl or no fentanyl at cesarean section. The percentage of newborns having normal scores is shown for each of four categories: overall assessment, awakeness, muscle tone, and reflex quality.

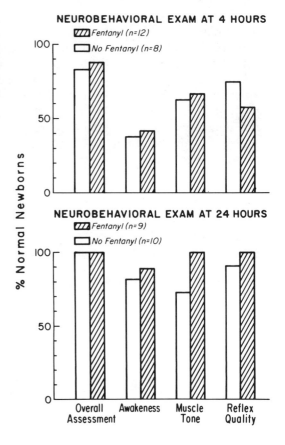

robehavioral results is in terms of the concentration of fentanyl in the fetus at delivery. Since the average fetal fentanyl concentration was 0.8 ng/ml, newborns were divided into those with cord plasma levels above and below 0.8 ng/ml. Neurobehavioral examination at four hours (Figure 18.2) showed the percentage of normals in each of four score categories. The babies with higher fentanyl levels had lower ratings for awakeness but showed few differences in the other three categories. At 24 hours there were no differences except for awakeness again, but the newborns given fentanyl scored slightly higher than the controls. The findings of an effect at four hours is not surprising since the elimination half-life for fentanyl in the adult is four hours [14] and may be considerably longer in the newborn, but there are no data on this latter point. The half-life of meperidine in the newborn may be five to six times longer than in the healthy adult [15].

NEW NARCOTICS

Studies on the placental transport of newer narcotics have been carried out in the term pregnant ewe. In these studies, the drug is administered intravenously as a bolus to the awake ewe, and serum samples are drawn simultaneously from the maternal and fetal arteries over four hours, then analyzed for drug concentrations using radioimmunoassay. Results of separate sheep studies using fentanyl, sufentanil, and alfentanil are shown in Figure 18.3. Placental passage appears similar in these closely related compounds despite differences in their lipid solubility, degree of ionization, and protein binding. Although the numbers are small, the fetal-maternal ratios for alfentanil are slightly higher than those for sufentanil and fentanyl. This may be a result of the high fraction of un-ionized alfentanil at physiological pH.

FIGURE 18.2. Neurobehavioral examination at 4 hours *(top)* and 24 hours *(bottom)* comparing newborns with umbilical cord fentanyl concentrations less than and more than 0.8 ng/ml at delivery. The percentage of newborns having normal scores is shown for each of four categories: overall assessment, awakeness, muscle tone, and reflex quality.

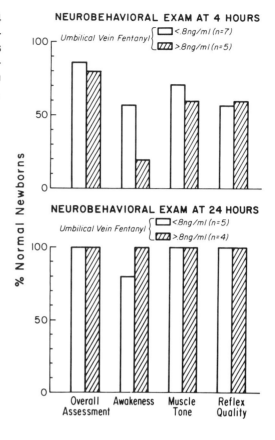

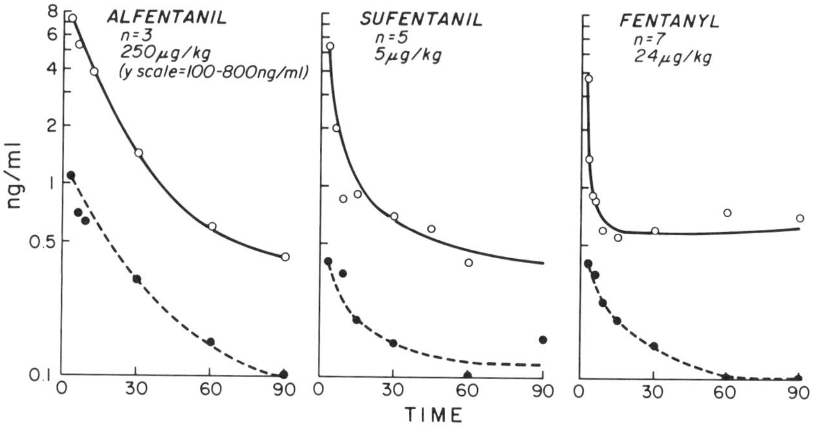

FIGURE 18.3. Washout curves for maternal *(solid line)* and fetal *(dashed line)* serum narcotic concentrations following an intravenous bolus of alfentanil 250 µg/kg *(left panel)*, sufentanil 5 µg/kg *(center panel)*, and fentanyl 24 µg/kg *(right panel)*. Study was done on awake term pregnant sheep.

The high lipid content of brain and the high lipid solubility of fentanyl result in brain concentrations of fentanyl being higher than serum concentrations, as has been shown in dogs [16]. Therefore serum fentanyl concentrations do not measure the brain's content or accumulation of drug. The low cord fentanyl levels could also be somewhat misleading if protein binding is less in the fetus than the mother, because then there would be more free drug in the fetus, which could result in higher tissue concentration. Fetal protein binding of drugs is lower than maternal and is dependent upon fetal maturity [17].

PLACENTAL TRANSPORT FACTORS

Factors affecting placental transport of drugs include molecular weight, lipid solubility, degree of ionization, protein binding, and placental maturation and metabolism. The commonly used narcotic drugs have molecular weights between 200 and 800, which should present no barrier to simple diffusion. Lipophilia could be an important factor influencing placental transport of drugs since the more lipid-soluble drugs cross membranes more easily. Some heptane or lipid/water solubility coefficients at pH 7.40 are: morphine (0.00001), Demerol (3.4), alphaprodine (10.0), fentanyl (20.0), and methadone (45.0).

The placental passage of fentanyl as reflected in fetal-maternal ratios averaged 0.31, which is the same as for meperidine but less than anticipated in view of the higher lipid solubility of fentanyl. This suggests the possibility of significant placental uptake and/or metabolism of fentanyl. There are no relevant data on this aspect, but tissue uptake in rabbits indicates high concentrations of fentanyl in lungs, kidney, and liver compared to plasma. It is more likely that rapid fetal tissue uptake of fentanyl accounts for the low cord concentrations at the time of sampling. The half-life of the fast component of a fentanyl decay in humans is one to two minutes. This means a very rapid redistribution of the drug out of the vascular compartment. A third, but unlikely, possibility for the low fetal-maternal ratio is a placental barrier. This would be most unusual, since other narcotics, both alkaloid and synthetic, readily cross the placenta.

The degree of ionization of a compound is an important physical characteristic determining transport across a membrane. The dissociation constant is pH dependent; and since most of the narcotics have a dissociation constant (pKa) value around 8.0, much of the drug is ionized and not available to cross the placenta. As the blood pH becomes more alkaline such as with hyperventilation, however, which is common during pregnancy, less drug is ionized or more drug becomes free. Alfentanil is unique in that it is highly un-ionized at physiologic pH.

Protein binding may be very different among narcotics, ranging from ±20% for morphine to ±93% for alfentanil. It is likely that higher protein binding indicates less placental passage. This is not simple, however, as individual narcotics may bind to different proteins. Of all the factors, plasma protein binding may be the most significant limitation for placental transport.

Finally, placental factors could be significant. On a weight basis, the placenta's ability to metabolize is less than either maternal or fetal liver, which suggests that it is not a major factor. Maturation of the placenta can affect diffusion rates as well as permeability; and evidence indicates that maturation, hence drug transfer, is greatest at term. To date, there is a paucity of information on this aspect with regard to narcotic compounds.

CONCLUSIONS

It is apparent that much work needs to be done in the area of both placental drug transport and newborn status after narcotics are given to the mother. In particular, we need to learn if the frequently used pregnant sheep model is accurate and translatable to human beings. Sheep placentas are multicotyledonous and do not have a hemichorial structure. Furthermore, sheep placentas contain five membranes within a thin uterine wall, compared to three membranes and a thick uterine wall in humans. First, a study must compare drug passage in sheep with subhuman primates when the drug is given in identical fashion and the variables such as time of pregnancy and anesthesia are controlled. Finally, it would be useful to administer two dissimilar narcotic drugs at the same time and measure placental passage. This might provide a clearer picture of which drug characteristics are important. It may be that lipid solubility and degree of protein binding make little difference in placenta transport and that all drugs that act on the central nervous system cross the placenta about equally.

This, of course, would focus more attention on the relative fetal brain uptake and removal of different compounds, and the desirability of using drugs with less affinity for brain tissue and thus more rapid brain clearance.

The ratio of brain to plasma concentration of drug is perhaps more important for drugs acting on the central nervous system. Morphine has a higher affinity for brain (brain/plasma partition of 0.046) than its lipid solubility would suggest. Compared to the brain/plasma partition of 10.5 for fentanyl, it turns out that the ratio of brain fentanyl to brain morphine would be only 230 : 1.

REFERENCES

1. Shnider SM, Wright RG, Levinson G, et al. Uterine blood flow and plasma norepinephrine changes during maternal stress in the pregnant ewe. Anesthesiology 1979;50:524–7.

2. Crawford JS, Rudofsky S. The placental transmission of pethidin. Br J Anaesth 1965;37:929–33.

3. Shnider SM, Moya F. Effects of meperidine on the newborn infant. Am J Obstet Gynecol 1964;89(8):1009–15.

4. Szeto HH, Clapp JF, Abrams R, et al. Brain uptake of meperidine in the fetal lamb. Am J Obstet Gynecol 1980;138(5):528–33.

5. Fung DL, Asling JH, Eisele JH, Martucci R. A comparison of alphaprodine and meperidine pharmacokinetics. J Clin Pharmacol 1980;20:37–41.

6. Shute E, Davis ME. The effect on the infant of morphine administered in labor. Surg Gynecol Obstet 1933;57:727–36.

7. Kupferberg HJ, Way EL. The pharmacologic basis for the increased sensitivity of the newborn rat to morphine. J Pharmacol Exp Ther 1963;141:105–12.

8. Grimwade J, Walker D, Wood C. Morphine and the fetal heart rate. Br Med J 1971;3:373.

9. Petrie RH, Yeh SY, Murata Y, et al. The effect of drugs on fetal heart rate variability. Am J Obstet Gynecol 1978;130(3):294–9.

10. Szeto HH, Clapp JF III, Larrow RH, Hewitt J, Inturrisi CE, Mann LI. Disposition of methadone in the ovine maternal-fetal unit. Life Sci 1981;28(19):2111–17.

11. Szeto HH, Mann LI, Bhakhavathsalan A, Liu M, Inturrisi CE. Meperidine pharmacokinetics in the maternal-fetal unit. J Pharmacol Exp Ther 1978;206(2):448–59.

12. Eisele JH, Wright R, Rogge P. Newborn and maternal fentanyl levels at cesarean section. Anesth Analg (Cleve) 1982;61(2):179.

13. Scanlon JW, Ostheimer GW, Lurie AO, Brown WU, Weiss JB, Alper MH. Neurobehavioral responses and drug concentrations in newborns after maternal epidural anesthesia with bupivacaine. Anesthesiology 1976;45(4):400–5.

14. Schleimer R, Benjamini E, Eisele J, Henderson G. Pharmacokinetics of fentanyl as determined by radioimmunoassay. Clin Pharmacol Ther 1978;23(2):188–94.

15. Caldwell J, Wakile LA, Notarianni LJ, et al. Maternal and neonatal disposition of pethidine in childbirth—a study using quantitative gas chromatography-mass spectrometry. Life Sci 1978;22:589–96.

16. Ainslie SG, Eisele JH, Corkill G. Fentanyl concentrations in brain and serum during respiratory acid-base changes in the dog. Anesthesiology 1979;51:9–13.

17. Ehrenebo M, Agurell S, Jalling B, Boreus LO. Age differences in drug binding by plasma proteins: studies on human fetuses, neonates and adults. Eur J Clin Pharmacol 1971;3:189–93.

19 THE SAFE USE OF SHORT-ACTING OPIOIDS IN OBSTETRIC ANESTHESIA

Gerard W. Ostheimer

Dr. Walter Channing was the first professor of midwifery and medical jurisprudence at Harvard Medical School; he also founded the Boston Lying-In Hospital. In May of 1847 he performed a delivery during which Dr. Nathan Coley Keep gave ether to produce analgesia for the first time in the recorded obstetric history of the United States. (It is possible that Dr. Crawford Long had administered ether to relieve the pain of childbirth sometime between 1842 and this date, but verification is lacking.) As was the usual way with professors at that time, Channing reported his work with ether over the next year in a "Treatise on Etherization in Childbirth" [1]. I quote from his preface:

My great, I had almost said my sole, object in this circular,—in short, in my whole efforts—was to ascertain here at home, in the birthplace of etherization, what has been the precise results of many experiments, made by many physicians, of the employment of the remedy of pain. My object was to learn if this use of it has been *safe,*—safe both to *mother* and to *child;* and thus, as far as such results might reach, to contribute something towards settling the most important point concerning its further use, namely, that of its *safety.*

Our concern with the use of short-acting opioids in obstetrics must be to determine whether they are safe for both the mother and the fetus, soon to be newborn. To evaluate a narcotic in women of child-bearing potential, we must first study women undergoing gynecologic surgery. Then the drug can be used as a supplement to nitrous oxide in a parturient who has just delivered, usually by cesarean section. Questions to be addressed in the peripartum period include whether stress-free labor and delivery really is the optimal situation for both mother and fetus; whether these drugs can be safely used for epidural analgesia during labor and the postdelivery period; whether they can be used for general anesthesia at cesarean delivery; what their effects are during labor since they easily cross the placenta; whether they will be secreted in breast milk; and what effect they will have on the newborn's neurobehavioral status. A related question is the effect of the short-acting narcotics on in vitro fertilization, both on the procedure itself and in terms of any potential for causing abnormalities in the fetus.

Finally, the interaction with endorphins

can be studied to evaluate the effects of stress on both mother and fetus. In this connection, Goodlin [2] used naloxone to block endorphin release and studied an infant's response in utero and its reaction to stress in the newborn environment. It would appear that the fetus needs a level of endorphins during labor and delivery so it can adapt to its new environment, and this work suggests that perhaps stress is good for the fetus.

A number of tests developed to evaluate the status of infants at birth and early neonatal period can be used to assess the effects of obstetric anesthesia. The remainder of this chapter describes these tests and what they can demonstrate about the sequelae of maternally administered analgesia and anesthesia.

RELATIONSHIP OF OBSTETRIC ANESTHESIA AND SHORT-TERM EFFECTS ON THE NEONATE

The Apgar score [3] has been the traditional and most frequently used method for evaluating the well-being of the newborn and the effects of obstetric medication. Devised by Dr. Virginia Apgar to focus attention on the neonate, this scoring system, although subjective, has proved to be rapid and reproducible. The five evaluations—heart rate, respiratory effort, reflex irritability, muscle tone, and color—are essentially vital signs. It is an excellent screening test for vital functions during the first few minutes of life; however, it detects only the most severe neonatal narcotization from excessive or poorly timed maternal medications, and the subtle effects of drugs are likely to be overlooked.

As a predictor of normal neurologic development, the Apgar score is a crude tool. Drage and associates [4] found that full-term newborns with Apgar scores of 0 to 3 at 5 minutes of age had a greater frequency of neurologic abnormalities at 1 year of life than similar newborns with scores of 7 or more. Only 4.2% of the full-term newborns with

five-minute Apgar scores less than 4 were abnormal at 1 year of age, however.

Historically, all the mothers in Apgar's original reports had received some form of pain relief. In fact, Dr. Apgar collected her data from anesthetic records, so babies whose mothers did not receive anesthesia were not evaluated in the initial studies. Many drugs used in obstetrics that were thought to have no effect on the newborn when evaluated by Apgar score have been found to exert discrete influences when neurobehavioral testing is performed.

Neurobehavioral Assessment Techniques

Neurobehavioral assessment is not a standard part of the newborn examination but has been used to assess the infant's response to its environment. Several tests have been introduced over the years. Graham and associates [5] developed one of the earliest, which includes evaluation of motor strength, sensory responses to visual and auditory stimuli, tactile adaptive responses, pain thresholds, and irritability. The characteristic response by the infant is scored, whereas in Rosenblith's [6] modification of Graham's scale, the best performance is noted and the pain threshold test is eliminated. Prechtl and Beintema [7] introduced a test that evaluates the presence or absence of a series of reflexes, including the sleep or awake state, postural movement, general activity, tremor, skin color, breathing, and twitching. This extensive evaluation is primarily neurologic and not behavioral.

Desmond and her colleagues [8] described a characteristic series of changes in vital signs and behavior of term neonates during the first six hours of life. An initial period of reactivity occurring immediately after birth is followed by an unresponsive interval between 1 and 4 hours of age, which in turn is followed by a second period of reactivity. Desmond and associates concluded that the effects of drugs given in labor and delivery may not be apparent during the first period of reactivity because of the stimulation of the delivery process, but would become evident during the unresponsive interval. Recovery from drug effects begins after delivery when placental circulation to the newborn ceases and the infant begins to eliminate the drugs directly or as metabolites. A good beginning characterized by a good Apgar score does not rule out the possibility of problems arising during the first few hours of life.

Brazelton [9] developed a neurobehavioral examination that, while based on Prechtl and Beintema's test, is primarily an attempt to score the infant's response to its environment. The newborn's reactions to all stimuli depend upon its state of consciousness. This examination specifically evaluates state before each item of the examination; thus its variability becomes an important dimension. Studies show variable results during the first day of life. The examiner requires considerable training to reach a satisfactory degree of reliability [10].

The potential of Brazelton's scale for evaluating the abnormal newborn gives the examination a broad spectrum of applicability, and its usefulness for comparisons in and across cultures has been demonstrated. The examination has been used to study a variety of perinatal influences including maternal medication, narcotic withdrawal syndrome, neonatal hyperbilirubinemia and phototherapy, intrauterine malnutrition, and subsequent neonatal performance after maternal oxytocin challenge testing. Data have been reported comparing the Brazelton score as predictor of one-year neurologic outcome with the standard NIH Collaborative Study neurologic examination [11]. The Brazelton scale detected equal numbers of neurologically impaired children and had far fewer false positive results, so fewer subsequently normal children were thought to be abnormal in the neonatal period. This scale also correlates well with the Bayley Mental Quotients at 10 weeks of age.

In 1974, in an attempt to study the effects on the newborn of epidural anesthesia administered to the parturient during labor and delivery, Scanlon and his associates [12] devised a neurobehavioral examination, the Scanlon Early Neonatal Neurobehavioral Scale (ENNS), which includes an evaluation of the newborn's state of consciousness before each individual observation. Response decrement behavior (habituation) to pinprick, resistance against passive motion (pull to sitting, arm recoil, truncal tone, and general body tone), rooting, sucking, Moro response, habituation to light and sound, placing, alertness, and general assessment are graded on a numeric scale of 0 to 3. A judgment is then made on the lability of state exhibited by the newborn during the examination. None of the items tested are continuous scales. For several scores (particularly tone), both extremely high and extremely low scores may be abnormal. Therefore a summation or total score can be misleading. Statistical techniques should be applied to measure differences in median scores. Several nonparametric tests are useful, such as chi square and the Fischer exact test; F testing and matched-pair median subtests covariant analysis are also appropriate.

Amiel-Tison, Barrier, and Shnider [13] devised a scoring system to evaluate adaptive capacity and neurologic function in full-term infants. Their Neonatal Neurologic and Adaptive Capacity Score (NACS) is performed more quickly than other examinations, puts more emphasis on neonatal tone, and does not use noxious stimuli. An editorial accompanying publication of the NACS [14] is severely critical of both the examination and the statistical approach used by the authors. From the article it is not possible to assess in a valid manner whether the NACS can "differentiate between the infant who has drug-induced depression and one whose depression results from asphyxia, birth trauma, or neurologic disease," as the authors claim it can, since data on the latter group are not included. A more serious flaw in the paper is the evaluation of inhalation analgesia for vaginal delivery as a basis for comparing the NACS and ENNS. Why did the authors not use epidural anesthesia, the same technique used in the initial ENNS study? The efficacy of the NACS must be determined by future investigators.

All these neurobehavioral assessments provide only an early screening of neonatal activity. Few long-term studies are available to determine if the findings on a screening neurobehavioral examination correlate significantly with later mental and neurologic development of the infant.

Effects of Maternal Hypotension and Anesthetic Technique on the Neonate

Corke and associates [15] evaluated the neurobehavioral status of infants born to mothers with and without hypotension (systolic arterial pressure less than 90 torr) after spinal anesthesia. The occurrence of hypotension in the mother was reflected by acidosis in the infant at delivery even when the hypotension was corrected within two minutes. When the babies were examined with the ENNS between 2 and 4 hours of age, no neurobehavioral differences were found in either group. We postulated that if the hypotension were allowed to continue, evidence might be found of changes in central nervous system function.

Hollmen and colleagues [16] evaluated the effect of epidural anesthesia with 1.5% lidocaine with 1:200,000 epinephrine and general anesthesia using thiopental, nitrous oxide–oxygen, and succinylcholine on the neurologic activity of newborns following cesarean section. In six obstetric patients, mean arterial blood pressure fell below 70 torr after epidural anesthesia. In four of the infants whose mothers had hypotension after epidural anesthesia, pH values 15 minutes after delivery were below 7.20. There was a significant correlation between maternal hypotension and weak rooting and sucking reflexes in the newborns at 1 and 2 days of age. All infants of high-risk obstetric patients in this series had abnormal neurologic activity independent of the anesthetic tech-

nique used. This work by Hollmen's group extends our work and confirms the hypothesis that maternal hypotension, if not corrected, will cause alterations in the infant's neurobehavioral status. Perhaps these changes in the newborn would be more readily apparent if ephedrine was not used to correct the hypotension, since it readily passes the placenta and may cause jitteriness and shivering in the neonate.

RELATIONSHIP OF OBSTETRIC ANESTHESIA AND LONG-TERM EFFECTS ON THE NEONATE

Two groups of investigators have demonstrated that obstetric anesthesia does not produce adverse long-term effects on the neonate. Ounsted and her associates [17] prospectively studied 570 infants within three days of delivery and at regular intervals for four years. At 4 years of age, medical, behavioral, and developmental assessments were performed to evaluate motor skills, language, and comprehension. Strong associations were found among emergency cesarean sections, fetal distress during labor, and asphyxia at birth. The impact of obstetric anesthesia was also examined [18]. Methods of pain relief were categorized as general anesthesia, epidural anesthesia, systemic analgesia (usually with meperidine), or none, which included local infiltration; some patients received a combination. No significant differences were found in the developmental status of the children at 4 years of age according to the method used to relieve pain in the mother.

Van den Berg and colleagues [19] investigated the association of obstetric medications with scores of cognitive development at age 5 years using the Peabody Picture Vocabulary Test (PPVT) and the Raven Progressive Colored Matrices. The PPVT is a language-based achievement test that correlates with scholastic ability. The Raven test is based on logic and consists of sets of configuration problems arranged in order of increasing difficulty. No significant effect of obstetric anesthesia or analgesia on child development was found.

CONCLUSIONS

Clearly, the key to achieving the best possible intrauterine environment for the fetus is to maintain adequate uteroplacental perfusion and thus prevent fetal acidosis and hypoxia. Short periods of hypotension may unmask fetal compromise that can be demonstrated biochemically, whereas longer hypotensive intervals will produce altered biochemical and neurobehavioral results up to 48 hours after delivery. Judicious use of analgesia and anesthesia can be complicated by maternal hypotension secondary to aortocaval compression or sympathetic blockade. These changes decrease uteroplacental perfusion, producing fetal hypoxia and acidosis and placing the fetus in jeopardy. Our mission in obstetric anesthesia remains the same as the objective stated by Dr. Walter Channing some 140 years ago: pain relief in obstetrics must be safe for both mother and child. Perhaps some of the new opioids will help us to achieve that goal.

REFERENCES

1. Channing W. A treatise on etherization in childbirth. Illustrated by 581 cases. Boston: William D. Ticknor and Company, 1848.
2. Goodlin RC. Naloxone and its possible relationship to fetal endorphin levels and fetal distress. Am J Obstet Gynecol 1981;139:16–9.
3. Apgar V. A proposal of a new method of evaluation of the newborn infant. Anesth Analg (Cleve) 1953;32:260–7.
4. Drage JS, Kennedy C, Berendes H, Schwartz BK, Weiss W. The Apgar score: index of infant morbidity. Dev Med Child Neurol 1966;8:141–8.
5. Graham FK, Pennayer MM, Caldwell BM, Hartman AP. Relationship between clinical status and behavior test performance in a newborn group with histories suggesting anoxia. J Pediatr 1957;50:177–89.
6. Rosenblith JF. The modified Graham behavior test for neonates: test-retest reliabil-

ity, normative data, and hypotheses for future work. Biol Neonate 1961;3:174–92.
7. Prechtl JFR, Beintema D. The neurological examination of the full-term infant. Clin Dev Med (Lond) 1964;No. 12.
8. Desmond MM, Franklin RR, Vallbona C, et al. The clinical behavior of the newly born. I. The term baby. J Pediatr 1963;62:307–25.
9. Brazelton TB. Neonatal behavioral assessment scale. Clin Dev Med (Lond) 1973;No. 50.
10. Scanlon JW. Clinical neonatal neurobehavioral assessment: methods and significance. In: Marx GF, ed. Clinical management of mother and newborn. New York: Springer-Verlag, 1979:65–83.
11. Tronick E, Brazelton TB. Clinical uses of the Brazelton neonatal behavioral assessment scale. In: Friedlander BZ, Sterritt GM, Kirk GW, eds. Exceptional infant. III. Assessment and intervention. New York: Brunner/Mazel, 1975.
12. Scanlon JW, Brown WU Jr, Weiss JB, Alper MH. Neurobehavioral responses of newborn infants after maternal epidural anesthesia. Anesthesiology 1974;40:121–8.
13. Amiel-Tison C, Barrier G, Shnider SM, et al. A new neurologic and adaptive capacity scoring system for evaluating obstetric medications in full-term newborns. Anesthesiology 1982;56:340–50.
14. Tronick E. A critique of the neonatal neurologic and adaptive capacity score (NACS). Anesthesiology 1982;56:338–9.
15. Corke BC, Datta S, Ostheimer GW, et al. Spinal anaesthesia for caesarean section: the influence of hypotension on neonatal outcome. Anaesthesia 1982;37:658–62.
16. Hollmen AI, Jouppila R, Koivisto M, et al. Neurologic activity of infants following anesthesia for cesarean section. Anesthesiology 1978;48:350–6.
17. Ounsted M, Scott A, Moar V. Delivery and development—to what extent can one associate cause and effect? J R Soc Med 1980;73:786–92.
18. Ounsted M, Scott A, Moar V. Pain relief during childbirth and development at 4 years. J R Soc Med 1981;74:629–30.
19. van den Berg BJ, Levinson G, Shnider SM, et al. Evaluation of long-term effects of obstetric medication on child development. Abstracts of the Society for Obstetric Anesthesia and Perinatology, Boston, 1980:52.

20 CONTINUOUS-INFUSION ALFENTANIL FOR SURGICAL ANESTHESIA

Charles H. McLeskey

Dr. Lowenstein opened this conference with the prediction that in the future, increasing numbers of drugs will be given by continuous infusion. Alfentanil has an onset of action approximately three times faster than that of fentanyl; it also has a more rapid β elimination half-life. Both factors suggest that alfentanil could make a valuable contribution to our anesthetic regimens when given by continuous infusion for maintenance anesthesia. We have administered alfentanil in this manner (preceded by a loading dose) to provide anesthesia for patients undergoing a wide variety of surgical procedures. This chapter discusses the results.

THE ALFENTANIL PROTOCOL

We investigated patients' cardiovascular responses to the stresses of intubation and subsequent incision if anesthesia was induced with alfentanil combined with thiopental. Next, we sought to determine the effective dose range for alfentanil when given by continuous infusion, together with nitrous oxide, for maintenance anesthesia. We were searching for the so-called therapeutic window for alfentanil. We studied 33 patients in ASA classes I through III who were scheduled to undergo surgical procedures lasting from 60 to 120 minutes. All were premedicated with 10 mg of diazepam and monitored appropriately for the surgical procedure.

Our methodology was as follows. After a defasciculating dose of pancuronium, a loading dose of alfentanil was administered, 25 μg per kilogram of body weight, followed by a second 25-μg/kg dose one minute later; anesthetic induction was completed with a reduced dose of thiopental, approximately 2 mg/kg. This regimen was chosen because early in the study I was not sure what dose of alfentanil was needed for induction. To be certain our patients would be amnestic for the stresses of laryngoscopy and intubation, I combined alfentanil with the reduced dose of thiopental. Intubation was then facilitated with succinylcholine.

After intubation, 60% nitrous oxide was administered. Pancuronium was given as needed for the procedure. An alfentanil infusion was then begun, with one-third of the patients receiving an initial infusion of 1 μg/kg/min and the other groups receiving either 1.5 or 2 μg/kg/min. For the infusion, 40 ml of alfentanil as it comes from the manufacturer was added to 460 ml of 5% dextrose in water. The solution was administered with a Valleylab infusion pump. The initial infusion was adjusted to a rate of 0 to 3.0 μg/kg/min as determined by patient needs. If the patient experienced tachycardia or hypertension, the infusion rate was increased; if bradycardia or hypotension developed, the rate was reduced. At the conclusion of the surgical procedure, nitrous oxide and alfentanil were discontinued and muscle relaxants were reversed. The patients were extubated and taken to the recovery room.

Blood pressure and heart rate measurements were recorded at five-minute intervals during the infusion period, at the time of incision, and during induction of anesthesia, as illustrated by the upward-pointing arrows in Figure 20.1. Statistical significance of changes from control during the study was determined by analysis of variance.

In Table 20.1, grouped data for systolic blood pressure, diastolic blood pressure, and heart rate are shown for the following periods: control measurements, after administration of the alfentanil loading dose, after

thiopental was given to complete the induction, after endotracheal intubation, and after the incision.

BENEFITS OF THE CONTINUOUS-INFUSION TECHNIQUE

Induction of anesthesia with a loading dose of alfentanil and reduced dose of thiopental was effective in preventing a stress response to either incision or endotracheal intubation. In spite of these noxious stimuli, blood pressure and heart rate remained at approximately control values or below throughout the procedure. In addition, clinically significant hypotension did not result from this induction regimen. Our patients had been scheduled to have one- to two-hour operations; however, the average duration was approximately three hours and two patients had procedures that lasted almost ten hours. Alfentanil infusion rates were left unchanged in a minority of the patients. In most, we adjusted the rate upward or downward depending upon variable surgical needs or patient sensitivity.

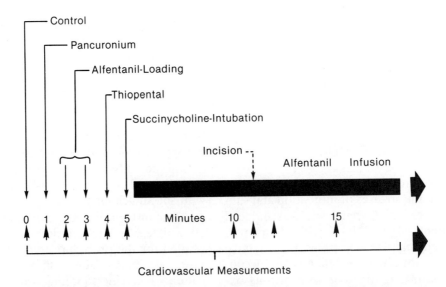

FIGURE 20.1. Hemodynamic changes during continuous alfentanil infusion.

TABLE 20.1.   Mean hemodynamic values during alfentanil infusion

Determination	Control	After Alfentanil	After Thiopental	Postintubation	Postincision
Systolic BP	133.5	125.5*	106.5*	122.2*	120.8*
Diastolic BP	83.0	78.5*	69.2*	77.3*	79.3
Heart rate	81.5	79.1	78.2*	82.5	73.4*

*$p < 0.05$ compared to control.

The percentage of time that all study patients, grouped together, were administered the various infusion rates (µg/kg/min) during surgery was as follows:

0.5	1.0	1.5	2.0	2.5	3.0
16%	30%	28%	21%	4%	1%

No single infusion rate was applicable for all patients; rather, rates ranging from 1 to 2 µg/kg/min were those most commonly employed.

Emergence from anesthesia was rapid in most patients and seemed not to vary with the duration of infusion. For instance, those who had extremely long infusions appeared to emerge as rapidly as those who had rather short periods of infusion. No patients had recall.

Side effects of the technique included chest wall rigidity in approximately 30% of patients during induction. Naloxone was used to assist with emergence from anesthesia in 4 of the 33 patients. The need for naloxone was greatest early in the study and most likely reflects our initial inexperience with the alfentanil technique. Later, as we became more familiar with the pharmacokinetics of alfentanil, the requirement for naloxone was almost nil.

CONCLUSIONS

Our conclusions are, first, that the combination of alfentanil and thiopental is effective for induction in that it prevents cardiovascular stress responses to endotracheal intubation and incision. Second, there appears not to be a single universally applicable infusion rate for alfentanil. Rather, the effective range of commonly employed infusion rates varied from 1 to 2 µg/kg/min. The third and perhaps most important conclusion, at least in my estimation, is that this anesthetic regimen has great potential and applicability for a wide variety of surgical procedures of different lengths.

21 A DISCUSSION ON A LOADING ALFENTANIL BOLUS AND CONTINUOUS INFUSION TECHNIQUE FOR GENERAL SURGERY

Simon de Lange

A bolus dose of alfentanil, when combined with a reduced dose of thiopental, can prevent significant elevations in heart rate and in systolic and diastolic blood pressures (compared to preinduction control values) during intubation and incision. Dr. McLeskey made these observations in 33 adult patients undergoing a variety of surgical procedures. In addition, by using three different infusion rates of alfentanil and varying them according to clinical indications, he attempted to find an ideal rate for general surgery. None was established; however, a significant percentage of patients appeared to be stable at 1.0 or 1.5 μg per kilogram of body weight per minute. Anesthesia was maintained with 60% nitrous oxide and recovery was rapid after stopping the infusion and the inhalational agent. This chapter indicates the advantages and disadvantages of the technique used, with reference to current alfentanil studies.

INDUCTION OF ANESTHESIA

An advantage of using both alfentanil and thiopental for induction of anesthesia is that doses of both drugs can be reduced. Thus the cardiovascular depressant effects of thiopental are limited, but good analgesia is achieved during intubation because of the rapid onset of action of alfentanil. A similar technique has become established with fentanyl, but this opioid is not ideal for the purpose since its peak analgesic effect occurs 5 to 10 minutes after intravenous injection [1]. Also, the short duration of action of alfentanil compared to fentanyl results in significantly less postoperative respiratory depression after short surgical procedures [1,2].

Although the alfentanil bolus of 50 μg/kg of body weight used by Dr. McLeskey resulted in a slight but significant decrease in systolic and diastolic blood pressures, the fall of these measurements after thiopental, 2 mg/

114

kg, was much more marked. Thiopental is a myocardial depressant and capacitance vessel dilator, and may cause hypotension during induction of anesthesia [3,4]. Alfentanil without supplementation is an anesthetic agent [5]. When used for induction of anesthesia, it produces little change in cardiovascular dynamics in patients undergoing cardiac or general surgical procedures [6]. In contrast to thiopental, alfentanil induction allows endotracheal intubation with stable hemodynamics [7].

If alfentanil alone had been used for anesthetic induction in Dr. McLeskey's study, the cardiovascular and central nervous system (CNS) depressant action of thiopental would have been avoided. In addition, combination of the two agents precluded full assessment of alfentanil as an induction agent. Since the operative time was expected to exceed one hour, induction with alfentanil would have been possible; for shorter operations, to avoid postoperative respiratory depression, a combined induction technique with a reduced dose of alfentanil and etomidate could have been used, as etomidate has little cardiovascular depressant action [8]. In studies where the alfentanil induction dose is predetermined from the patient's weight, the important relationship of dose to consciousness is not taken into account.

We found considerable variation in the induction dose of alfentanil calculated on a weight basis [6,7,9]. This was partly due to the use of different premedicant drugs and varying surgical populations. The pharmacokinetic profile of alfentanil does not appear to be correlated to the weight or age of the subject, and it was forecast that prediction of dosage based on these factors may not be useful [10]. We confirmed these findings for both the induction and the total operative dose required during coronary artery surgery [9,11]. Yet in our surgical group there was reasonably good correlation between the titrated induction dose and the total operative dose of alfentanil [9]. Thus the alfentanil dose required to induce unconsciousness may

serve as a useful indicator of further operative requirements.

RIGIDITY

In Dr. McLeskey's study there was a relatively low incidence (10%) of muscle rigidity after induction of anesthesia. Rigidity of the thoracic and abdominal muscles and occasionally the extremities is a major side effect of alfentanil induction [6,7]. In our own studies, we have observed a frequency of occurrence of between 27% and 75%; the incidence appears to depend on speed of intravenous administration, dosage and type of premedication used, surgical population, and possibly the use of a defasciculating dose of muscle relaxant [6,7,9,11,12]. The defasciculating dose of pancuronium, 25 µg/kg, used in Dr. McLeskey's study was relatively large and may have been a contributing factor to the low frequency of rigidity.

We use pancuronium, 20 µg/kg, and although we consider that this dose may reduce the intensity, we currently believe that it does not reduce the frequency of muscle rigidity. A higher dose may well be effective in this respect, but a few of our patients have complained of diplopia and muscle weakness before induction and we are unwilling to increase our standard dose. In contrast, with increasing experience and appropriate timing of the alfentanil and muscle relaxant sequence, we find that we can dispense with the defasciculating dose completely without an increase in the frequency of muscle rigidity or of its intensity when it occurs (de Lange S, de Bruijn NP, unpublished data, 1983).

Other factors that may reduce the incidence of muscle rigidity are benzodiazepine premedication and the rate of intravenous alfentanil administration. For instance, when the induction dose of alfentanil was given in 30 seconds, 75% of our patients developed muscle rigidity [12]. We have suggested that a heavy benzodiazepine premedication may reduce the incidence of muscle rigidity [6], but the sedative effect of a standard 10-mg dose of diazepam was not recorded in Dr. McLeskey's study.

Muscle rigidity may be a dose-related phenomenon since it occurs less frequently when smaller induction doses are effective [6,9,11]. By reducing the alfentanil induction dose required and by its CNS depressant action, thiopental was probably the most important factor in the low incidence of muscle rigidity observed in Dr. McLeskey's study. This is a definite advantage of the combined technique used provided it is important that this side effect be minimized. Opioid-induced muscle rigidity does not usually present a problem, however, since it can be controlled easily and completely by a fully curarizing dose of muscle relaxant [6,7].

THE STRESS RESPONSE

It is common practice during induction of anesthesia to compensate for hemodynamic depressant drug action by evoking the patient's own stress response to laryngoscopy and intubation. In Dr. McLeskey's study it was noted that both systolic and diastolic pressures were significantly decreased but then restored by the patient's autonomic reflex response to the stimulus of laryngoscopy and intubation. These hemodynamic fluctuations were probably accompanied by release of catecholamines, so it was not possible to state that the stress response to intubation was prevented also. The hemodynamic stress response to incision may have been ablated, but not necessarily the metabolic stress response. To verify these assumptions, levels of catecholamines and other stress hormones should be measured during and after these noxious stimuli.

INFUSION RATE

No single optimum infusion rate of alfentanil was identified by McLeskey. This may be expected, for in an analogous manner, no concentration of a volatile inhalational agent is ideal throughout surgery. Anesthetic requirements depend on the severity of the surgical intervention and are modified by patient variables as well as the cardiovascular depressant action of the volatile inhalational agent. Alfentanil has a very wide therapeutic index [13]. In contrast to volatile inhalational agents, where the use of high concentrations is limited by cardiovascular depression, high alfentanil infusion rates may be used without a similar untoward effect [9].

This technique might provide optimum stability for general surgical procedures, but the patient would require ventilatory support for several hours postoperatively. Thus infusion rates should be adjusted so that adequate reflex suppression is provided but postoperative respiratory depression is not incurred. Studies in patients undergoing cardiac surgery indicate that different concentrations of alfentanil may be required to block the cardiovascular stress response to various intensities of surgical stimulation in one patient, but a given concentration might block the response of a standard surgical stimulus in most patients [9]. This is probably the same during general surgery. To determine optimum infusion rates at any one time during surgery, the type of procedure should be standardized and patient variability limited. This was not done in the study under review, so that the results are difficult to interpret.

In a similar study we limited the patients to those in ASA class I and the procedures to lower abdominal gynecologic surgery [12]. Nitrous oxide was the only anesthetic agent other than alfentanil used throughout anesthesia. In a manner analogous to adjusting the concentration of a volatile inhalational agent to clinical signs of inadequate anesthesia, we altered the rate of alfentanil infusion, started at 0.8 µg/kg/min, by upward or downward increments of 0.4 µg/kg/min (limits 0.4 to 2.5 µg/kg/min). These adjustments were related to precisely defined hemodynamic, somatic, and autonomic responses [12]. If these were large, and for rapid control, an alfentanil bolus of 7 μg/kg was given.

With this technique we could determine the minimal effective infusion rate and dosage required at different stages of similar procedures. These varied according to the intensity of the surgical stimulus: the highest mean alfentanil dosage, 2.07 ± 0.26μg/kg/min, was required from skin incision to intraabdominal retraction; the lowest mean dose, 0.58 ± 0.05 μg/kg/min, was used during microscopic pelvic surgery [12].

Information on the mean interval dosages required may provide more useful information on the management of alfentanil infusion in a given type of surgery than average rates throughout a wide variety of procedures, as described in McLeskey's study. Furthermore, by titrating alfentanil infusion rates and dosage to clinical response, an optimum alfentanil plasma concentration might be identified for a standard surgical stimulus, thus establishing a therapeutic window where good surgical anesthesia is provided but not at the cost of postoperative respiratory depression [14].

CLINICAL RESPONSE

In a study of this type it is important to observe the clinical response to surgery in as many ways as possible so that the infusion rate may be more accurately titrated: precise limits should be set on the cardiovascular response to stress or on any cardiac depression; or autonomic signs such as sweating and lacrimation are useful indications; and muscular response such as limb and eye movements should be observed [12]. With the cooperation of the surgeons, we minimized use of muscle relaxants so that a normal "train of four" was present 75% of anesthetic time. Thus somatic response provided a useful guide to depth of anesthesia. This response is negated if routine muscle relaxation is used, as in Dr. McLeskey's study. In addition, if the clinical response to surgery is not precisely defined, subsequent workers may not

be able to reproduce and benefit from the experimental technique described.

RECOVERY TIME TO VENTILATION

Emergence from anesthetic with Dr. McLeskey's technique was rapid, but it was not recorded at which time the alfentanil infusion was stopped in relation to the end of surgery. In our study we were able to discontinue the infusion 16 ± 1.2 minutes before the final skin suture, yet maintain satisfactory anesthesia [12].

Measurements of adequate ventilation were not defined by Dr. McLeskey, nor were use of narcotic antagonists and the time required to establish adequate ventilation recorded. These are important facts in assessing the technique. We too observed that emergence from anesthesia was rapid, and adequate ventilation, as defined by precise values, was established (without the use of a narcotic antagonist) 4 ± 0.5 minutes after stopping nitrous oxide at the end of the operation [12].

REFERENCES

1. Hull CJ, Jacobson L. A clinical trial of alfentanil as an adjuvant for short anaesthetic procedures. Br J Anaesth 1983;55:173S–8S.
2. Helmers JHJH, van Leeuwen L, Adam AA, Giezen J, Deen L. A double-blind comparison of the postoperative respiratory depressant effects of alfentanil and fentanyl. Acta Anaesthesiol Belg 1982;33:13–21.
3. Conway CM, Ellis DB. The haemodynamic effects of short-acting barbiturates. Br J Anaesth 1969;41:534–42.
4. Eckstein JW, Hamilton WK, MacCammond JM. The effects of thiopental on peripheral venous tone. Anesthesiology 1961;22:525–8.
5. McDonnell TE, Bartowski RR, Williams JJ. ED$_{50}$ of alfentanil for induction of anesthesia in unpremedicated young adults. Anesthesiology 1982;57:A352.
6. Nauta J, de Lange S, Koopman D, Spierdijk J, van Kleef J, Stanley TH. Anesthetic

induction with alfentanil: a new short-acting narcotic analgesic. Anesth Analg (Cleve) 1982;61:267–72.

7. Nauta J, Stanley TH, de Lange S, Koopman D, Spierdijk T. van Kleef J. Anaesthetic induction with alfentanil: comparison with thiopental, midazolam and etomidate. Can Anaesth Soc J 1983;30:53–60.

8. Kettler D, Sonntag H. Intravenous anesthetics: coronary blood flow and myocardial oxygen consumption. Acta Anaesthesiol Belg 1974;25:704–11.

9. de Lange S, de Bruijn NP. Alfentanil-oxygen anaesthesia: plasma concentrations and clinical effects during variable-rate continuous infusion for coronary artery surgery. Br J Anaesth 1983;55:183S–9S.

10. Bower S, Hull CJ. Comparative pharma-cokinetics of fentanyl and alfentanil. Br J Anaesth 1982;54:871–7.

11. de Lange S, Stanley TH, Boscoe MJ. Alfentanil-oxygen anaesthesia for coronary artery surgery. Br J Anaesth 1981;53:1291–6.

12. Ausems ME, Hug CC Jr, de Lange S. Variable-rate infusion of alfentanil as a supplement to nitrous oxide anesthesia for general surgery. Anesth Analg (NY) 1983;62:982–6.

13. Cookson RF, Niemegeers CJE, van den Bussche G. The development of alfentanil. Br J Anaesth 1983;55:147S–55S.

14. Ausems ME, Hug CC Jr. Plasma concentration of alfentanil required to supplement nitrous oxide anaesthesia for lower abdominal surgery. Br J Anaesth 1983;55:191S–7S.

Part III DISCUSSION

DR. M. M. GHONEIM: I would like to comment on the presentations given by Dr. Rosow and Dr. Brown. We performed a study on human volunteers, and the results were opposite to what they found. We compared 7.5 or 15 μg/kg of alfentanil with 1.5 or 3 μg/kg of fentanyl. We found huge differences in the effects of the two drugs. It is hard for me to imagine that the differences were due entirely to our dosage of 15 μg versus their use of 20 μg.

I think alfentanil is definitely shorter-acting than fentanyl. And I think, Dr. Rosow, that you obtained similar rates of recovery from the two drugs because you also administered fairly high doses of barbiturates and nitrous oxide with the alfentanil. Barbiturates have strong effects on recovery, and your conclusions, I'm sure, were influenced by the conditions under which you did the study. But by no means can you conclude that alfentanil has the same duration of action as fentanyl.

DR. CARL E. ROSOW: Your study was useful to us, Dr. Ghoneim. You performed a double-blind comparison of two doses of each drug, and you stated that alfentanil had a greater potency than the figure we had been given earlier. On the basis of your findings, I felt comfortable administering a larger dose of alfentanil than I would have thought I could give safely. Also, I was surprised at how brief the duration of alfentanil was. But you used awake volunteers. They really are not comparable to our unconscious patients, and I would be hesitant to make very many comparisons of the effects seen in the two groups.

Also, we normally give anesthesia with barbiturates and nitrous oxide, and under those conditions we just weren't able to detect a clinical difference between the durations of the two drugs. You used a very sensitive measure—response to a carbon dioxide challenge—in your analysis. We lack the capability to track a parameter like that. If a clinical difference does exist, I'm afraid we would be unable to detect it.

DR. GHONEIM: My point was whether you might have found a difference if you had changed the amount of barbiturate, or the amount of alfentanil or fentanyl.

DR. THEODORE H. STANLEY: An important issue here is drug mixing or drug interaction, and barbiturates may potentiate not only the duration but the effectiveness of alfentanil.

DR. ROSOW: A related question is what one should use as an indication for administering more narcotic. For example, I have never been comfortable treating increases in blood pressure with a narcotic; I think it's a misinterpretation of the pharmacodynamics of the drug. I think what most of us do is to titrate with a barbiturate for small pressure increases, but if we find ourselves giving a bit more barbiturate than we want to, we add more narcotic.

DR. ELI M. BROWN: What we were trying to do in our study was to compare the two drugs by substituting alfentanil in a technique we have used for years with fentanyl. The technique was one used for pelvic laparoscopy in outpatient surgery. We simply replaced the fentanyl with alfentanil and used it in exactly the same way, but we could not detect any differences.

Now, you may be right. Perhaps we could induce anesthesia with 150 or 200 μg of alfentanil and use just alfentanil, nitrous oxide, and pancuronium—that way we would not have to use a barbiturate for induction. But I don't know what that would show, or what advantages we would gain. My patients certainly would not awaken any faster, and I doubt that there would be less nausea and vomiting. I just can't see what the advantage would be to substituting that technique for our present one.

DR. GHONEIM: I did not mean that I would recommend giving pure narcotic anesthesia. My point is that when we compare the two drugs by themselves, alfentanil is shorter acting than fentanyl.

DR. STANLEY: You used multiple doses in your study, Dr. Rosow. The pharmacokinetics of these drugs are based on single doses. Could that partially explain some of the effects you observed?

DR. ROSOW: Yes, it could. We might have found some significant differences, but I don't know whether they would be clinically meaningful.

DR. J. HULL: I want to take issue with something Dr. Eisele said. I may not have heard you right, Dr. Eisele, but did you state that alfentanil would be less likely than fentanyl to cross the placental barrier because it is more highly ionized?

DR. JOHN H. EISELE, JR.: Yes.

DR. HULL: At pH 7.4 alfentanil is 10% ionized, not 10% un-ionized. Also, 50% of fentanyl is present in the red blood cells, while 10% of alfentanil enters the red cells. If we look at the proportions of the two drugs in whole blood, not just in plasma, we find that at pH 7.4 the amount

119

unbound, un-ionized alfentanil is more than twice that of fentanyl. Therefore it will cross the placental barrier much more quickly.

DR. EISELE: That would be true, I agree, but I don't have all the facts on the degree of ionization. My statement was based on Dr. Hug's Table 9.3, which indicated that alfentanil is 89% ionized at pH 7.4.

DR. HULL: No, you've got it the wrong way around, I'm afraid.

DR. EISELE: Then clearly the opposite explanation would fit: since alfentanil is highly unionized, it will move more easily across the placental barrier.

DR. HULL: Absolutely.

DR. TONY L. YAKSH: I'd like to know if anesthetic doses of morphine, alfentanil, and sufentanil produce a similar degree of muscle stiffness or rigidity. Also, do we know whether naloxone reverses muscle rigidity as readily as it reverses the "anesthesia," or respiratory depression, produced by these narcotics?

DR. ROSOW: Naloxone reverses rigidity quite rapidly. However, the amount of rigidity we see is highly variable and seems to be related to the presence or absence of other agents used in the anesthetic regimen.

DR. STANLEY: It's also very species related. Some species simply do not become rigid after opioids, while others do.

DR. YAKSH: The reason I asked that question is because in many animals, if delta ligand drugs are given at doses that produce really good anesthesia, we don't see rigidity. Instead, we see flaccidity. This happens in rats, and at high enough doses it occurs in cats. Morphine at high doses produces a rigidity that has been shown to result from excitation of flexors and extensors. High doses of delta ligands, on the other hand, tend to produce flaccidity. It's interesting because, to my knowledge, met-enkephalin is the only delta ligand, or agent with delta ligand properties, that is systemically active. I honestly don't know if met-enkephalin in high doses would even produce anesthesia. If it could, would it produce flaccidity because of its delta ligand properties, or would it be like morphine and produce rigidity? It might, in fact, produce flaccidity.

DR. EDWARD LOWENSTEIN: I'd like to comment on the decreased blood pressure Drs. Bartkowski and Murphy observed in elderly patients given alfentanil and fentanyl. Since histamine is not released with these drugs, the diminution does not appear to be a histamine response. However, we have known for more than a decade that morphine inhibits sympathetic nervous activity. It is tempting to attribute the decreases in blood pressure observed in elderly patients to this same mechanism, which may be characteristic of all opioids. I wonder, Dr. Bartkowski, whether you have considered the possible mechanism for this effect.

DR. RICHARD R. BARTKOWSKI: We have certainly thought about what the mechanism might be. It seems that the decreases in blood pressure occur only when opioids are administered rapidly. When they are given slowly, cardiovascular stability seems to be maintained in a wide range of patients. Why should blood pressure drop only when the drugs are given rapidly? I don't know.

DR. STANLEY: For alfentanil, the answer might be that the onset of action is three to four times faster than with fentanyl. By giving an equally potent dose, one is permitting enormously rapid entry of drug into the brain.

DR. LOWENSTEIN: The same thing is true experimentally with morphine: this sympatholysis is seen only with rapid infusion or rapid administration.

DR. SIMON DE LANGE: I'd like to comment about administering a large bolus dose of alfentanil very rapidly. Alfentanil generally shows between 83% and 93% plasma binding, depending on its concentration. When alfentanil concentration rises above 1 µg/ml, plasma protein binding begins to fall. At high concentrations, 10 µg/ml, plasma binding is only about 60%. When a bolus dose is given very quickly, I think the amount in blood becomes supersaturated and very high concentrations of the free, un-ionized drug reach the brain.

DR. PAUL WHITE: We did a study involving outpatients in which we compared fentanyl and alfentanil by either the conventional intermittent bolus or continuous infusion techniques. We found that with the infusion technique, it was easier to titrate alfentanil than fentanyl. We also found significantly shorter recovery times with alfentanil. We used clinical parameters, for example, time to wakening, orientation, ambulation, and discharge, as well as psychomotor tests (such as the Trieger dot test and a variety of sedation analog scales). The difference we observed may be related to how the drugs were administered as well as the inherent pharmacodynamic differences between fentanyl and alfentanil. Rather than injecting large bolus doses of the opioid compounds, we used a continuous titration method, which minimized the amount of drug administered.

IV SHORT-ACTING OPIOIDS

22 THE USE OF SHORT-ACTING NARCOTICS IN NEUROSURGICAL ANESTHESIA

Robert D. McKay

In 1969, Michenfelder et al [1] described the ideal agent for general anesthesia in neurosurgery as one that should be potent, nonirritating, nonexplosive, stable, and nontoxic. It should permit rapid, smooth induction and emergence (without coughing, retching, or vomiting); it should abolish laryngeal and pharyngeal reflexes at light levels of anesthesia; and it should be compatible with epinephrine. It should not increase intracranial pressure or unduly depress the cardiovascular or other organ systems of the body. Today, as in 1969, no one agent meets all of these criteria. The use of short-acting narcotics, either alone or in combination with other drugs, may satisfy many of these requirements.

EXPERIENCE WITH NARCOTICS IN NEUROSURGICAL PROCEDURES

The administration of narcotics can be associated with a rise in intracranial pressure; this rise can be particularly dangerous in patients with preexisting intracranial hypertension. Keats and Mithoefer [2] showed in 1955 that this increase in intracranial pressure is caused by the elevation in carbon dioxide partial pressure (P_{CO_2}) due to respiratory depression. Changes in intracranial pressure tend to parallel changes in cerebral blood flow. Miller et al [3] studied the effects of droperidol, 5 to 10 mg, and fentanyl, 0.1 mg, both separately and combined, in patients about to undergo craniotomy. Both Innovar (the combination) and fentanyl significantly increased cerebrospinal fluid (CSF) pressure and P_{CO_2}; droperidol alone resulted in no change. Michenfelder and Theye [4] studied the cerebral effects of fentanyl and droperidol, both separately and combined, in dogs in which normocapnia was maintained. Droperidol, 0.3 mg per kilogram of body weight, resulted in a significant decrease in cerebral blood flow and increase in cerebrovascular resistance accompanied by a slight reduction in cerebral metabolic requirement for oxygen ($CMRO_2$) and mean arterial pressure. Fentanyl, 6 μg/kg, resulted in a significant decrease in cerebral blood flow to 55% of control and $CMRO_2$, with an increase in cerebrovascular resistance; these changes lasted about 30 minutes. The administration of Innovar demonstrated partially additive effects of the two drugs; cerebral blood flow was decreased for 60 minutes, while the reduction in $CMRO_2$ lasted 40 minutes. Carlsson et al [5] studied the influence of high-dose fentanyl on cerebral blood flow and metabolism. Fentanyl produced a significant dose-related depression of 40% in both cerebral blood flow and $CMRO_2$. Two rats given fentanyl, 200 μg/kg, showed seizure activity in the electroencephalogram, however. This was accompanied by increases of $CMRO_2$ toward control level.

In general, the effects of fentanyl on intracranial and cerebral perfusion pressures have been difficult to determine because of differences in patient populations, surgical stress, concurrent drug therapy (for example, nitrous oxide, barbiturates, muscle relaxants, and droperidol), Pco_2, and blood pressure, as well as methodology of measuring intracranial pressure. Fitch et al [6] studied the effects of droperidol, 5 mg, and fentanyl, 0.1 mg, in nine anesthetized normocapnic patients with intracranial space-occupying lesions. They found a significant decrease in CSF pressure as well as mean arterial pressure; cerebral perfusion pressure decreased insignificantly. The addition of halothane, 1%, in these patients resulted in a significant increase in CSF pressure even beyond original control values; this was accompanied by significant reductions in both mean arterial and cerebral perfusion pressures. Misfeldt et al [7] studied the effects on intracranial pressure of droperidol, 7.5 to 12.5 mg, and then fentanyl, 0.2 to 0.3 mg, in anesthetized normocapnic patients with intracranial mass lesions. After administration of droperidol, there was an insignificant increase in intracranial pressure with a significant decrease in both mean arterial and cerebral perfusion pressures. The addition of fentanyl resulted in an unchanged intracranial pressure but further reductions in mean arterial and cerebral perfusion pressures. Hypocapnia decreased both intracranial and mean arterial pressures and increased cerebral perfusion pressure. Moss et al [8] studied the effects of fentanyl, 0.2 mg, on intracranial, mean arterial, and cerebral perfusion

pressures in patients with intracranial lesions. There was no significant change in the first, but the last two were significantly reduced. Thus administration of fentanyl to patients with decreased intracranial compliance tends to result in either a modest decrease or no change in intracranial pressure. Changes in cerebral perfusion pressure are more likely to reflect changes in mean arterial pressure, particularly when droperidol is used or when hypotension is already present.

Maintenance of circulatory stability during stress such as laryngoscopy and intubation, described with fentanyl, can be important in preventing increases in intracranial pressure, particularly when cerebral autoregulation is impaired. Martin et al [9] showed that fentanyl, 8 μg/kg, combined with thiopental, 3 mg/kg, was superior to thiopental, 6 mg/kg, in preventing significant increases in mean arterial pressure, heart rate, and pulmonary capillary wedge pressure during laryngoscopy and intubation. The use of short-acting narcotics is also associated with preservation of cerebral autoregulation, as shown by McPherson et al [10] who studied alfentanil. Smith and Marque [11] studied cerebral edema formation in response to cryogenic cerebral injury in dogs during several anesthetic techniques. With both barbiturates and Innovar there was significantly less brain edema than in the control group or in the group anesthetized with volatile anesthetics.

Fentanyl has been used as anesthetic in the dose range of 75 to 150 μg/kg [12]. The application of this high-dose fentanyl technique to neurosurgical operations evolved through efforts to eliminate nitrous oxide to reduce the risk of venous air embolism, particularly during operations in which the patient was in the seated position. Sufentanil is a synthetic narcotic with greater potency and shorter duration of action than fentanyl. When used alone in high doses (20 μg/kg) during neurosurgical procedures, it appears to provide a relatively stress-free intraoperative course, satisfactory operating conditions, and a hemodynamically stable postoperative course, including early awakening and extubation when compared to a high-dose fentanyl technique [13]. In such cases, the careful titration of naloxone postoperatively permits early detailed neurologic examinations.

The effects of narcotics and naloxone on the ischemic brain are controversial. Baskin and Hosobuchi [14] reported the use of naloxone, 0.4 mg, in two patients with cerebral ischemia and one patient with cerebral infarction; the patients with ischemia showed neurologic improvement, while the patient with cerebral infarction did not. Morphine worsened the neurologic deficit; this effect could be reversed by naloxone. These same authors also found naloxone to reverse induced ischemic neurologic deficit in the gerbil [15]. Other authors, however, found naloxone not to be effective in another cerebral ischemia model using the gerbil [16]. Hayes et al [17] reported the use of naloxone in a severe head injury model in the cat. They found the naloxone reversed hypotension and improved oxygenation; intracranial pressure was increased although cerebral perfusion pressure was also increased. More studies are needed to shed light on the role of endogenous opiates in cerebral ischemia and head injury.

In the absence of cerebral ischemia, Innovar, being a cerebral vasoconstrictor, is associated with higher stump pressures and lower cerebral blood flows than halothane or enflurane during carotid endarterectomy. In the presence of ischemia, however, these differences are abolished or attenuated such that the stump pressures tend to be low and similar [18].

VALUE OF SUFENTANIL IN NEUROSURGICAL ANESTHESIA

Since induction with barbiturate and maintenance with nitrous oxide are frequently used in combination with narcotics for neurosurgery, we compared the anesthetic and hemodynamic effects of sufentanil–nitrous oxide to those of fentanyl–nitrous oxide–oxygen after induction with thiopental in 30 patients undergoing craniotomy.

There are no differences in heart rate between the two groups. Blood pressure values are shown in Figure 22.1. Similar hemodynamics occurred in both groups except immediately after intubation, five minutes after intubation, and after incision, when the blood pressure in the fentanyl group was significantly higher than that of the sufentanil group. Blood pressure was generally more labile in the fentanyl group, in which patients had a significantly ($p < 0.05$) greater requirement for volatile anesthetics (14 of 15 fentanyl versus 8 of 15 sufentanil). Brain relaxation (assessed by the surgeons, who were unaware of the anesthetic in use) was satisfactory in more patients receiving sufentanil (12 of 15) than fentanyl (7 of 15) despite similar PCO_2. Ten patients in the fentanyl group received thiopental to treat either inadequate brain relaxation or arterial hypertension; the dose required (4.5 ± 1.1 mg/kg) was significantly ($p < 0.05$) higher than the dose of thiopental required (1.1 ± 0.1 mg/

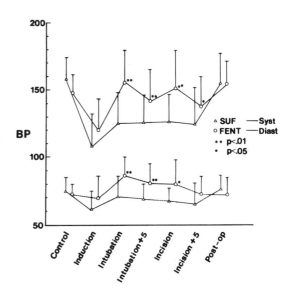

FIGURE 22.1. Systolic and diastolic blood pressure in the 30 patients who received sufentanil or fentanyl during craniotomy.

kg) in seven sufentanil patients. The two groups had a similar incidence of intraoperative hypotension, postoperative analgesic requirement, recovery times, and postoperative narcotic reversal requirements.

Results of our study show that sufentanil is a useful drug to administer with thiopental and nitrous oxide in the anesthetic management of patients undergoing craniotomy. Sufentanil was associated with more hemodynamic stability and better brain relaxation than fentanyl. In comparison of the drugs, it is possible that equipotent doses were not used. Sufentanil is considered to be 5 to 10 times as potent as fentanyl and we used roughly a threefold greater total fentanyl dose. Our mean induction dose of fentanyl (14 μg/kg) was almost five times our mean induction dose of sufentanil (3 μg/kg), however; yet intubation and incision produced less cardiovascular response in the sufentanil group.

We also compared sufentanil to enflurane in patients undergoing carotid endarterectomy. Those who received sufentanil had less hypertension with intubation and less postoperative requirement for sodium nitroprusside to treat hypertension. There was no significant difference in cerebral blood flow between the groups. Hypertension was induced during carotid clamping; inducing hypertension in the sufentanil group more frequently required phenylephrine than in the enflurane group.

DISADVANTAGES OF NARCOTICS IN NEUROSURGICAL PROCEDURES

There are some potential disadvantages to the use of narcotics during neurosurgical anesthesia. Intraoperative awareness may be a problem, but this can usually be avoided by premedication, as well as concurrent administration of other drugs. More common is the risk of chest wall rigidity, which could increase intracranial pressure by causing hypercapnia. Chest wall rigidity, however, can be easily controlled by the early use of muscle relaxants.

Postoperative complications of short-acting narcotics in neurosurgical anesthesia primarily relate to inadequate or too rapid reversal with a narcotic antagonist. Failure to reverse when indicated or inadequate reversal of narcotics could result in respiratory depression leading to hypercapnia, which could increase intracranial pressure. On the other hand, too rapid reversal with naloxone may be associated with hypertension, nausea, and vomiting; Estilo and Cottrell [19] reported a case of cerebral aneurysm rupture secondary to the use of naloxone. These complications of reversal should be avoided by close observation of the patient in an intensive care setting and titration of drugs under the care of personnel who are aware of the effects of these medications.

CONCLUSION

In summary, the short-acting narcotics have become a cornerstone in the anesthetic management of patients with decreased intracranial compliance. Studies using higher doses of short-acting narcotics as the sole anesthetic drug have been very promising. Sufentanil appears to be as good as or slightly better than fentanyl.

The author expresses his gratitude to Pam D. Varner, M.D., Peter L. Hendricks, M.D., Mary L. Adams, B.S., and J.G. Reves, M.D. for assistance in preparing this manuscript; Paula Dennis for preparing illustrations; and Judy Farrar for typing the manuscript.This study was supported by Janssen Pharmaceuticals, grant number JRD 33, 800/015A.

REFERENCES

1. Michenfelder JD, Gronert GA, Rehder K. Neuroanesthesia. Anesthesiology 1969; 30:65–100.
2. Keats AS, Mithoefer JC. The mechanism of increased intracranial pressure induced by morphine. N Engl J Med 1955;252:1110–13.
3. Miller R, Henry CT, Stark DCC. Effect of Innovar, fentanyl and droperidol on the

cerebrospinal fluid pressure in neurosurgical patients. Can Anaesth Soc J 1975;22:502–8.

4. Michenfelder JD, Theye RA. Effects of fentanyl, droperidol and Innovar on canine cerebral metabolism and blood flow. Br J Anaesth 1971;43:930–6.

5. Carlsson C, Keykhah M, Smith DS, Harp JR. Influence of high-dose fentanyl on cerebral blood flow and metabolism. Acta Physiol Scand 1981;113:271–2.

6. Fitch W, Barker J, Jennett WB, McDowall DG. The influence of neuroleptanalgesic drugs on cerebrospinal fluid pressure. Br J Anaesth 1969;41:800–6.

7. Misfeldt BB, Jorgensen PB, Spotoft H, Ronde F. The effects of droperidol and fentanyl on intracranial pressure and cerebral perfusion pressure in neurosurgical patients. Br J Anaesth 1976;48:963–8.

8. Moss E, Powell D, Gibson RM, McDowall DG. Effects of fentanyl on intracranial pressure and cerebral perfusion pressure during hypocapnia. Br J Anaesth 1978;50:779–84.

9. Martin DE, Rosenberg H, Aukburg SJ, et al. Low-dose fentanyl blunts circulatory responses to tracheal intubation. Anesth Analg (Cleve) 1982;61:680–4.

10. McPherson RW, Johnson RM, Traystman RJ. The effects of alfentanil on the cerebral vasculature. Anesthesiology 1982;57(3):A354.

11. Smith AL, Marque JJ. Anesthetics and cerebral edema. Anesthesiology 1976;45(1):64–72.

12. Shupak RC, Harp JR. Reversible narcotic coma for neuroanesthesia. Anesthesiology 1981;55:A230.

13. Shupak RC, Harp JR, Buchheit WA. High-dose sufentanil vs. fentanyl anesthesia in neurosurgery. Anesthesiology 1982;57(3):A350.

14. Baskin DS, Hosobuchi Y. Naloxone reversal of ischemic neurological deficits in man. Lancet 1981;2:272–5.

15. Hosobuchi Y, Baskin DS. Reversal of induced ischemic neurologic deficit in gerbils by the opiate antagonist naloxone. Science 1982;215:69–71.

16. Holaday JW, D'Amato RJ. Naloxone and ischemic neurologic deficits in the gerbil: is there an effect? Science 1982;218:592–4.

17. Hayes RL, Galinat BJ, Kulkarne P, Becker DP. Effects of naloxone on systemic and cerebral responses to experimental concussive brain injury in cats. J Neurosurg 1983;58:720–8.

18. McKay RD, Sundt TM, Michenfelder JD, et al. Internal carotid artery stump pressure and cerebral blood flow during carotid endarterectomy: modifications by halothane, enflurane and Innovar. Anesthesiology 1976;45:390–9.

19. Estilo AE, Cottrell JE. Naloxone, hypertension, and ruptured cerebral aneurysm (letter to the editor). Anesthesiology 1982;54:352.

23 THE PLACE OF SHORT-ACTING NARCOTICS IN NEUROSURGICAL OPERATIONS

Elizabeth A. M. Frost

Dr. McKay in Chapter 22 has told us what every neuroanesthesiologist's dream might be for the ideal neuroanesthetic agent: one that is potent, nonexplosive, nontoxic; one that will allow us to perform rapid induction without alteration of any of the intracranial dynamics. We would like to see compatibility with epinephrine, as this drug is frequently infiltrated to the scalp by the neurosurgeon. We would also like to see diminution of pharyngeal and laryngeal reflexes at light levels of anesthesia, so the patient does not buck in response to insertion of the pin head-holder or during the skin incision. Last, but far from least, the patient should awaken rapidly so that the neurosurgeon can perform a reliable neurologic assessment.

With these ideals in mind, Dr. McKay examined some of the properties of the short-acting narcotic agents. He compared the anesthetic and hemodynamic effects of sufentanil, 2 to 3 µg per kilogram of body weight, and fentanyl, 10 to 20 µg/kg, in patients undergoing craniotomies for tumor excision. He showed that sufentanil offered greater hemodynamic stability during intubation and incision. Those, of course, are two instances that are usually accompanied by a hypertensive response. He also demonstrated greater stability of blood pressure intraoperatively with sufentanil. This finding would be of considerable value if it could be reproduced in patients with cerebrovascular disease. Dr. McKay indicated that greater stability was found in patients undergoing carotid endarterectomy who, because of their generalized hypertensive disease, do frequently experience a rather erratic intraoperative course.

Dr. McKay's anesthetic management was hardly pure pharmacologically, however. He used several other drugs, and I wonder just how many drug interactions took place. Were we to examine a purer technique using one agent rather than combinations of tranquilizers with relaxants, barbiturates, and inhalational agents, would there indeed be any differences in the findings?

IMPORTANCE OF PATHOPHYSIOLOGY IN CHOICE OF ANESTHETIC TECHNIQUE

The investigators indicate that sufentanil may be superior in effecting adequate brain relaxation, but this property is very difficult to define. Neurosurgical evaluation is subjective. Physiologic variation in the intracranial arena is momentary and subject to many factors. I think that perhaps the most important issue is the pathology involved. Brain tumors may be surrounded by a hyperemic area that may or may not respond to pharmacologic vasoconstriction.

It has become apparent, I believe, that rational neuroanesthetic care must be guided by the relevant pathology. We are not confronted by a homogeneous situation. Having something wrong inside (GOK, or "God only knows" syndrome) does not mean that we can use the same anesthetic technique in each case. We have to look very carefully at the pathology in order to make a reasonable choice of the agents or the technique to employ.

Disease states characterized by decreased blood flow may well be aggravated by agents that further decrease the flow, so that patients who have diffuse atheromatous cerebrovascular disease may do better with a technique that maintains or increases flow, such as inhalational agents. On the other hand, if these patients have concomitant systemic hypertension that is poorly controlled, the intraoperative stability afforded by sufentanil would indeed be advantageous, especially if autoregulation is no longer intact. Patients with aneurysms or arteriovenous malformations, in whom maintenance of stable transmural pressure is very important, might well do better and be better protected by a narcotic infusion.

Although most clinicians commonly use the words *swelling* and *edema* interchangeably, these terms can be more precisely applied to distinct temporal processes [1]. Brain swelling, for instance, is defined as an increase in cerebral blood volume. It probably is caused by cerebral vasoparalysis with a resulting hyperemia, and may occur in the immediate period following blunt head trauma or for several hours or days after gunshot wounds. It is also commonly found in areas surrounding brain tumors and in global head injuries in children. (The pathophysiology of head injury in children is very different from that in adults.) Prolonged hyperemia in these cases leads to vasogenic edema and increased intracranial pressure. The enhanced computerized tomographic (CT) scan shows increased brain density and compressed ventricles [2]. These are the cases in which patients have increased blood flow and probably would respond—do indeed respond—very well to narcotic techniques.

Brain edema, on the other hand, is defined as increased water content in the extravascular spaces of the brain. The white matter density of edematous brain is less than that of normal brain on CT scan. Water content, quantitatively determined by tissue density, is higher. Brain edema, either focally or unilaterally, develops in the later stages of head injuries (after a few hours), or after stroke. According to the Monro-Kellie doctrine, cerebral blood volume is decreased, because as the brain water content increases in the skull (a closed box), the volume of the other two intracranial components, cerebrospinal fluid and blood, is reduced.

VALUE OF THE NARCOTICS IN NEUROSURGICAL ANESTHESIA

In our study of 132 patients who sustained head injuries, improvement in outcome was demonstrated in those with missile injury who were anesthetized with fentanyl rather than with inhalation agents [3]. Patients who were operated on four to six hours after sustaining blunt injury fared significantly better if inhalation agents were used, that is, we were working in a time period when blood flow was decreased and a hypoperfusion state had

developed. This suggests that prior knowledge of cerebral blood flow, which may be
quite variable depending on pathology, is
critical to appropriate choice of anesthetic
technique [4]. Interestingly, we noted that,
in all groups, patients who received only nitrous oxide had significantly poorer out-
comes. This finding may be explained partially by animal studies in which nitrous oxide
increased cerebral metabolism out of proportion to the increase in cerebral blood flow
[5]. Clinical reports have also documented
intracranial pressure elevation in neurosurgical patients associated with nitrous oxide
anesthesia [6,7]. Addition of short-acting
narcotics such as fentanyl has an attenuating
action on this deleterious response of raised
intracranial pressure.

We demonstrated some other beneficial
effects of short-acting narcotics in the intensive care of neurosurgical patients. Central
neurogenic hyperventilation, for instance, is
a fairly common respiratory abnormality after
severe head injury [8]. It is recognized by a
pattern of rapid, deep, sustained hyperventilation resulting in severe hypocapnia, which
shifts the oxygen dissociation curve to the
left and causes hypoxia. The intense work of
breathing causes an increased metabolic rate
and further aggravates the hypoxic situation. This pattern is frequent in midbrain
compression secondary to transtentorial her-
niation and carries a poor prognosis; however, some improvement may be obtained
by controlling respiration. The use of nondepolarizing muscle relaxants has been, to
date, probably one of the easiest ways of
trying to control respiration in these otherwise usually very healthy, muscular people.
But it is disadvantageous in that neurologic
assessment is no longer possible.

We have found that small intravenous
doses of fentanyl, 25 to 50 μg, depress respiration sufficiently to allow establishment
of an intermittent mandatory ventilation
mode. The dose is repeated approximately
every hour. Alternatively, continuous infusion of fentanyl, 0.5 to 0.75 μg/kg/hr, may
be used. Adequate neurologic assessment is

still possible. A further advantage is that intracranial pressure is stable during the tracheal suctioning and other respiratory maneuvers.

We have also demonstrated the efficacy
of fentanyl in reducing intracranial pressure
refractory to other commonly employed
therapeutic techniques. Major ventricular
arrhythmias are rare after head injury and
are usually associated with severe intracranial hypertension. Small doses of fentanyl may
be used to reduce intracranial pressure, possibly by improving cerebral perfusion pressure, and thus reestablish regular sinus
rhythm. Prognosis is generally poor, however, and patients rarely survive when they
are this severely injured.

CONCLUSION

While I do not know if we can actually claim
that the shorter-acting narcotics are a cornerstone of neuroanesthetic care, I would go
so far as to say that they are certainly a valuable addition to the pharmacologic armamentarium for the patient with neurologic
disease. Particular value, I believe, is to be
found for disease states that are characterized by increased cerebral blood flow, and
for respiratory control in the intensive care
setting.

REFERENCES

1. Fishman RA. Brain edema. Br Med J
    1976;1:1438–9.
2. Zimmerman RA, Bilaniuk LT, Bruce D, et
    al. Computed tomography of pediatric head
    trauma. Acute general cerebral swelling. Ra-
    diology 1978;126:403–8.
3. Frost EAM, Kim B, Thiagarajah, et al.
    Anesthesia and outcome in severe head in-
    jury. Br J Anaesth 1981;53:3–310.
4. Obrist WD, Dolinskas CA, Gennarelli TA,
    Zimmerman RA. Relation of cerebral blood
    flow to CT scan in acute head injury. In Popp
    AJ, Neural Trauma. New York: Raven Press,
    1979:41–50.

5. Sakabe T, Kuramoto T, Inoue S, et al. Cerebral effects of nitrous oxide in the dog. Anesthesiology 1978;48:195–200.

6. Laitinen LV, Johansson GG, Takkanen L. The effect of nitrous oxide in pulsatile cerebral impedance and cerebral blood flow. Br J Anaesth 1967;39:781–5.

7. Merricksen HT, Jorgensen PB. The effect of nitrous oxide on intracranial pressure in patients with intracranial disorders. Br J Anaesth 1973;45:486–92.

8. Lee ME, Klassen AE, Heaney LM, Resch JA. Respiratory rate and pattern disturbances in acute brain stem infarction. Stroke 1976;7:382–5.

24 SUFENTANIL: A REVIEW

Nabil R. Fahmy

Sufentanil citrate (Sufenta, Janssen) is a new potent synthetic opioid analgesic related to fentanyl. The chemistry of sufentanil was described by van Bever et al in 1976 [1]. It is a thienyl derivative of the 4-anilinopiperidine compound fentanyl (Figure 24.1). Structurally, it is the citrate salt of N-[4-(methoxymethyl)-1-[2-(2-thienyl) ethyl]-4-piperidinyl]-N-phenylpropanamide. Its molecular weight is 578.68. It is a white crystalline powder that is soluble in water and organic solvents. The drug is supplied in 1-, 2-, and 5-ml (colorless) glass ampules; each milliliter contains 50 µg of sufentanil citrate.

ANIMAL PHARMACOLOGY

Pharmacodynamics

Sufentanil has properties characteristic of a pure opioid agonist (analgesia, respiratory depression, gastrointestinal spasm, physical dependence, reversal of its actions by naloxone, and convulsions in toxic doses). It has a high affinity for the µ opioid receptors, an effect that is about ten times greater than that of fentanyl [2]. Sufentanil produces the Straub tail, mydriasis, hyperactivity, and analgesia in the mouse; in the rat, it produces catatonia and analgesia [3]. Administration of the drug to dogs causes sedation, respiratory depression, and reversal of apomorphine-induced vomiting [3].

Studies using the tail-withdrawal reflex in rats indicate that sufentanil is 4520 times more potent than morphine [3]. It has a high therapeutic index, the ratio of the median lethal dose to the median effective dose (LD_{50}/ED_{50}) being 25,211, whereas morphine and fentanyl have LD_{50}/ED_{50} ratios of 69 and 277 respectively [3]. These animal studies suggested that the greater potency of sufentanil would permit the use of very high doses with a low frequency of adverse reactions. De Castro postulated that, in clinically useful doses, sufentanil would significantly suppress the cardiovascular and endocrine responses to surgical stress [4].

The electroencephalographic (EEG) effects of sufentanil are similar to those of fentanyl [5,6]. Both drugs shift the dominant frequencies (alpha and theta activity) toward the low-frequency, high-voltage delta wave activity. These changes are reversed by naloxone. The magnitude of the EEG effect was similar after 0.01 mg of sufentanil or 0.1 mg of fentanyl [6]. Sufentanil decreased cerebral blood flow by 47% and cerebral metabolic rate by 36% in Wistar rats, effects that are similar to those of fentanyl [7].

FIGURE 24.1. Structural formula for sufentanil.

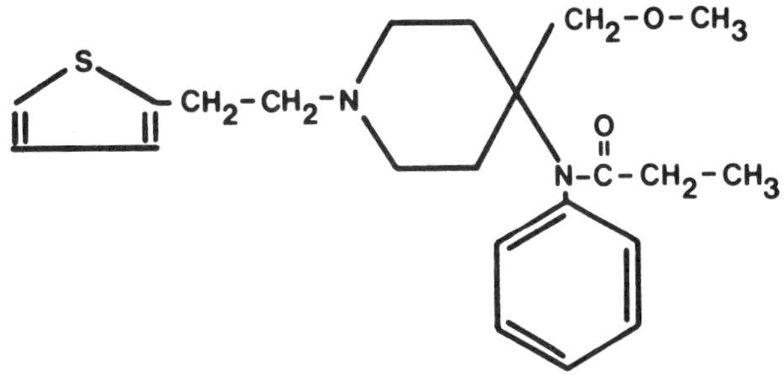

Pharmacokinetics

Because sufentanil is a highly lipophilic compound, it is rapidly and extensively distributed to all tissues. Administration of radiolabeled sufentanil to rats (Janssen Pharmaceutica, data on file) has shown that peak tissue levels were reached in 2 minutes in brain, lung, liver, kidney, and myocardium; in 8 to 15 minutes in the thymus, spleen, testes, and gastrointestinal tract; and after 30 minutes in the pancreas and fatty tissue. After 24 hours 86.8% of radiolabeled sufentanil was excreted, and 99.4% was eliminated after 96 hours (37.8% in urine and 61.8% in the stool). In the dog, however, 60% of the compound appeared in the urine and 40% in the feces. Unchanged sufentanil accounted for only 1.5% to 2.5% of the dose in either species.

Sufentanil is rapidly metabolized by N-dealkylation and O-demethylation to essentially inactive compounds (Janssen Pharmaceutica, data on file). The O-demethylated metabolite has approximately 10% the activity of the parent compound. The metabolic pathway in human beings has yet to be determined.

Toxicity

Acute toxicity and death in animal species (mice, rats, guinea pigs, and dogs) result from respiratory depression and/or central nervous system excitation. Long-term administration causes death from prolonged inanition and weight loss. The drug does not have embryotoxic or teratogenic effects in rats or rabbits (Janssen Pharmaceutica, data on file).

HUMAN PHARMACOLOGY

Pharmacodynamics

In humans, sufentanil produces profound analgesia that is five to ten times that of fentanyl [4]. Respiratory depression also follows its use. In addition, gastrointestinal spasm can lead to constipation, delayed gastric emptying time, and elevation of intrabiliary pressure. Repeated administration can lead to tolerance and physical dependence. Animal studies have demonstrated that the dependence liability of sufentanil is similar to that of fentanyl [8].

The analgesic property of sufentanil is employed primarily in anesthesia either as the analgesic component of balanced anesthesia [9–11] or in combination with oxygen and muscle relaxants (sufentanil-oxygen anesthesia) in cardiac surgical procedures [12–14]. Intramuscular sufentanil has been compared with morphine for the relief of facial pain [15]. Moderate doses (4 to 8 µg/kg of body weight) are used for balanced anesthesia. The drug is compatible with the commonly used hypnotics and muscle relaxants [9–11].

High-dose Sufentanil-Oxygen Anesthesia for Cardiac Surgical Procedures

High doses of opioids (morphine, 1 to 3 mg/kg; fentanyl, 50 to 100 µg/kg) have been advocated for the anesthetic management of patients undergoing cardiac surgery [16,17]. These drugs are expected to produce hypnosis and/or anesthesia, hemodynamic stability, and blockade of the cardiovascular and endocrine effects of surgical stress. Recall of intraoperative events has been reported in cardiac patients anesthetized with high doses of morphine (1 to 3 mg/kg) and fentanyl [18,19]. To eliminate awareness during anesthesia, such patients are often premedicated with scopolamine or a benzodiazepine (diazepam or lorazepam). The addition of diazepam or nitrous oxide during operation has produced important hemodynamic changes when combined with high doses of morphine or fentanyl [20,21].

High doses of fentanyl or sufentanil produce loss of consciousness. Patients undergoing mitral valve operations who were premedicated with diazepam required 11 µg/kg of fentanyl to lose the response to voice and pinprick [17]. Healthy patients undergoing coronary artery bypass grafting needed 18 to 25 µg/kg [22,23]. In a study comparing sufentanil and fentanyl in a similar group of patients premedicated with oral lorazepam, 0.08 mg/kg, loss of response to verbal commands occurred after 4.2 ± 0.8 µg/kg of sufentanil or 28 ± 9 µg/kg of fentanyl [14]. The production of amnesia with these drugs is not universal [18,19]. Awareness during sufentanil-oxygen anesthesia has not yet been reported.

Electroencephalographic effects of small doses of fentanyl, 0.4 to 0.6 mg total, and sufentanil, 0.04 to 0.06 mg total, have been described in humans in combination with droperidol, 15 to 20 mg, and nitrous oxide [6]. The only important result in that study was a tenfold increase in the high-voltage slow delta waves. Fentanyl in a dose of 50 to 70 µg/kg produced a characteristic massive increase in delta waves [24]. The EEG responses to sufentanil, 15 µg/kg, were indistinguishable from those seen after fentanyl, 50 to 70 µg/kg [25]. This is in keeping with the similarity in the pharmacologic profiles of the two compounds. The constancy of the delta band contribution to total power suggests that this may serve as a useful index of anesthetic depth during high-dose opioid anesthesia [25]. It is interesting to note that

natural sleep (non-rapid eye movement) also increases slow-wave activity of the EEG.

Hemodynamic Effects

In a group of cardiac surgical patients under basal neuroleptanesthesia, sufentanil in a dose of 0.3 µg/kg produced greater decreases in systemic arterial pressure, peak rate of rise of intraventricular pressure (dP/dt), and myocardial oxygen consumption than fentanyl, 3 µg/kg [26]. In a double-blind comparison of sufentanil, 2 µg/kg, and fentanyl, 20 µg/kg, used as anesthetic supplements, no significant differences were found in their hemodynamic effects [11]. Similarly, there were no significant differences between the effects of fentanyl, 7 µg/kg, and sufentanil, 0.7 µg/kg, on systemic or coronary hemodynamics in patients without cardiac disease [27].

Studies on sufentanil in patients undergoing coronary artery bypass graft surgery indicate that the drug, like fentanyl, produces few hemodynamic changes [12–14,26,28]. The patients included in these studies had good left ventricular function, were premedicated with a benzodiazepine, and were receiving high doses of β blockers. In these studies, mean blood pressure and systemic vascular resistance were either unchanged or decreased; heart rate, cardiac output, and right atrial and pulmonary capillary wedge pressures were unchanged; and pulmonary arterial pressure was unchanged or increased. Reports of large decreases in systemic arterial pressure and vascular resistance have appeared in the literature, however [9].

Tachycardia, hypertension, and increased cardiac output can follow the combined use of sufentanil and pancuronium [29]. These effects have not been observed with the use of succinylcholine or metocurine [30]. Similarly, the combination of pancuronium and fentanyl can produce tachycardia that is not influenced by the concurrent use of β-adrenergic blocking drugs.

Endocrine and Metabolic Effects

Considerable interest has been shown in recent years in the ability of opioid analgesics to modify endocrine and metabolic responses to surgical trauma [31–33]. Major operative procedures can elicit the release of large amounts of "stress" hormones, which include cortisol, adrenocorticotropic hormone (ACTH), growth hormone, catecholamines, aldosterone, renin, and vasopressin. In addition, the concentrations of various metabolic substrates (e.g., glucose, lactate, triglycerides, and nonesterified fatty acids) are altered by surgical trauma. Both morphine and fentanyl can modify the endocrine and metabolic responses to cardiac and noncardiac operations. Even small doses of morphine inhibit ACTH release and block the pituitary-adrenal and substrate mobilization response to surgery [31]. Morphine, 1 mg/kg, reduces the cortisol response to abdominal surgery [32], while a dose of 4 mg/kg abolishes the cortisol and growth hormone responses to cardiac surgery prior to cardiopulmonary bypass [32,34]. The increases in plasma catecholamine concentrations that occur in patients anesthetized with high-dose morphine for cardiac surgery can, however, by increasing myocardial oxygen consumption, be potentially harmful in those with severe coronary artery disease [35]. Fentanyl, 50 µg/kg, given as a supplement to thiopental and nitrous oxide–oxygen anesthesia in gynecologic surgery, abolishes the hyperglycemic response and reduces the cortisol and growth hormone responses more than halothane–nitrous oxide–oxygen [33]. Similar findings have also been reported during gastric operations [36].

High-dose fentanyl anesthesia prevents endocrine changes and substrate mobilization during the prebypass period of cardiac surgery; the large increases during cardiopulmonary bypass are not altered [22, 37, 38]. Furthermore, the continuous administration of fentanyl for 12 to 18 hours after surgery also fails to prevent postoperative endocrine and metabolic responses [38].

Thus although both morphine and fentanyl have a favorable influence on endocrine and metabolic responses to surgery, they are not capable, at least in doses currently employed, of completely abolishing them. Bovill et al [39] evaluated the endocrine and metabolic responses to cardiac operations in 10 patients who received 20 µg/kg of sufentanil and air-oxygen anesthesia. With the exception of prolactin, there were no significant changes in the concentration of any of the hormones or substrates measured before cardiopulmonary bypass. Concentrations of insulin and growth hormone were unchanged but those of plasma cortisol increased significantly one hour after the start of operation. During and after bypass, blood glucose and antidiuretic hormone levels increased. Thus sufentanil prevented the endocrine and metabolic responses to surgery before cardiopulmonary bypass but was ineffective in preventing these responses during or after bypass.

Pharmacokinetics

Bovill et al [40] have studied the pharmacokinetic profile of two dose levels of sufentanil, 0.5 and 5 µg/kg. The plasma concentration of the drug fell rapidly after injection, and by 30 minutes 98% of sufentanil had left the plasma. Plasma concentrations in those who received 0.5 µg/kg were less than 0.1 ng/ml (the limit of sensitivity of the assay) by three hours, precluding meaningful kinetic analysis in this group. In the 5-µg/kg group, the decay curves were triexponential. The calculated kinetic variables obtained from that study are given in Table 24.1, which also contains the kinetic values for fentanyl [41].

It is apparent from these pharmacokinetic data that sufentanil has a more rapid onset and shorter duration of action than fentanyl [14,28,42]; the smaller volume of distribution and high clearance contribute to the shorter terminal half-life of sufentanil. There is also less of a tendency for the drug to ac-

TABLE 24.1. Comparison of pharmacokinetic data for sufentanil (in surgical patients) and fentanyl (in volunteers)*

Determination	Sufentanil 5 μg/kg	Fentanyl 6.4 μg/kg
$T_{1/2}\pi$ (min)	0.7	1.7
$T_{1/2}\alpha$ (min)	13.7	13.4
$T_{1/2}\beta$ (min)	149	219
Vc (L/kg)	0.104	0.356
Vd (L/kg)	2.48	3.99
Cl (ml/kg/min)	11.3	12.7

$T_{1/2}\pi$, $T_{1/2}\alpha$, $T_{1/2}\beta$ = uptake, distribution, and terminal elimination half-times.

Vc = apparent volume of central compartment; Vd = apparent volume of distribution at steady state; Cl = plasma clearance.

*Data from McClain and Hug [41].

cumulate after repeated doses, and a shorter duration of postoperative respiratory depression is expected [14,28,42].

Sufentanil is more bound to human plasma proteins than is fentanyl (92.5% versus 84.4%) [43]. Plasma protein binding is independent of the concentration over the whole therapeutic range. Protein binding is significantly affected by changes in plasma pH. Binding of sufentanil to plasma proteins decreases by 28% when plasma pH rises from 7.4 to 7.8 and increases by 29% when pH is lowered from 7.4 to 7.0.

Infusions of sufentanil have been administered to patients undergoing coronary artery bypass grafting. De Lange et al [14] found that consciousness was lost in 1.3 ± 0.3 minutes with the infusion of 300 μg/min. Administration of slower rates (18.9 ± 6.5 μg/kg) by Smith et al [28] caused loss of consciousness (determined by loss of response to verbal commands) after three minutes. In the same study, recovery of consciousness was significantly faster with sufentanil than with morphine or fentanyl. Responses to command in the postoperative period occurred after 180 ± 124.1, 137.9 ± 95.9, and 35.7 ± 33.5 minutes with morphine, fentanyl, and sufentanil, respectively.

CLINICAL USES OF SUFENTANIL

Sufentanil has been approved for use as an analgesic during anesthesia. In this context, it can be employed as the analgesic component of nitrous oxide–relaxant (balanced) anesthesia or as the sole anesthetic drug with oxygen.

Nitrous Oxide–Relaxant–Sufentanil Anesthesia

Sufentanil in doses ranging from 2 to 9 μg/kg is an excellent analgesic supplement to nitrous oxide–relaxant anesthesia. Although an occasional decrease in pressure may occur, sufentanil administration is usually associated with a stable hemodynamic state. For operations lasting 4 to 6 hours, an initial dose of 5 μg/kg is usually sufficient. Postoperative respiratory depression is usually of a moderate degree and ventilatory assistance is seldom needed. However, some patients may require reversal of opioid-induced respiratory depression with small doses of naloxone (0.1 to 0.2 mg).

In a study in which we compared sufentanil with fentanyl, we found that the requirements for the former drug were approximately 19% of those for the latter drug in operations of comparable duration. In addition, the stress hormone responses to surgery were significantly attenuated with sufentanil (Fahmy, unpublished data, 1984).

Sufentanil has been used successfully for orthopedic, general surgical, and neurosurgical procedures.

Side Effects

Truncal rigidity, hypotension, postoperative respiratory depression, nausea and vomiting, and renarcotization have all been observed after the administration of sufentanil.

CONCLUSION

Sufentanil is a potent opioid analgesic that is useful as an adjunct to nitrous oxide–relaxant anesthesia and as the sole anesthetic agent in high doses. It is more potent than fentanyl, probably by five to six times. It is more effective than fentanyl in suppressing hormonal responses to surgical stress, and has a faster onset and shorter duration of action. Its side effects are not qualitatively different from those of fentanyl.

REFERENCES

1. van Bever WFM, Niemegeers CJE, Schellekens KHL, Janssen PAJ. N-4-substituted 1-(2 arylethyl)-4-piperidinyl-N-phenylpropanamides, a novel series of extremely potent analgesics with unusually high safety margins. Arzneim Forsch 1976;26:1548–51.

2. Stahl KD, van Bever WFM, Janssen PAJ, Simon EJ. Receptor affinity and pharmacological potency of a series of narcotic analgesics, antidiarrheal and neuroleptic drugs. Eur J Pharmacol 1977;46:199–205.

3. Niemegeers CJE, Schellekens KHL, van Bever WMF, Janssen PAJ. Sufentanil, a very potent and extremely safe intravenous morphine-like compound in mice, rats and dogs. Arzneim Forsch 1976;26:1551–6.

4. de Castro J. Use of sufentanil in analgesic anesthesia. Anesth Reanim Prat 1976; 6:96–114.

5. Wauquier A, van den Broeck WAE, Niemegeers CJE, Janssen PAJ. Effects of morphine, fentanyl, sufentanil and the short-acting morphine-like analgesic alfentanil on the EEG in dogs. Drug Dev Res 1981;1:167–79.

6. Kubicki S, Freund G, Henschel FW, Schoppenhorst M. Fentanyl und Sufentanil im elektroenzephalographischen Vergleich. Anaesthesist 1977;26:333–42.

7. Keykhah M, Smith D, Carlsson C, Englebach I, Harp J. Effects of sufentanil on cerebral blood flow and oxygen consumption. Anesthesiology 1982;57:A248.

8. Colpaert FC, Niemegeers C, Janssen PAJ, van Ree J. Narcotic cueing properties of intraventricularly administered sufentanil, fentanyl, morphine and met-enkephalin. Eur J Pharmacol 1978;47:115–9.

9. Ghoneim MM, Dhanaraj J, Choi WW. Comparison of four opioid analgesics as supplements to nitrous oxide anesthesia. Anesth Analg (NY) 1984;63:405–12.

10. van de Walle J, Lauwers P, Adriaensen H. Double-blind comparison of fentanyl and sufentanil in anaesthesia. Acta Anaesthesiol Belg 1976;27:129–38.

11. Rolly G, Kay B, Cockx F. A double-blind comparison of high doses of fentanyl and sufentanil in man. Influence on cardiovascular, respiratory and metabolic parameters. Acta Anaesthesiol Belg 1979;30:247–54.

12. Sebel PS, Bovill JG. Cardiovascular effects of sufentanil anesthesia. Anesth Analg (Cleve) 1982;67:115–9.

13. de Lange S, Boscoe MJ, Stanley TH, de Bruijin N, Philbin DM, Coggins CH. Antidiuretic and growth hormone responses during coronary artery surgery with sufentanil-oxygen and alfentanil-oxygen anesthesia in man. Anesth Analg (Cleve) 1982; 61:434–8.

14. de Lange S, Boscoe MJ, Stanley TH, Pace N. Comparison of sufentanil-O_2 and fentanyl-O_2 for coronary artery surgery. Anesthesiology 1982;56:112–18.

15. Cathelin M, Vignes R, Malki A, Viars P. Le citrate de sufentanil administré par voie intramusculaire. Activité analgésique chez l'homme conscient. Anesth Analg (Paris) 1981;38:21–5.

16. Lowenstein E, Hallowell P, Levine FH, Daggett WM, Austen G, Laver MB. Cardiovascular response to large doses of intravenous morphine in man. N Engl J Med 1969;281:1389–93.

17. Stanley TH, Webster LR. Anesthetic requirements and cardiovascular effects of fentanyl-oxygen and fentanyl-diazepam-oxygen anesthesia in man. Anesth Analg (Cleve) 1978;57:411–6.

18. Hilgenberg JC. Intraoperative awareness during high-dose fentanyl-oxygen anesthesia. Anesthesiology 1981;54:341–3.

19. Mummaneni N, Rao TLK, Montoya A. Awareness and recall during high-dose fen-

tanyl-oxygen anesthesia. Anesth Analg (Cleve) 1980;59:948–9.

20. Lappas DG, Buckley MJ, Laver MB, Daggett WM, Lowenstein E. Left ventricular performance and pulmonary circulation following addition of nitrous oxide to morphine during coronary artery surgery. Anesthesiology 1975;43:61–9.

21. Tomichek RC, Rosow CE, Philbin DM, Moss J, Teplick RS, Schneider RC. Diazepam-fentanyl interaction: hemodynamic and hormonal effects in coronary artery surgery. Anesth Analg (Cleve) 1983;62:881–4.

22. Stanley TH, Philbin DM, Coggins CM. Fentanyl oxygen anaesthesia for coronary artery surgery: cardiovascular and antidiuretic hormone responses. Can Anaesth Soc J 1979;26:168–72.

23. Lunn JK, Webster LR, Stanley TH, Woodward A. High-dose fentanyl anesthesia for coronary artery surgery. Plasma fentanyl concentration and influence of nitrous oxide on cardiovascular responses. Anesth Analg (Cleve) 1979;58:390–5.

24. Sebel PS, Bovill JG, Wauquier A, Rog P. Effects of high-dose fentanyl anesthesia on the electroencephalogram. Anesthesiology 1981;55:203–11.

25. Bovill JG, Sebel PS, Wauquier A, Rog P. Electroencephalographic effects of sufentanil anaesthesia in man. Br J Anaesth 1982;54:45–52.

26. Hempelmann G, Seitz W, Piepenbrock S, Schleussner E. Vergleischende Untersuchungen zu kardialen und vasculären Effekten des neuen Analgetikums Sufentanil (R30,730) und Fentanyl. Prakt Anaesth 1978;13:429–37.

27. Larsen R, Sonntag H, Schenk HD, Radke J, Hilfiker O. Die Wirkungen von Sufentanil und Fentanyl auf hämodynamik Coronardurchblutung und myocardialen Metabolismus des Menschen. Anaesthesist 1980;29:277–9.

28. Smith NT, Dec-Silver H, Harrison WK, Sanford TJ, Gillig J. A comparison among morphine, fentanyl and sufentanil anesthesia for open-heart surgery: induction, emergence and extubation. Anesthesiology 1982;57:A291.

29. Khoury GF, Estafanous FG, Zurick AM, Lytle B. Sufentanil/pancuronium versus su-

fentanil/metocurine anesthesia for coronary artery surgery. Anesthesiology 1982;57:A47.

30. Khoury GF, Estafanous FG, Samonte AF, Cosgrove DM. Evaluation of sufentanil-O_2 versus halothane-N_2O/O_2 anesthesia for coronary artery surgery. Anesthesiology 1982;57:A290.

31. Briggs FN, Munson PL. Studies on the mechanism of stimulation of ACTH secretion with the aid of morphine as a blocking agent. Endocrinology 1955;57:205–19.

32. George JM, Reier CE, Lanese RR, Power JM. Morphine anesthesia blocks cortisol and growth hormone responses to surgical stress in humans. J Clin Endocrinol Metab 1974;38:736–41.

33. Hall GM, Young C, Holdcroft A, Alaghband-Zadeh J. Substrate mobilization during surgery—a comparison between halothane and fentanyl anaesthesia. Anaesthesia 1978;33:924–30.

34. Brandt MR, Korshin J, Prange Hansen A, et al. Influence of morphine anaesthesia on the endocrine-metabolic response to open-heart surgery. Acta Anaesthesiol Scand 1978;22:400–12.

35. Hasbrouck JD. Morphine anesthesia for open heart surgery. Ann Thorac Surg 1970;10:364–9.

36. Cooper GM, Paterson JL, Ward LD, Hall GM. Fentanyl and the metabolic response to gastric surgery. Anaesthesia 1981;36:667–71.

37. Kono K, Philbin DM, Coggins CH, et al. Renal function and stress response during halothane or fentanyl anesthesia. Anesth Analg (Cleve) 1981;60:552–6.

38. Walsh ES, Paterson JL, O'Riordan JBA, Hall GM. Effects of high-dose fentanyl anaesthesia on the metabolic and endocrine response to cardiac surgery. Br J Anaesth 1981;53:1155–65.

39. Bovill JG, Sebel PS, Fiolet JWT, Touber JL, Kok K, Philbin DM. The influence of sufentanil on endocrine and metabolic responses to cardiac surgery. Anesth Analg (Cleve) 1983;62:391–7.

40. Bovill JG, Sebel PS, Blackburn CL, Heykants J. Kinetics of alfentanil and sufentanil: a comparison. Anesthesiology 1981;55:A174.

41. McClain DA, Hug CC Jr. Intravenous fen-

tanyl kinetics. Clin Pharmacol Ther 1980;28: 106–14.

42. Kay B, Rolly G. Duration of action of analgesic supplements to anaesthesia. A double-blind comparison between morphine, fentanyl and sufentanil. Acta Anaesthesiol Belg 1977;28:25–32.

43. Meuldermans WEG, Hurkmans RMA, Heykants JJP. Plasma protein binding and distribution of fentanyl, sufentanil, alfentanil and lofentanil in blood. Arch Int Pharmacodyn Ther 1982;257:4–19.

25 COMPARISON OF OPIOIDS IN BALANCED ANESTHESIA

Joan W. Flacke, Benjamin J. Kripke, Byron C. Bloor, and Werner E. Flacke

We are currently investigating the hemodynamic and hormonal effects of moderate doses of sufentanil and fentanyl as analgesic supplements during anesthesia [1]. In contrast to Dr. Nabil Fahmy's investigation,* our comparison is being carried out under double-blind conditions utilizing lower doses of these two drugs. It is worth remembering that the dose-response curves for the hemodynamic effects of opioid narcotics, assuming that the threshold dose has been given, are very flat. This is, of course, totally unlike the situation with inhalational anesthetics, and perhaps causes us sometimes to overdose our patients with opioids (either inadvertently or otherwise) just because of the apparent lack of adverse effects. This flatness of the dose-response curves is evident once again in the remarkable similarity of Dr. Fahmy's results to preliminary findings in our investigation, carried out in a different group of surgical patients, in a different manner, and with different doses of fentanyl and sufentanil.

The extensive studies of de Castro in dogs [2] have shown that with increased potency of an opioid analgesic, its safety margin also increases. In other words, the ratio of the dose causing toxic (side) effects to the dose needed to achieve the desired (therapeutic) effects is increased. Clinically this has been shown also to be the case with the large doses of narcotics that we use in cardiovascular surgery [3,4]. But does this hold true for the small to moderate amounts that are used as part of the anesthetic for operations such as those we and Dr. Fahmy have studied? In this situation, will there be any differences among opioids in their ability to bring about desirable effects, such as cardiovascular stability and suppression of autonomic nervous responses to surgery, as opposed to undesirable actions, such as histamine release, muscle rigidity, hypotension, hypertension, and/or postoperative problems of respiratory depression, nausea, and vomiting?

INVESTIGATION OF NARCOTICS IN BALANCED ANESTHESIA

To answer some of these questions as objectively as possible, we are comparing, under

---

*Sufentanil as an analgesic supplement in general surgical procedures. Presented by Nabil H. Fahmy, M.D., at the Symposium on Opioids in Anesthesia, The Cleveland Clinic, May 26–27, 1983.

double-blind conditions, sufentanil, fentanyl, morphine, and meperidine as components of balanced anesthesia in patients undergoing general as well as orthopedic surgical procedures. Otherwise our study protocol is similar to that of Dr. Fahmy. After the patients gave consent and were randomly assigned into four groups, they were premedicated with diazepam and droperidol. Intraarterial blood pressure and heart rate were measured and recorded continuously, and arterial blood samples were taken at intervals to determine plasma norepinephrine, epinephrine, and histamine levels. Our patients were also pretreated with pancuronium and had anesthesia induced with one of the four opioids, and then were given thiopental and succinylcholine. In our patients the narcotic drug was titrated over 6.5 ± 0.3 (mean ± SEM) minutes in intravenous increments up to a maximum loading dose of 0.15 ml/kg of body weight. If unconsciousness or side effects were encountered, the total calculated induction dose was not given. The opioids were supplied in syringes labeled: "Narcotic. Equivalent in Potency to Meperidine 33 mg/ml." Actual drug concentrations in the syringes are shown in Table 25.1. We too decided on a potency ratio of 5:1 for sufentanil versus fentanyl.

In patients studied thus far, all 10 who received morphine and all but 1 of the 11 who received fentanyl tolerated the entire induction dose; however, 6 of 12 given meperidine did not, and in 5 cases this was because of side effects (hypotension, rigidity). Six of 13 patients given sufentanil also did not receive the entire induction dose, but this was due in every case to the occurrence of unconsciousness with lesser amounts of the drug, indicating perhaps a faster onset of action and/or underestimation of the potency of sufentanil in relation to the other agents. Mean (± SEM) induction doses actually administered were 0.6 ± 0.2 mg/kg morphine and 4.3 ± 0.3 mg/kg meperidine; sufentanil and fentanyl dosages were 1.4 ± 0.04 and 7.1 ± 0.5 μg/kg respectively, as opposed to 4 to 5 μg/kg and 20 to 25 μg/kg given to Dr. Fahmy's patients. Thus he induced with

about three times as much drug as we did, perhaps in anticipation of longer operations. So far the mean operating time for our patients is 158 ± 13 minutes, or about one-half as long as in his study.

Times to intubation and incision were 11 ± 2 and 33 ± 1 minutes respectively, without intergroup differences. Induction was evaluated by the anesthesiologist, and by the patient when interviewed 24 hours later. The majority of ratings were "good" or "satisfactory" with the exception of the meperidine group, in which the anesthesiologist gave "fair" or "bad" ratings to more than 50% of the patients because of side effects. Patients' evaluations for meperidine were satisfactory, however.

The maintenance protocol was again similar to that of Dr. Fahmy, with 60% nitrous oxide; however, pancuronium was the muscle relaxant used. Narcotic supplements of 0.01 to 0.05 ml/kg were given whenever blood pressure or heart rate increased to greater than 15% above control values or other signs of inadequate analgesia occurred. If we were unable to control these with supplementary doses of the opioid (sometimes plus small doses of thiopental), a potent inhalational agent was added, and no more cardiovascular or catecholamine data from that patient were included in the study analysis for the operative period.

To date, total opioid doses used in our investigation are 2.4 ± 0.5 μg/kg sufentanil, 15.1 ± 1.2 μg/kg fentanyl, 1.2 ± 0.1 mg/kg morphine, and 8 ± 0.5 mg/kg meperidine (Table 25.1); thus doses per kg per hour after the induction dose are similar to Dr. Fahmy's and in accordance with those reported in the literature [5,6]. In spite of these fairly substantial amounts of narcotic, 3 of 10 patients who received morphine and 5 of 12 given meperidine required the addition of a potent inhalational agent. Only one who was given fentanyl and none who received sufentanil needed this supplementation. The least thiopental was used in patients receiving sufentanil and the most in those receiving meperidine, but the difference was not significant.

TABLE 25.1. Course and side effects of anesthesia with various narcotic agents

Drug	N	Concentration	Total Dose Given*	Inhalation Agents	Total No. of Side Effects (max = N × 7)		Naloxone			
					Disturbing	Nondisturbing	No.		Average Dose* (μg/kg)	
							IV	IM	IV	IM
Sufentanil	13	10 μg/ml	2.4 ± 0.5 μg/kg	0	6	10	5	0	1.8 ± 0.4	0
Fentanyl	11	50 μg/ml	15.1 ± 1.2 μg/kg	1	6	10	3	0	3.2 ± 1.2	0
Morphine	10	4 mg/ml	1.2 ± 0.1 mg/kg	3	8	10	9	3	3.5 ± 1.2	5.1 ± 0.8
Meperidine	12	33 mg/ml	8.0 ± 0.5 mg/kg	5	17	17	5	1	5.3 ± 1.0	2.8

*Mean ± SEM.

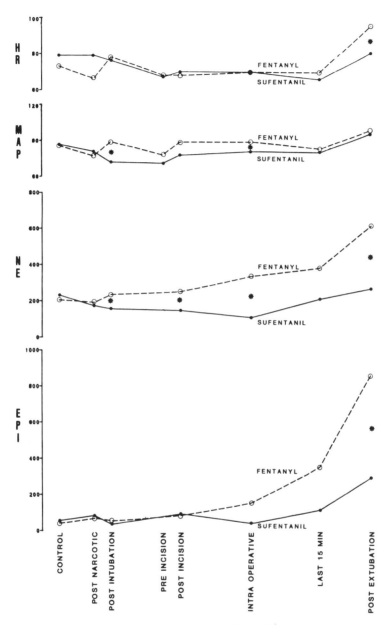

FIGURE 25.1.   Mean values for heart rates (HR), in beats/min; mean arterial blood pressure (MAP), in mm Hg; and plasma norepinephrine (NE) and epinephrine (EPI) levels, in pg/ml, shown for patients receiving sufentanil *(solid line)* and fentanyl *(dashed line)*. Sampling periods are as indicated. The intraoperative point for the hemodynamic data is a minute-by-minute average of values for the first 75 minutes after incision. For catecholamines it is the average value from all blood samples collected during this time period. * = significant differences ($p < 0.05$) between groups.

INTRAOPERATIVE AND POSTOPERATIVE EFFECTS

We looked specifically for seven side effects: hypotension or hypertension, bradycardia or tachycardia, muscle rigidity, histamine release, and nausea and/or vomiting in the recovery room. If these occurred, they were rated as disturbing or nondisturbing (Table 25.1). Patients in our fentanyl and sufentanil groups exhibited less hypotension (38% of the sufentanil and 45% of the fentanyl group) and rigidity (23% of sufentanil and 9% of fentanyl patients) than did those of Dr. Fahmy, but they received lower drug doses, as mentioned. The overall frequency of both severe and nonsevere side effects has been highest in the meperidine group, which had 40% of maximally possible side effects (maximum possible side effects = 7 times the number of patients in the group). Fewest side effects were observed in the fentanyl and sufentanil patients, with about 20% of the maximum possible number (only 7% of them disturbing) in both groups.

Blood pressures and heart rates rose to a greater extent at intubation and ran consistently higher throughout the operative period with morphine and meperidine than with fentanyl or sufentanil. Mean values for the latter are shown in Figure 25.1. Asterisks denote significant differences between values for the two drugs. Mean arterial pressures were lowest after intubation and during the intraoperative period with sufentanil, as were heart rates after extubation. Plasma norepinephrine levels were consistently higher with fentanyl than with sufentanil. Epinephrine levels remained low in both groups until the intraoperative period and then were higher with fentanyl, but not significantly so until after extubation.

These hemodynamic and catecholamine results are very similar to those reported by Dr. Fahmy except for the slower heart rates in both of his groups, perhaps related to the difference in muscle relaxant used. Also, his fentanyl patients had higher blood pressures than ours, so he found no difference in this parameter between groups. At the end of the operation our patients showed signs of cardiovascular and autonomic stimulation also (Figure 25.1).

After discontinuation of nitrous oxide, our patients responded faster than those of Dr. Fahmy: 5 ± 0.9 minutes for our sufentanil patients versus 18 for his, and 6 ± 0.7 versus 24 minutes for the fantanyl groups. Time to extubation was also shorter in our study: 7 ± 1 versus 30 minutes for sufentanil and 9 ± 2 versus 37 minutes for fentanyl. This difference probably reflects the lower doses used. Need for naloxone (Table 25.1) was similar in the two studies for sufentanil patients (38% of ours, 36% of Fahmy's), but only 27% of our fentanyl patients required reversal compared with 45% of his. Of interest is the fact that our patients who received sufentanil needed lower doses of naloxone than those given fentanyl in spite of the fact that the mean time since the last narcotic supplement was only 46 minutes in the former group as opposed to 84 minutes in the latter. The frequency of naloxone use was greater in the morphine and meperidine patients and total doses given were much higher. Several patients required repeated injections (Table 25.1).

CONCLUSION

Preliminary findings in a double-blind comparison of four opioids as components of balanced anesthesia demonstrate a smoother anesthetic course with fewer side effects, greater cardiovascular and autonomic stability, and less postoperative respiratory depression with sufentanil and fentanyl than with morphine and meperidine. In addition, our findings with the former two drugs were essentially in agreement with the study of Dr. Fahmy.

REFERENCES

1. Flacke JW, Kripke BE, Bloor BC, Flacke WE, Katz RL. Intraoperative effectiveness

of sufentanil, fentanyl, meperidine, or morphine in balanced anesthesia: a double-blind study. Anesth Analg 1983;62:259–60.

2. de Castro J, van de Water A, Wouters L, et al. Comparative study of cardiovascular, neurological and metabolic side-effects of eight narcotics in dogs. Acta Anaesthesiol Belg 1979;30:1–96.

3. de Lange S, Boscoe MJ, Stanley TH, Pace N. Comparison of sufentanil-O$_2$ and fentanyl-O$_2$ for coronary artery surgery. Anesthesiology 1982;56:112–18.

4. Smith NT, Dec-Silver H, Harrison WK, Sanford TJ, Gillig J. A comparison among morphine, fentanyl, and sufentanil anesthesia for open-heart surgery. Induction, emergence, and extubation. Anesthesiology 1982;57:A291.

5. van de Valle J, Lauwers P, Adriaensen H. Double-blind comparison of fentanyl and sufentanil in anaesthesia. Acta Anaesthesiol Belg 1976;27:129–38.

6. Kay B, Rolly G. Duration of action of analgesic supplements to anaesthesia. Acta Anaesthesiol Belg 1977;28:25–32.

26 SHORT-ACTING NARCOTICS FOR CARDIOVASCULAR ANESTHESIA IN CHILDREN

Paul R. Hickey

The current popularity of high-dose, short-acting narcotics is spreading into pediatric practice. As is unfortunately customary, there are few studies of these drugs to document their efficacy and safety in children. Studies of new agents are especially necessary in very young children, whose physiology and pharmacology differ substantially from those of the adult.

Current textbooks of pediatric anesthesia either fail to mention use of short-acting narcotics [1] or suggest use of fentanyl in small doses of 1 to 2 µg/kg of body weight [2,3]. Small doses of fentanyl as part of a balanced anesthetic technique have been the only use of short-acting narcotics in pediatric anesthesia. Some textbooks of cardiovascular anesthesia do suggest use of high-dose fentanyl as a primary anesthetic in children undergoing cardiac procedures [4,5], but provide no documentation of its effects. Anesthesia with high-dose, short-acting narcotics in adults has proved advantageous in ways also useful in the pediatric population. Fentanyl [6,7], sufentanil [8,9], and alfen-tanil [10,11] provide hemodynamic stability on induction, even in patients with significant limitations of cardiovascular reserve. These narcotics blunt responses to tracheal intubation [12,13] and are variably effective in blocking hormonal and cardiovascular responses to surgical stress [14,15]. As reflected in current adult practice, these attributes of short-acting narcotics are especially important during procedures that destabilize patients with diminished cardiovascular reserve.

PROBLEMS IN PEDIATRIC ANESTHESIA

In the pediatric population there are several subgroups with consistently diminished cardiovascular reserve. Neonates and infants under 6 months of age have significantly less cardiovascular reserve than older children, as shown by the high frequency of cardiovascular depression and hypotension during halothane induction of normal neonates and infants [16,17]. In addition to this age-related compromise, there is further compromise of reserve by congenital heart disease, diaphragmatic hernia, gastroschisis, and other serious congenital abnormalities when sick infants arrive in the operating room.

Significant problems with arterial oxygenation in many of these patients have made pediatric anesthesiologists reluctant to use nitrous oxide in this population. Given the intolerance to potent inhalational agents, "anesthesia" using air, oxygen, and muscle relaxants, occasionally supplemented with small doses of meperidine or morphine, has been all too frequently used in the past in sick infants. In preverbal patients, consumer complaints about this practice are not expressed.

In young, unstable patients undergoing major procedures, high-dose, short-acting narcotics would seem to be almost ideal anesthetics. Stability on induction, potent analgesia, blunting of responses to stimulation, and use with 100% oxygen in hypoxemic patients are major advantages in young children. One disadvantage of this technique in children is the same as in adults. Even with short-acting narcotics such as fentanyl and sufentanil, use of high-dose techniques significantly prolongs the elimination half-life of these drugs [18,19], usually necessitating postoperative ventilation. This problem may be overcome by using alfentanil, which has a much shorter half-life [19].

Other disadvantages of the high-dose narcotic technique in pediatric anesthesia are intravenous access and lack of information. Intravenous access is sometimes a problem in neonates and infants, but clearly must be established at some point in the anesthesia. Preanesthetic intravenous insertion, even in a crying child, may be more humane and prudent than attempting inhalation induction. A more serious obstacle to this technique is lack of pediatric experience with these drugs in high doses. The dearth of published studies in the pediatric population exacerbates this problem, necessitating uncertain extrapolation of adult data to young children.

REVIEW OF PEDIATRIC STUDIES

The original study of high-dose fentanyl in young children was published by Robinson and Gregory in 1981 [20]. Anesthesia using fentanyl, pancuronium, and air-oxygen was studied in 10 premature infants undergoing ligation of patent ductus arteriosus. Doses of fentanyl ranged from 30 to 50 μg/kg, given as a bolus. The circulatory system was stable throughout the procedures as was arterial oxygenation, reflected in transcutaneous oxygen tension (PO_2). Induction with this regimen resulted in only a 5% decrease in heart rate and systolic blood pressure, both of which returned to levels slightly above normal with surgical stimulation. The infants were all awake and breathing spontaneously within one hour of their return from the operating room.

Subsequently, high-dose fentanyl anesthesia in a group of 20 infants under 1 year of age with complex congenital heart disease was studied by Hansen and Hickey in 1982 [21]. This group included sick (ASA classes III and IV) infants with congestive heart failure and/or severe cyanosis. Lesions included tetralogy of Fallot, transposition of the great arteries, complete atrioventricular canal, and large ventricular septal defects. Fentanyl in doses of either 50 or 75 μg/kg was used as the sole anesthetic together with pancuronium and oxygen. No difference in response was noted between the doses of fentanyl. Induction was smooth and prompt in these unstable patients, with only mild, clinically insignificant changes in heart rate and blood pressure. Hemodynamic responses to intubation were completely blocked, and hemodynamic responses to surgical incision and sternotomy were blocked to a variable degree. A few patients required supplementation with nitrous oxide during the periods of maximal surgical stimulation. These tended to be the more vigorous and less ill infants. Transcutaneous PO_2 levels rose progressively during induction, intubation, and surgical stimulation. Patients were responsive in the intensive care unit 290 minutes after fentanyl was given.

A subsequent study of sufentanil in a similar group of infants undergoing cardiac surgery at the same institution showed similar results [21]. Sufentanil, in doses of 5 to 10 μg/kg, given with pancuronium and oxygen, was well tolerated. Only minimal changes in hemodynamics were seen on induction, and hemodynamic responses to intubation were completely blocked. Transcutaneous Po_2 rose progressively from baseline through induction, intubation, and stimulation. Hemodynamic responses to incision and sternotomy were again variably blocked, but somewhat more reliably than with fentanyl. Time from administration of the drug to responsiveness in the intensive care unit was similar to that found for fentanyl.

A group of cyanotic patients anesthetized with fentanyl or sufentanil in these studies also showed progressive increases in transcutaneous Po_2, confirmed by arterial blood gas determinations. These patients are generally only able to increase arterial Po_2 by increasing their pulmonary blood flow and decreasing right-to-left shunting.

Fentanyl pharmacokinetics have subsequently been studied in a similar but slightly older group of children during cardiac surgery [22]. The children were given 50 μg/kg of fentanyl as a bolus followed by continuous fentanyl infusion of 0.15 or 0.30 μg/kg/min. Plasma fentanyl levels were decreased by 78% during bypass. Mean half-life of the distribution phase ($t_{1/2}\alpha$) was 12 minutes, and of the elimination phase ($t_{1/2}\beta$) 141 minutes. Total body clearance was 12.8 ml/kg/min and volume of distribution at steady state was 1385 ml/kg. Observed plasma levels in this study were up to 300% higher than those found in a similar study in adults [23]. Half-lives and total body clearances were all within reported ranges for adult values, whereas the volumes of distribution were significantly lower, probably accounting for the increased plasma levels observed in these children.

A previous study of fentanyl pharmacokinetics in children with heart disease using 5- to 25-μg/kg boluses of fentanyl was reported in 1981 [24]. In this study, induction was done with either halothane or ketamine.

A triexponential curve-fitting technique was used, and the investigators found a mean half-life for uptake ($t_{1/2}\pi$) of 6 minutes, a $t_{1/2}\alpha$ of 9 minutes, and a $t_{1/2}\beta$ of 165 minutes. Total body clearance was 12.4 ml/min/kg and volume of distribution was 2660 ml/kg.

Use of fentanyl in the postoperative period to stabilize the cardiopulmonary system in critically ill neonates after repair of congenital diaphragmatic hernia was recently reported by Vacanti et al [25]. After a fentanyl-pancuronium anesthetic, a continuous infusion of fentanyl at 3 μg/kg/hr together with pancuronium was used to help control pulmonary artery hypertension and resulting right-to-left shunting through the ductus arteriosus in these neonates. A survival of 71% was achieved in these patients in contrast to 10% in a control group whose treatment for postoperative pulmonary hypertension and right-to-left shunting in the postoperative period was more conventional.

THE VALUE OF NARCOTICS IN PEDIATRIC ANESTHESIA

In the studies cited it is clear that high-dose fentanyl and sufentanil are excellent basal anesthetics in young, sick children with unstable cardiovascular and pulmonary systems. Pathophysiology in these children is different from that in adults. Nevertheless, the hemodynamic stability with induction and partial blunting of responses to tracheal intubation and surgical stimulation reported in adults have been confirmed in children with congenital heart disease.

The pharmacokinetics of fentanyl in children with congenital heart disease are similar to those in adults except for the volume of distribution. The significantly higher plasma levels achieved in children should be noted, although the meaning of these higher levels is unclear. In the neonatal and infant periods, pharmacokinetics may be expected to vary considerably from those of the adult [26,27]. Thus until further studies of pharmacokinetics have been done in healthy children, narcotic dosing with short-acting agents in young patients will necessarily continue to be empiric.

While use of short-acting narcotics for anesthesia in adults has neglected the pulmonary circulation, the pediatric studies suggest a somewhat different focus for the use of short-acting narcotics in young children. The data on transcutaneous Po_2 levels using fentanyl and sufentanil in young children with congenital heart disease suggest stabilization of the pulmonary vascular system with consequent increases in pulmonary flow and decreases in right-to-left shunting. Similarly, data on the use of fentanyl to control pulmonary hypertension in the postoperative period after repair of congenital diaphragmatic hernia to decrease right-to-left ductal shunting support this suggestion.

Stability of the pulmonary circulation and minimizing of shunting across both foramen ovale and ductus arteriosus are important issues in the anesthetic management of all neonates. Similarly, pulmonary vascular resistance and intracardiac shunts are critical in the anesthetic management of all patients with congenital heart disease, whatever their age. These considerations emphasize the need for further exploration of the effects of short-acting narcotics on the pulmonary circulation.

The need for postoperative ventilation after high-dose narcotics might be avoided by the use of alfentanil infusions. This would retain the advantages of profound analgesia with cardiovascular stability for shorter, simpler procedures in unstable children. Although no studies of alfentanil in children have been published, clinical studies are currently being done at several institutions.

CONCLUSIONS

Only a few studies on the use of high-dose, short-acting narcotics in children have been done thus far. Clearly, further work is needed to confirm their findings, extending them to children without congenital heart disease.

The data presently available show that high doses of short-acting narcotics provide excellent hemodynamic stability on induction and blunt the hemodynamic responses to stimulation in very sick infants and neonates. Older children with severe congenital heart disease have also shown remarkable stability with these drugs.

Data on the stabilizing effects of these narcotics on the pulmonary circulation are only suggestive at present, but they presage a potentially wide application of these drugs for neonatal care in both the operating room and the intensive care unit. This attribute of the short-acting narcotics makes them especially suitable for cyanotic patients with congenital heart disease.

It is now clear that short-acting narcotics in high doses have a significant role in the armamentarium of the pediatric anesthetist and have the potential for an even greater role in the future.

REFERENCES

1. Smith RM. Anesthesia for infants and children. St. Louis: CV Mosby, 1980.
2. Jackson Rees G, Grey TG. Paediatric anesthesia: trends in current practice. Woburn, MA: Butterworths, 1981.
3. Brown TCK, Fisk GC. Anaesthesia for children. Oxford: Blackwell Scientific Publications, 1979.
4. Tarhan S. Cardiovascular anesthesia and postoperative care. Chicago: Year Book Medical Publishers, 1982.
5. Ream AK, Fogdall RP. Acute cardiovascular management: anesthesia and intensive care. Philadelphia: JB Lippincott, 1982.
6. Sebel PS, Bovill JG, Boekhorst RAA, Rog N. Cardiovascular effects of high-dose fentanyl anaesthesia. Acta Anaesthesiol Scand 1982;26:308–15.
7. Stanley TH, Webster LR. Anesthetic requirements and cardiovascular effects of fentanyl-oxygen and fentanyl-diazepam-oxygen anesthesia in man. Anesth Analg (Cleve) 1978;57:411–16.
8. Sebel PS, Bovil JG. Cardiovascular effects of sufentanil anesthesia. Anesth Analg (Cleve) 1982;61:115–19.

9. de Lange S, Stanley TH, Boscoe MJ. Comparison of sufentanil-O_2 and fentanyl-O_2 anesthesia for coronary artery surgery. Anesthesiology 1980;53:S64.

10. de Lange S, Stanley TH, Boscoe MJ. Alfentanil-oxygen anaesthesia for coronary artery surgery. Br J Anaesth 1981;53:1291–6.

11. Spierdijk J, van Kleef J, Nauta J, Stanley TH, de Lange S. Alfentanil: a new narcotic induction agent. Anesthesiology 1980;53:S32.

12. Martin DE, Rosenburg H, Aukburg SJ, et al. Low-dose fentanyl blunts circulatory responses to tracheal intubation. Anesth Analg (Cleve) 1982;61:680–4.

13. Black TE, Kay B, Healy TEJ. Alfentanil prevents the stress response to intubation. Anesthesiology 1983;59:A87.

14. Stanley TH, Philbin DM, Coggins CH. Fentanyl-oxygen anaesthesia for coronary artery surgery: cardiovascular and antidiuretic hormone responses. Can Anaesth Soc J 1979;26:168–71.

15. de Lange S, Boscoe MJ, Stanley TH, et al. Antidiuretic and growth hormone responses during coronary artery surgery with sufentanil-oxygen and alfentanil-oxygen anesthesia in man. Anesth Analg (Cleve) 1982;61:434–8.

16. Friesen RH, Lichtor J. Cardiovascular depression during halothane anesthesia in infants: a study of three induction techniques. Anesth Analg (Cleve) 1982;61:42–5.

17. Lichtor JL, Beker BE, Ruschhaupt DG. Myocardial depression during induction in infants. Anesthesiology 1983;59:A452.

18. McClain DA, Hugg CC. Intravenous fentanyl kinetics. Clin Pharmacol Ther 1980;28:106–14.

19. Bovill JG, Sebel PS, Blackburn CL, et al. Kinetics of alfentanil and sufentanil: a comparison. Anesthesiology 1981;55:A174.

20. Robinson S, Gregory GA. Fentanyl-air-oxygen anesthesia for ligation of patent ductus arteriosus in preterm infants. Anesth Analg (Cleve) 1981;60:331–4.

21. Hickey PR, Hansen DD. Fentanyl- and sufentanil-oxygen-pancuronium anesthesia for cardiac surgery in infants. Anesth Analg (Cleve) 1984;63:117–24.

22. Crean P, Goresky G, Koren G, et al. Fentanyl pharmacokinetics in children with congenital heart disease. Anesthesiology 1983;59:A448.

23. Sprigge JS, Wynands JE, Whalley DG, et al. Fentanyl infusion anesthesia for aorto-coronary bypass surgery: plasma levels and hemodynamic responses. Anesth Analg (Cleve) 1982;61:972–8.

24. Baskoff JD, Stevenson RL. Fentanyl pharmacokinetics in children with heart disease. Anesthesiology 1981;55:A194.

25. Vacanti JP, Crone RK, Murphy J, et al. Treatment of congenital diaphragmatic hernia with chronic anesthesia to control pulmonary artery hypertension. Anesthesiology 1983;59:A436.

26. Rane A, Wilson JT. Clinical pharmacokinetics in infants and children. Clin Pharmacokinet 1976;1:2–24.

27. Morselli PL. Clinical pharmacokinetics in neonates. Clin Pharmacokinet 1976;1:81–98.

27 SHORT-ACTING NARCOTICS IN PEDIATRIC ANESTHESIA

Burton S. Epstein

As Dr. Hickey notes in the preceding chapter, there are few reports on the use of narcotics in children, and we sense a fear of studying the drugs in infants. Instead, as is frequently the case, information derived from adult investigations eventually finds its way to application in children. I commend Drs. Hickey and Hansen for formally studying high-dose sufentanil and fentanyl before advocating their use in very high-risk (ASA classes III and IV) infants under 1 year of age who are undergoing repair of complex congenital heart defects. My purpose in this chapter is to comment briefly on Dr. Hickey's presentation before turning to the role of short-acting narcotics in pediatric anesthesia in general, since anesthesia for cardiac surgery is not among my specialties.

NARCOTICS IN PEDIATRIC CARDIAC SURGERY

Two potential major side effects of narcotic anesthesia, bradycardia and chest wall rigidity, were not observed with the technique Dr. Hickey described. Presumably this was because of their use of atropine and pancu-

ronium before induction as well as the slow incremental administration of the narcotic and additional pancuronium spaced over 5 to 10 minutes during induction of anesthesia.

With the fentanyl doses employed, however, systolic and diastolic blood pressure rose with incision and sternotomy. Also, according to Dr. Hickey's original manuscript, several patients in both groups experienced large increases in systolic and diastolic pressures, and nitrous oxide was required to produce clinically adequate anesthesia. One can only speculate on the possible implications of these observations. (a) Did the addition of nitrous oxide produce cardiovascular depression that would not have occurred with fentanyl and sufentanil alone? (b) If patients in the study group had been older, would postoperative awareness have been an issue? (c) Would use at least 100 µg of fentanyl per kilogram of body weight, or the equivalent dose of sufentanil, obviate the need for nitrous oxide to prevent a hypertensive response to incision or sternotomy?

Nicholson [1] used an induction dose of up to 100 µg/kg of fentanyl. This was highly successful in maximizing hemodynamic stability and minimizing the need for supplemental agents; it also eliminated awareness, as judged from discussion with patients over 4 years of age. In her study, an additional 20-µg/kg dose of fentanyl was administered before cardiopulmonary bypass.

Since Drs. Hickey and Hansen did not discuss further observations after their analysis of cardiovascular responses to incision and sternotomy, I cannot comment about their conduct of anesthesia or problems they may have encountered during the remainder of any of the procedures. I presume additional narcotic might have been given before or after bypass if the fentanyl technique was used during surgery. In a group of patients with significant cardiac dysfunction in whom non-anesthetic-related indications for postoperative ventilatory support exist, the precise onset of postoperative awareness does not seem a matter for concern. As is usually the case, most of the patients were kept sedated and intubated overnight until they became hemodynamically stable. This is good medical practice that represents an advantage, rather than a disadvantage, of the technique.

With regard to Dr. Hickey's observation that oxygenation was improved in cyanotic infants, I am reminded of comments by Richard Levin [2] of Children's Memorial Hospital in Chicago (pp. 43–44):

Cyanotic children become unconscious from hypoxia induced by crying and excitement, and their state of consciousness and oxygenation may be improved after receiving morphine. The latter depresses metabolism and also dilates the pulmonary outflow tract and vasculature, decreasing the right to left intracardiac shunt.

This mechanism is analogous to Dr. Hickey's finding with regard to temporal artery puncture and transcutaneous oxygen tension.

Regardless of the mechanism involved, the fact that Drs. Hickey and Hansen observed improved oxygenation after fentanyl is fascinating. Their use of the transcutaneous oxygen analyzer prior to insertion of an arterial line is to be commended. I am confident that we can expect additional reports from their

group of safe administration of anesthesia in children with complex cardiac problems.

NARCOTICS IN GENERAL PEDIATRIC ANESTHESIA

Based on review of the literature on narcotics in pediatric anesthesia, I believe the following list presents an accurate summary of the intraoperative indications for the use of narcotics in children, either as part of a balanced technique or when postoperative ventilation is not expected to be problematic.

1. Premature infant—ligation of patent ductus arteriosus
2. Critically ill neonate
3. Infant less than 6 months of age
4. Electrocorticography and the wake-up technique
5. Increased intracranial pressure
6. Heart surgery
7. At termination of surgery to minimize pain and/or coughing

Robinson and Gregory [3] used high-dose fentanyl in ligation of a patent ductus arteriosus in premature infants for the same reason that narcotics have been advocated in critically ill neonates or in infants less than 6 months of age: to reduce the hypotension that commonly follows the use of potent inhalational agents [4]. Narcotics are used in electrocorticography and in wake-up techniques employed for Harrington rod insertion when the patient's immediate cooperation is needed. As Drs. McKay and Frost discussed (Chapters 22 and 23), narcotics are used to reduce intracranial pressure in children, just as they are in adults. Their use in heart surgery was reviewed earlier in the conference.

USE OF NARCOTICS TO REDUCE POSTOPERATIVE PAIN

A topic that has not been addressed at this gathering is the use of narcotics at the termination of surgery, particularly to minimize pain in the postoperative period. At present, among the drugs currently approved for this use, fentanyl is the prototype for patients expected to have a short stay in the hospital postoperatively. I would like to share some of my feelings about children's problems in short-stay recovery units after outpatient anesthesia.

Short-stay surgical patients represent 40% of the population undergoing surgery at our institution. Over a three-year period there is monotonous repetition of the reasons for overnight hospitalization. In the majority of instances the cause is pain, vomiting, or both. Certainly, the outpatient procedures done in children's hospitals or in general hospitals in which children are anesthetized—operations such as herniotomy, adenoidectomy, circumcision, and orchidopexy—are commonly associated with pain. I believe too little emphasis has been placed on the pain children frequently experience after these procedures. We cannot ignore it—benign neglect is not in order. Studies comparing newborns anesthetized with regional block for circumcision versus those who did not receive an anesthetic demonstrated systemic responses to the trauma in the latter group, even among newborns [5]. I would plead that we try to quantify, even crudely, a system for evaluating pain, discomfort, anxiety, or whatever occurs in the recovery phase. The severity might be assessed by some kind of numeric scoring system based on crying, excitement, anxiety, the patient's claim that he has pain, and the character of the pain.

We have successfully used such a system of assessing postoperative medication requirement to compare the efficacy of injection of a local anesthetic for regional block to that of a narcotic such as fentanyl or alfentanil. In one study, when a patient scored above a designated cut-off point, we administered alfentanil. In a regimen that I call low-dose in deference to Dr. Stanley, 5 μg/kg of intravenous alfentanil successfully reduced pain and anxiety in approximately a minute during the immediate recovery period after adenoidectomy. It is incredible how fast this drug works to calm an otherwise uncontrollable patient who may do damage to himself in the recovery room. For 80% of our patients who required alfentanil based on their discomfort score, no further doses of the drug were needed [6].

In this regard, I think we anesthesiologists do not appreciate enough that it is important to calm a child down and get him in contact with his parents as quickly as possible after operation. Sometimes parents can be the calming influence that precludes the need for longer-acting drugs to reduce anxiety, pain, or discomfort.

We rigidly adhere to five discharge criteria for short-stay surgery: (a) stable vital signs, (b) ability to cough and gag, (c) ability to walk, (d) clear state of consciousness, and (e) ability to retain oral fluids. In our series, in which alfentanil was given in one or a maximum of two 5-μg/kg doses, these criteria were met in approximately four hours, at which time patients were discharged home.

CONCLUSION

The pediatric population we are seeing today includes sick patients such as the ones Dr. Hickey described. Frequently, too, it includes patients who will go home the same day and who may have pain that we ought to treat. Through efforts of the participants in this symposium, we can continue to improve our ability to render appropriate treatment to these special patients entrusted to our care.

REFERENCES

1. Nicholson SC. High-dose fentanyl (HDF) in the pediatric patient. An update for the clinician on anesthesia for infants and children (abstract). Children's Hospital of Philadelphia, 1983.
2. Levin RM. Pediatric anesthesia handbook. New York: Medical Examination Publishing Co., 1980.

3. Robinson S, Gregory GA. Fentanyl-air-oxygen anesthesia for ligation of patent ductus arteriosus in preterm infants. Anesth Analg (Cleve) 1981;60:331.
4. Diaz JH, Lockhart CH. Is halothane really safe in infancy? (abstract). Anesthesiology 1979;51:S313.
5. Williamson PS, Williamson ML. Physiologic stress reduction by a local anesthetic during newborn circumcision. Pediatrics 1983;71:36.
6. Oh TH, Abramowitz MD, Epstein BS. Alfentanil: a new analgesic for postoperative pain control in children. Abstracts of the American Academy of Pediatrics, 1982.

28 INTRATHECAL AND EPIDURAL SHORT-ACTING NARCOTICS

Luke M. Kitahata, J. G. Collins, and Maki Matsumoto

During the past several years, the subarachnoid or epidural application of opioids to produce analgesia for pain of both acute and chronic origin has enjoyed wide popularity in clinical practice. Compared with systemic administration of opioids and/or spinal administration of local anesthetics, spinal opioid administration produces effective analgesia that is predominantly segmental and free of sympathetic and motor depression. The amount of opioid used can be far smaller than that used for intravenous administration, yet clinically important analgesia lasts much longer than that seen after intravenous administration.

The segmental extent of analgesia from a given volume of opioid solution is roughly the same as the segmental distribution of analgesia after a similar dose of local anesthetic. A variable degree of systemic uptake or redistribution of the drug in the cerebrospinal fluid to supraspinal sites results in some central effects: shift of the carbon dioxide response curve to the right; variable degrees of analgesia in areas outside the segmental distribution of blockade; and a mild and variable degree of central depression and somnolence in susceptible subjects. The cen-

tral effects are markedly less after epidural injection than after intravenous administration of opioids [1]. The net effect of powerful segmental analgesia combined with relatively slight impairment of respiratory sensitivity offers a marked advantage over systemically administered opioids.

The side effect of greatest concern after spinal or epidural opioid administration is respiratory depression. It has been suggested that the use of more lipid-soluble opioids (e.g., shorter-acting drugs such as fentanyl) may decrease the potential occurrence of the problem. This chapter reviews some of the clinical studies in which the short-acting narcotics have been employed and discusses the pharmacokinetics of spinal administration of these drugs in light of those clinical studies as well as recent animal studies.

EXPERIENCE WITH INTRATHECAL AND EPIDURAL NARCOTICS

A summary of some recent reports of the clinical use of fentanyl is contained in Table 28.1 [2–10]. The clinical reports have indi-

TABLE 28.1. Summary of recent reports on the clinical use of epidural fentanyl

Dose (μg)	Onset (min)	Duration (hr)	Analgesia	Side Effects	Patient Population	Reference
100	4–10	1½–2	Satisfactory	None	20 postoperative (cesarean section)	2
100	5	2	Satisfactory	Slight sedation	20 postoperative	3
100		2–7	Satisfactory	None	12 postoperative (general surgery)	4
80		2–3	Satisfactory	Mild itching	35 first stage labor	5
60		5.7 (avg.)	Satisfactory	None	25 postoperative (general surgery)	6
100			Satisfactory	None	40 obstetric patients, 20 postoperative (thoracic surgery)	7
150–200			Satisfactory (first stage) Unsatisfactory (second stage)	None None	38 in labor	8
Continuous infusion						
60/hr		48–72	Satisfactory	Nausea 4/10	10 postoperative (abdominal surgery)	9
50/hr		24	Satisfactory	Nausea (at 50 μg/hr)	30 postoperative (general surgery)	10
25/hr	5–10	(24–30)		None (at 25 μg/hr)		

cated that the onset of analgesia after fentanyl administration is 4 to 10 minutes and peak effects are seen at 20 to 30 minutes, with a duration of analgesia lasting 2 to 7 hours. Although the duration of analgesia is shorter than that seen with longer-acting narcotics, few notable side effects were seen after epidural fentanyl. No respiratory depression was reported except for some reduction in the respiratory rate, but without changes in partial pressure of carbon dioxide (Pco_2) [3]. Mild itching and slight sedation were reported in one study each. Using continuous epidural infusion, Bailey and Smith [10] reported nausea and vomiting in some of their patients with fentanyl (50 µg/hr), but neither symptom was noted when they used 25 µg/hr. Welchew and Thornton [9] reported nausea in 4 of 10 patients when 60 µg/hr was infused. Both of these infusion studies had high success rates for analgesia.

An important consideration when discussing the spinal or epidural use of short-acting narcotics is a realization that predictions of onset and duration of action of these drugs is based upon pharmacokinetic studies after their systemic administration. As is clear from case reports, the time course of analgesic action in spinal and epidural use is not in keeping with that seen after intravenous administration. The same holds true for the agents that are considered to be longer acting. This is an extremely important point, because comparisons or assumptions based upon systemic pharmacokinetic data may not necessarily be valid when applied to effects seen after spinal or epidural administration of these drugs. We know, for example, that duration of analgesia after spinal administration is significantly longer than that produced by systemic administration. We also know that transport of these drugs to other areas of the central nervous system relies heavily upon cerebrospinal fluid movement, a factor that is not always taken into consideration when assessing the pharmacokinetics of systemically administered narcotics.

RESULTS OF ANIMAL STUDIES

A comparison of results from animal work carried out in our laboratories points out some clear differences between characteristics and actions of these drugs given spinally versus systemically. According to the most recent edition of *The Pharmacological Basis of Therapeutics,* by Goodman and Gilman [11], fentanyl is approximately 80 times as potent as morphine. When, however, one compares the relative potency of morphine and fentanyl as measured by the ability of each drug, when administered spinally, to suppress noxiously evoked activity of dorsal horn neurons, the potency ratios are different. We recently reported data [12,13] indicating that both morphine and fentanyl administered spinally are capable of suppressing noxiously evoked activity of wide dynamic range in the dorsal horn of the spinal cord. Examination of the data reveals that similar levels of suppression of neuronal activity were produced by 0.25 mg of spinally administered morphine and 15 µg of spinally administered fentanyl. Clearly, after spinal administration, at least as measured by neurophysiologic data, the potency ratios are not 80:1 but are rather 16:1.

In addition to differences in potency, obvious differences in the onset and duration of the short-acting narcotics have been obtained from our animal studies. Figures 28.1 and 28.2 present data that clearly point out the differences between the timing of effects after spinal versus systemic administration of short-acting opioids. These data were obtained from a continuing study of the effects of alfentanil on noxiously evoked activity of dorsal horn neurons. We found that, at the level of the spinal cord, spinal administration of alfentanil produces suppression of noxiously evoked activity that has a slower onset but a longer duration of action than that seen after systemic administration. An example of the suppression of noxiously evoked activity of a single, wide dynamic range neuron

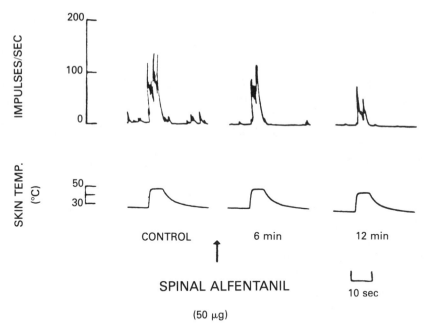

FIGURE 28.1. Effects of 50 μg of spinally administered alfentanil on the noxiously evoked activity of a single, wide dynamic range neuron. A radiant heat stimulus of 51°C for 8 seconds presented to this cell's receptive field caused significant activation. Spinally administered alfentanil caused suppression of this activity over time. See text for details.

is seen in Figure 28.1. Control stimulation caused activation of this neuron. After spinal administration of 50 μg of alfentanil there was significant suppression of this neuron, which took a fairly long time to develop such that at 12 minutes the activity had been reduced to 29% of control. Indeed, subsequent to that time supression became even greater, so that 30 minutes after administration of spinal alfentanil the noxiously evoked activity had been suppressed to 10% of control.

In contrast to spinal administration of this drug, the effects of systemic administration are seen in Figure 28.2. These data were obtained from a neuron after complete recovery from the effects of spinally administered alfentanil. Systemic administration of 25 μg/kg of alfentanil also caused significant suppression of this neuron. The suppression was

much more rapid in onset and also was of much shorter duration. Six minutes after systemic administration the evoked activity was reduced to 12% of control; however, by 12 minutes recovery had already begun. This is a typical pattern that we have seen in all neurons in which we have compared spinal versus intravenous administration of alfentanil.

CONCLUSION

It is clear that there is an important role for the shorter-acting opioids in spinal or epidural analgesia. This role, however, cannot be defined based upon pharmacokinetic values that have been obtained from systemically administered drugs, but rather must be determined from spinal administration of the

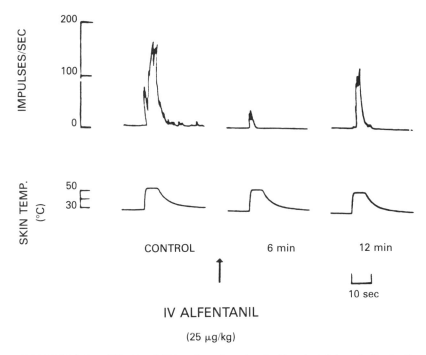

IV ALFENTANIL

(25 μg/kg)

FIGURE 28.2. Effects of 25 μg/kg of systemically administered alfentanil on the noxiously evoked activity of a single, wide dynamic range neuron. See Figure 28.1 and text for details. Note the short onset and duration of effect as compared with spinal alfentanil.

drugs especially in light of the various factors that may influence onset and duration. For example, the short duration of action of alfentanil is due in large part to its small volume of distribution and rapid clearance from the body [14]. In contrast, the short duration of action of fentanyl is due in large part to rapid redistribution of the drug (i.e., comparable to thiopental). These differences in pharmacokinetics are important in terms of systemic administration but may not allow direct extrapolation to time course after spinal or epidural administration. Not only are we in need of pharmacokinetic data derived from spinal application, but an improved understanding of cerebrospinal fluid movement would be most helpful. We are in the early stages of an exciting era of pain control. We hope answers to some of these questions soon will be forthcoming.

Supported by NIH grant NS-09871.

REFERENCES

1. Bromage PR, Camporesi E, Leslie J. Epidural narcotics in volunteers; sensitivity to pain and to carbon dioxide. Pain 1980;9;145–60.

2. Wolfe MJ, Nicholas ADG. Selective epidural analgesia. Lancet 1979;2:150–1.

3. Rutter DV, Skewes DG, Morgan M. Extradural opioids for postoperative analgesia. A double-blind comparison of pethidine, fentanyl and morphine. Br J Anaesth 1981;53:915–19.

4. Houlton PG, Reynolds F. Epidural diamorphine and fentanyl for postoperative pain. Anaesthesia 1981;36:1144–5.

5. Justin DM, Francis D, Houlton PG, Reynolds F. A controlled trial of extradural fentanyl in labour. Br J Anaesth 1982; 54:409–14.

6. Torda TA, Pybus DA. Comparison of four narcotic analgesics for extradural analgesia. Br J Anaesth 1982;54:291–5.

7. Wolfe MJ, Davies GK. Analgesic action of extradural fentanyl. Br J Anaesth 1980; 52:357–8.
8. Carrie LES, O'Sullivan GM, Seegobin R. Epidural fentanyl in labour. Anaesthesia 1981;36:965–9.
9. Welchew EA, Thornton TA. Continuous thoracic epidural fentanyl. A comparison of fentanyl with intramuscular papaveretum for postoperative pain. Anaesthesia 1982; 37:309–16.
10. Bailey PW, Smith BE. Continuous epidural infusion of fentanyl for postoperative analgesia. Anaesthesia 1980;35:1002–6.
11. Gilman AG, Goodman LS, Gilman A, ed. The pharmacological basis of therapeutics, 6th ed. New York, Toronto, London: Macmillan, 1980.
12. Homma E, Collins JG, Kitahata LM, Matsumoto M, Kawahara M. Suppression of noxiously evoked WDR dorsal horn neuronal activity by spinally administered morphine. Anesthesiology 1983;58:232–236.
13. Suzukawa H, Matsumoto M, Collins JG, Kitahata LM, Yuge O. Dose response suppression of noxiously evoked activity of WDR neurons by spinally administered fentanyl. Anesthesiology 1983;58:510–13.
14. Bovill JS, Sebel PS, Blackburn CL, Heykants J. The pharmacokinetics of alfentanil (R 39209): a new opioid analgesic. Anesthesiology 1982;57:439–43.

29 PRELIMINARY STUDIES ON THE ANTINOCICEPTIVE EFFECTS OF INTRATHECAL ALFENTANIL IN ANIMAL MODELS

Tony L. Yaksh, Rabiah Noueihed, and Philippe A. Durant

Early work using a chronic spinal catheterization procedure demonstrated that an action of opioid alkaloids limited to the spinal cord of the unanesthetized animal would produce a significant attenuation in the animal's response to otherwise aversive thermal, chemical, pressure, or electrical stimuli applied to the caudal dermatomes of the body [1–5]. In contrast to the powerful effect on the animal's pain behavior, spinally administered opioids failed to have minimal effects on autonomic, motor, or nonnociceptive sensory function. Systematic examination of the effect of these agents on spinal pain processing demonstrated that the analgesic effects of the spinally administered agents were characterized by a predictable pharmacology that was indistinguishable from that accepted for an opiate receptor. That is, the effects were dose dependent, stereospecific, antagonized in a dose-dependent fashion by naloxone, and subject to the development of tolerance, with cross-tolerance being observed among different opioid alkaloids [6,7].

Aside from the lack of effect on somatic and motor systems produced by analgesic doses of spinal opiates, of particular interest to the clinician was the long-lasting effect produced by this route of administration with agents such as morphine. This was related to the time required to clear the agent from the spinal drug pool created by the intrathecal or epidural injection. The principal side effect of spinal opiates, life-threatening respiratory depression, has been thought to result from the supraspinal redistribution of this large pool of free drug in the spinal space. A drug cleared rapidly from the spinal space might be of value. It would permit adequate analgesia without the persistence of a large amount of free drug in the cerebrospinal fluid. Prolonged analgesia might thus be obtained by repeated spinal injections through percutaneous catheters or by infusion.

Recent interest has been directed at the derivative of fentanyl, alfentanil. In animal and human studies, this agent, given systemically at doses that produce maximum measurable analgesia, will produce the effect for an interval significantly shorter than that produced by an equiactive dose of fentanyl [see, for example, 8–10]. As drugs given intrathecally commonly have different functional characteristics than when given systemically, we sought to examine the characteristics of alfentanil administered intrathecally in rats and cats.

NOCICEPTIVE TESTS IN ANIMALS

To investigate the spinal action of alfentanil, rats and cats were prepared with intrathecal catheters. These methods are described in detail elsewhere [5]. Briefly, rats were anesthetized with halothane and the catheter (PE-10) was inserted 7.5 to 8 cm into the lumbar subarachnoid space by an opening in the cisternal membrane after exposure with a small midline incision in the back of the skull. The catheter was passed subcutaneously and externalized on the top of the skull. A similar procedure was followed for cats except that the catheter was passed 25 to 30 cm caudally from the cisternal membrane [11].

Nociceptive thresholds were assessed in the rat by the tail-flick and hot-plate tests, measurements demonstrating the effect of the intrathecal drug on spinal and supraspinally mediated response systems respectively. To prevent tissue damage, failure to respond by 60 or 6 seconds on the hot plate and tail flick respectively, resulted in termination of the test and assignment of that response latency. In the cat, the thermal nociceptive skin twitch reflex was employed. In this, the back was closely shaved about 2 cm on either side of midline from just below the fifth thoracic vertebra to the ischeal crest. A thermal probe maintained at 70°C was placed lightly on the skin, activating a timer. A brisk local movement of the underlying skin normally appeared in 1 to 2 seconds. Removal of the probe at this time terminated the timing and provided the response latency. Holding the probe on the skin beyond this interval normally results in vigorous escape attempts by the animal and signs of discomfort. In the absence of a response in 10 seconds, the test was terminated and that latency assigned.

In the rat, all intrathecal drugs were delivered in a volume of 10 μl followed by 10 μl of saline to flush the catheter. In the cat, drugs were injected in a volume of 250 μl with 100 μl to flush the catheter. Naloxone, administered systemically, was given intraperitoneally in a volume of 0.1 ml/100 gm.

ANIMAL RESPONSES TO ALFENTANIL, FENTANYL, AND NALOXONE

The intrathecal injection of alfentanil resulted in a rapid elevation of the latency of the spinally mediated tail flick and the coordinated escape response (hot plate) generated by the high-intensity thermal stimuli in the rat. As shown in Figure 29.1, 30 μg of alfentanil produced a maximum measurable response in both tests at the shortest time interval examined (three minutes). By 30 minutes, the measured response was not statistically different from preinjection levels. Intrathecal fentanyl, 10 μg, a dose that produced a near maximum increase in the tail-flick and hot-plate response latency, produced a time course in response latencies that resembled that for alfentanil. Analysis of variance indicated no statistically significant difference between the results observed after injection as a function of time (F = 1.12; p > 0.10).

The effects of both fentanyl and alfentanil in the rat on the hot plate and tail flick were both dose dependent. As shown in Figure 29.2, fentanyl was approximately three times more potent than alfentanyl on hot-plate and tail-flick (data not shown) latency.

To determine the effects of an opiate antagonist, naloxone, 1 mg per kilogram of body weight, was administered intraperitoneally. Because of the relatively short duration of action of both fentanyl and alfentanil after intrathecal administration, the antagonist was administered 10 minutes prior to the intrathecal injection of the agonists.

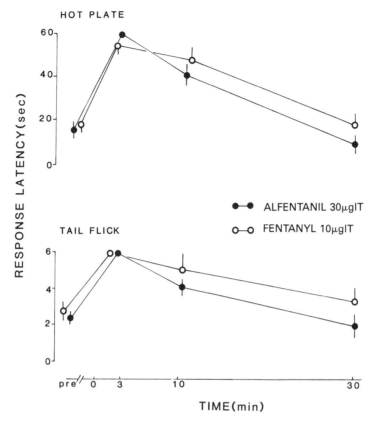

FIGURE 29.1.   Time course of escape latency on hot-plate and tail-flick tests before and after intrathecal fentanyl (10 μg) and alfentanil (30 μg). Each line represents the mean ± SE for four to six rats.

The effects of either agonist on the hot-plate and tail-flick (data not shown) response were totally antagonized.

Although systematic studies were not carried out, we observed that intrathecal alfentanil was also effective in blocking the thermally evoked skin twitch in the cat. As shown in Figure 29.3, 300 μg of intrathecal alfentanil resulted in rapid and complete antagonism of the reflex. As in the rat, the effect was observed at the shortest interval after treatment and lasted less than 60 minutes.

Intrathecal alfentanil in the doses administered had no effect on the motor function of the rat or cat as assessed by the strength or briskness of the placing, stepping, and righting reflexes.

CONCLUSIONS

Intrathecal administration of alfentanil produced a dose-dependent increase in the nociceptive threshold as gauged by thermally evoked nociceptive measurements in the rat and the cat. Based on the median effective dose (ED_{50}) values in the tail-flick test determined in the present and previous comparable studies carried out in the rat [5], the relative potency of alfentanil as compared to other representative opioid alkaloids after intrathecal injection in the rat was fentanyl > morphine > alfentanil > methadone. As shown in the rat, the pretreatment of the animal with naloxone resulted in a clear reversal of the antinociceptive effect.

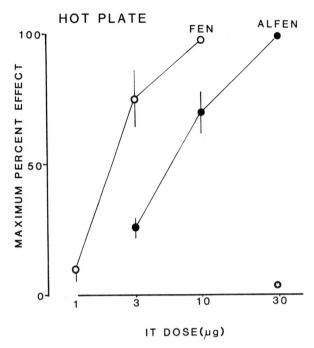

FIGURE 29.2.   Dose-response curves for intrathecal fentanyl (○———○ FEN) and alfentanil (●———● ALFEN) on the hot-plate response in the rat. (◉) represents the effect of 1 mg/kg of intraperitoneal naloxone administered 10 minutes prior to 30 μg of intrathecal alfentanil. The ordinate presents the maximum percent effect = (latency postdrug − latency predrug) ÷ (6 − latency predrug) × 100.

In the doses employed, no effect on motor function or behavior was observed. In other experiments not reported here, we systematically studied the high-dose toxicology of intrathecal alfentanil in the cat. At doses of 10 times that required to produce a maximum degree of antinociception as measured by the skin-twitch response (3000 μg), animals showed signs of agitation and excitement, presumably reflecting a supraspinal redistri-

FIGURE 29.3.   The time course of the change in latency on the thermally evoked skin twitch after intrathecal administration of 30 μg of alfentanil in the cat. Each point presents the mean and SE for five cats.

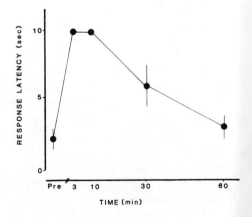

bution of the drug. All of the high-dose effects were readily antagonized by naloxone (Noueihed, Durant, and Yaksh, in preparation).

Perhaps most interesting was the time course of action of intrathecal alfentanil. Although there are insufficient points to estimate the time course with precision, comparison of the time required for the tail-flick response latency to return to within 1 standard deviation from baseline after intrathecal injection of a dose that produced a just maximal increase in the tail-flick response latency was morphine > fentanyl = alfentanil [5, present study]. It appears, therefore, that with approximately equiactive doses, alfentanil possesses a time course that is not statistically distinguishable from that observed with fentanyl.

As noted previously for opiate alkaloids, the results by which spinal drugs are cleared from the spinal space are bulk flow of the cerebrospinal fluid, clearance through root sleeves, and absorbance into the pial and parenchymal vasculature as the drug penetrates the cord. Early studies by Herz and Teschmacher [12] demonstrated a close correlation between lipophilicity (as measured by the lipid partition coefficient at physiologic pH) and (a) the rate of removal of the drug from brain and (b) the time of affect of the analgesia after intraventricular injection in animal models. This high correlation between time course of analgesia and drug lipophilicity has been demonstrated after spinal intrathecal administration in a variety of species, including primates [7].

The present results with alfentanil are therefore essentially consistent with these observations of Herz and Teschemacher. Bower and Hull [8] reported that the heptane-water coefficient of alfentanil at 37°C and pH 7.4 was 2.5, in contrast to fentanyl, which was 9.0. Thus alfentanil is only slightly less lipid soluble than fentanyl and predictably should have a similar or slightly longer duration of action—presumably because of a similar or slightly slower clearance from the spinal space. In lieu of kinetic studies this

suggestion must, however, be considered speculative. In the present studies the time course of the two agents given intrathecal was virtually identical.

These results concerning the duration of action of alfentanil appear somewhat in contrast to the data observed after systemic administration in mice where equiactive doses of alfentanil showed a significantly shorter duration of action than doses of fentanyl that produced the same magnitude of analgesic activity. Thus in the study of Williams et al [10], the time required for the analgesic effect to return to a half maximum was 8 minutes after 0.8 mg/kg of alfentanil and considerably greater than 16 minutes after 0.2 mg of fentanyl (approximately equiactive doses).

Bower and Hull [8] in their investigations of intravenous drug kinetics in human subjects, suggested that the apparent difference in duration of action of alfentanil and fentanyl could be attributed to the fact that the latter shows a greater volume of distribution and an elimination half-life that is double that of the former.

Although alfentanil may have a similar duration of action to fentanyl after intrathecal administration, it may be a promising candidate for spinal administration with continuous infusion, as it would not tend to show peripheral accumulation, as would fentanyl. These animal studies emphasize the limitation of extrapolating systemic drug response variables to the behavior of the drug given into the central nervous system spaces. Indeed, it should be noted that the question of the time course of these two drugs after epidural administration represents an additional question that is not addressed by this study. It is possible in view of the exposure of the agents to the large surface of the epidural venous plexus that different time courses, similar to those observed after systemic administration, may be observed. Clearly, the epidural, intrathecal, and parenteral routes of administration all present fundamentally different considerations in assessing the time course of a drug. Until more agents having differing pharmacokinetic properties are systematically studied by the different routes, generalizations are not warranted.

This work was supported in part by funds from the Mayo Foundation, Janssen Pharmaceutica, and grant DA02110 from the National Institutes of Health. We would like to thank Ms. Gail Harty for her assistance and Ms. Ann Rockafellow for preparing the manuscript.

REFERENCES

1. Yaksh TL, Kohl RL, Rudy TA. Induction of tolerance and withdrawal in rats receiving morphine in the spinal subarachnoid space. Eur J Pharmacol 1977;42:275–84.
2. Yaksh TL, Müller H, eds. Experimental and clinical studies of spinal opiate analgesia. Berlin: Springer-Verlag, 1982:1–147.
3. Yaksh TL, Reddy SVR. Studies on the analgetic effects of intrathecal opiates, α-adrenergic agonists and baclofen: their pharmacology in the primate. Anesthesiology 1981;54:451–67.
4. Yaksh TL, Rudy TA. Analgesia mediated by a direct spinal action of narcotics. Science 1976;192:1357–8.
5. Yaksh TL, Rudy TA. Studies on the direct spinal action of narcotics in the production of analgesia in the rat. J Pharmacol Exp Ther 1977;202:411–28.
6. Yaksh TL. Spinal opiate analgesia: characteristics and principles of action. Pain 1981;11:293–346.
7. Yaksh, TL. In vivo studies on spinal opiate receptor systems mediating antinociception. I. Mu and delta receptor profiles in the primate. J Pharmacol Exp Ther 1983;226:303–16.
8. Bower S, Hull CJ. Comparative pharmacokinetics of fentanyl and alfentanil. Br J Anaesth 1982;54:871–7.
9. Steegers PA, Booij LHDJ, Pelgrom R. Continuous infusion of alfentanil. Acta Anaesthesiol Belg 1982;33:81–7.
10. Williams JG, Brown JH, Pleuvry BJ. Alfentanil: a study of its analgesic activity and interactions with morphine in the mouse. Br J Anaesth 1981;54:81–5.
11. Yaksh TL. Analgetic actions of intrathecal opiates in cat and primate. Brain Res 1978;153:205–10.
12. Herz H, Teschemacher H. Activities and sites of antinociceptive action of morphine-like analgesics and kinetics of distribution following intravenous, intracerebral and intraventricular application. Adv Drug Res 1971;6:79–119.

V CARDIOVASCULAR EFFECTS OF OPIOID ANESTHESIA

30 CARDIOVASCULAR EFFECTS OF ALFENTANIL DURING INDUCTION AND AS A SUPPLEMENT DURING NITROUS OXIDE ANESTHESIA

Theodore H. Stanley, Wen Shin Liu, and Nathan Pace

Alfentanil (N-[1-[2-(4-ethyl-4,5-dihydro-5-oxo-1H-tetrazol-1-yl)ethyl]-4-(methoxymethyl)-4-piperidinyl]-N-phenylpropanamide monohydrochloride) is a new potent synthetic opioid, chemically and structurally related to fentanyl, which is currently undergoing clinical investigation in the United States. In the tail-withdrawal test in rats, alfentanil is approximately one-fourth to one-third as potent as fentanyl [1]. It has an onset of action three to four times as fast and a duration only one-third of fentanyl, yet its safety ratio (ratio of median lethal dose to median effective dose, LD_{50}/ED_{50}) in rats is 1080, versus 277 for fentanyl [1,2]. Hemodynamic studies in mechanically ventilated subjects suggest that cardiovascular stability is maintained after doses of alfentanil of 30 µg per kilogram of body weight in dogs and as high as 1 to 1.5 mg/kg in humans [2,3].

Alfentanil may thus provide advantages as an opioid supplement during nitrous oxide–narcotic–oxygen balanced anesthesia, be useful as an induction agent before employment of standard inhalation anesthetics, and have a place as a complete opioid anesthetic. This chapter reports our measurements of the hemodynamic effects, plasma cortisol and catecholamine responses, anesthetic requirements, and recovery times after alfentanil's use as an opioid supplement during nitrous oxide–narcotic–oxygen anesthesia and as an induction agent prior to halothane and nitrous oxide–oxygen.

THE STUDY PROTOCOL

The investigation was approved by the University of Utah Human Experimental Committee for patients in ASA physical status I or II who were scheduled to undergo orthopedic, gynecologic, or general surgical procedures of from 30 minutes to 2 hours. Informed consent was obtained and the patients were assigned to the induction or maintenance study at the time of the preoperative visit. Thirty patients served as experimental subjects in the induction study and 60 in the maintenance study. Once assigned to either study, the patients were further subdivided (random number table) into two groups within each study. Group 1 was scheduled to receive alfentanil and group 2, sodium thiopental in the induction study. Group 3 was scheduled to receive alfentanil–nitrous oxide and group 4 fentanyl–nitrous oxide in the maintenance study.

All patients were premedicated with diazepam, 0.1 mg/kg, and atropine, 0.3 to 0.6 mg, intramuscularly 90 minutes before the scheduled time of operation. Upon entrance to the operating room, an infusion of lactated Ringer's solution in 5% dextrose in water was started in an upper extremity peripheral vein, a precordial stethoscope was placed on the chest, a standard Riva Rocci blood pressure cuff applied to an arm, and a lead II electrocardiogram applied. After this, a 9.5-ml blood sample was obtained from a peripheral vein in the arm without an intravenous infusion using a 10-ml syringe filled with 0.5 ml heparin (1000 units/ml) in patients in groups 3 and 4. The 10-ml blood sample was divided into 4- and 6-ml subsamples. The 6-ml subsample (for catecholamine assay) was injected into a Vascutainer tube containing glutathione and EGTA (ethylene-glycol bis [β-aminoethyl] ether]-N,N'-tetra-acetic acid). Both samples were then placed in an ice-water bath for 10 minutes and centrifuged in a refrigerated centrifuge to separate plasma from cells. The plasma was removed with a Pasteur pipette, placed in a screw-topped vial, and frozen at $-20°C$ until analyzed. Control systolic and diastolic arterial blood pressures and heart rate were recorded five minutes after placement of all monitors.

Anesthetic induction commenced 5 to 10 minutes after control hemodynamic measurements. Patients were given 100% oxygen to breathe and two minutes later intravenous pancuronium, 1.5 mg/70 kg, to reduce muscle fasciculations from succinylcholine (and/or rigidity from alfentanil). Three minutes later patients in group 1 were given alfentanil, 150 µg/kg intravenously, over a period of 30 to 45 seconds; and patients in groups 2 and 4 received 3.5 mg/kg of sodium thiopental intravenously over a period of 15 seconds. Additional intravenous alfentanil, 2 to 4 mg, and thiopental, 50 to 100 mg, were given every 15 to 30 seconds beginning one minute after the start of anesthetic induction (in patients who were still conscious) until the patients were unresponsive to verbal command and had a negative eyelash reflex. After this, all patients were given succinylcholine, 1.5 mg/kg intravenously, and were intubated with a cuffed endotracheal tube. Two minutes after endotracheal intubation, patients in groups 1 and 2 received halothane, 0.1 to 1.5%, and nitrous oxide, 60%, in oxygen as the only other anesthetics for the remainder of the operation. Halothane concentrations were regulated to maintain systolic arterial blood pressure (measured every five minutes) within ± 15% of control values. Patients in group 3 were given alfentanil, 20 µg/kg intraveneously, and in group 4 fentanyl, 7 µg/kg intravenously, over a one-minute period two minutes after endotracheal intubation. Additional alfentanil, 0.5 to 1.0 mg, or fentanyl, 50 to 100 µg, was given intravenously to patients in groups 3 and 4 respectively whenever and as long as systolic arterial blood pressure and/or heart rate were greater than 15% above control values. Most patients were then slowly paralyzed with pancuronium, 0.5 to 1.0 mg/10 kg, initially and 1- to 2-mg increments every 45 to 60 minutes thereafter. Some patients required no additional muscle relaxant. At the end of the operations, muscle relaxation was antagonized with neostigmine, 2 to 5 mg, and atropine, 0.5 to 1.0 mg intravenously, and patients were extubated when tidal volume as estimated clinically was over 5 ml/kg and respiratory rate over 8 breaths per minute.

Arterial blood pressure and heart rate

were measured at the moment of unconsciousness (after thiopental or alfentanil) but before endotracheal intubation, two minutes after endotracheal intubation, and every five minutes thereafter for the remainder of the operation. In patients in groups 3 and 4, additional blood samples for cortisol and catecholamine analysis were obtained 15 minutes after endotracheal intubation, 30 and 60 minutes after beginning the operation, and 1 hour postoperatively. Blood samples were analyzed for plasma cortisol by radioimmunoassay (coefficient of variation = 8%; sensitivity = 0.1 μg/100 ml) [4] and for epinephrine and norepinephrine by radioenzymatic assay (coefficients of variation = 10 and 9%; sensitivity = 25 and 30 pg/ml respectively) [5,6]. No exogenous corticosteroids or catecholamines were given to patients at any time during the study period. Blood samples for plasma cortisol were collected in only the first 30 patients in groups 3 and 4, whereas catecholamine analyses were done in all 60 patients of these groups.

Upon arrival in the recovery room, patients were evaluated by a nurse, who was unaware of the anesthetic technique, for the presence or absence of an eyelash reflex and responses to simple commands (such as "open eyes") every two to three minutes. In addition, the time at which each patient was first correctly oriented to person, place, and time was noted. Recovery times were measured from the end of operation to a positive response. The presence of intraoperative awareness/lack of complete amnesia was determined at the first postoperative visit by questioning the patient with regard to the last recollection prior to anesthetic induction and first recollection following anesthetic recovery.

Statistical methods of analysis included chi square, t test, nonparametric tests, Fisher's exact test, one-way analysis of variance, analysis of covariance, Hotelling t square analysis, and multivariate analysis of variance for repeated measures with Scheffé contrasts. Statistical software was BMDP (UCLA, 1981) (P_1D, P_3D, P_7D, P_1V) and MGLM (multivariate general linear model program). A p value below 0.05 was taken to be statistically significant.

Patients in the four study groups were similar with respect to age and weight. Patients in groups 2 and 4 had slightly longer operations than those in groups 1 and 3, but there was no statistical difference in duration of anesthesia among any of the groups. Patients in group 1 received an average of 246 ± 25 μg/kg of alfentanil for induction of anesthesia, while patients in groups 2, 3, and 4 received 5.0 ± 0.3, 4.5 ± 0.2, and 4.6 ± 0.2 mg/kg of thiopental respectively (Table 30.1). There were no statistical differences in the thiopental induction requirements in groups 2, 3, and 4.

TABLE 30.1. Anesthetic requirements (mean ± SEM)

Requirement	Group 1: Alfentanil	Group 2: Thiopental	Group 3: Thiopental	Group 4: Thiopental
Dose of induction agent (mg/kg)	0.246 ± 0.025	5.0 ± 0.3	4.5 ± 0.2	4.6 ± 0.2
Halothane conc. for first 40 min (%)	0.79 ± 0.08*	1.37 ± 0.07	. . .	. . .
Alfentanil dose for entire operation (μg/kg)	246 ± 25	. . .	173 ± 16	. . .
Fentanyl dose for entire operation (μg/kg)	. . .	. . .	. . .	11.9 ± 0.6

*$t = 4.45$; df = 28; $p < 0.001$ when compared to group 2, multivariant analysis of variance.

EFFECTS OF ALFENTANIL USED FOR INDUCTION OR AS A SUPPLEMENT

Time to loss of eyelid reflex was one minute or less in all patients in groups 2, 3, and 4, but occurred in less than one minute in only 5 of 16 in group 1. Most of the patients having anesthesia induced with alfentanil lost their eyelid reflexes within two minutes (11 of 16), but two did not lose this reflex until six minutes and then only after additional alfentanil. Rate of anesthetic induction was significantly slower in group 1 than groups 2, 3, and 4 (Kruskal Wallis chi square, $p < 0.001$).

Patients in group 1 required significantly ($p < 0.001$) lower halothane concentrations than those in group 2 for the first 40 minutes of their operative procedures (Table 30.1). After anesthetic induction with sodium thiopental, patients in group 3 required 173 ± 5 μg/kg of alfentanil and those in group 4 11.9 ± 0.6 μg/kg of fentanyl for the remainder of the operation.

Anesthetic induction was associated with significant changes in hemodynamics in all groups except group 1 (Table 30.2). Control blood pressures and heart rates were similar in the four groups (Table 30.2). After administration of the anesthetic agent, heart

rate was significantly higher in groups 2, 3, and 4 than group 1. Two minutes after endotracheal intubation, systolic and diastolic blood pressures and heart rates were significantly higher in groups 2, 3, and 4 than group 1. Blood pressures and heart rates were similar to control values throughout the remainder of anesthesia and operation in all four groups.

Plasma norepinephrine was significantly decreased 15 minutes after anesthetic induction in groups 3 and 4 and remained decreased throughout the operation. Plasma epinephrine was slightly decreased in both groups 15 minutes after anesthetic induction and slightly increased throughout the operation. Epinephrine and norepinephrine became markedly elevated 1 hour after operation in both groups when compared to preoperative and intraoperative values. Plasma cortisol was not significantly changed in either group throughout the study period.

Recovery of eyelash reflex and response to commands were similar and shortest in groups 3 and 4 and longest in group 2 (Table 30.3). Recovery of eyelash reflex and response to command was intermediate in group 1. There was no significant difference in time to orientation among the four groups. These relationships remained true even when

TABLE 30.2. Arterial blood pressures and heart rates during anesthetic induction (mean ± SEM)

Determination	Group	Induction Agent	Control	After Induction Agent	2 min after Intubation
Systolic BP (torr)	1	Alfentanil	123 ± 5	126 ± 7	123 ± 6*
	2	Thiopental	127 ± 4	122 ± 5	144 ± 5
	3	Thiopental	113 ± 3	119 ± 3	140 ± 5
	4	Thiopental	117 ± 3	114 ± 4	140 ± 6
Diastolic BP (torr)	1	Alfentanil	77 ± 3	73 ± 4	67 ± 3†
	2	Thiopental	69 ± 2	69 ± 5	85 ± 5
	3	Thiopental	72 ± 2	76 ± 4	93 ± 3
	4	Thiopental	74 ± 2	77 ± 3	91 ± 3
Heart rate (beats/min)	1	Alfentanil	82 ± 4	86 ± 5*	81 ± 6†
	2	Thiopental	74 ± 4	92 ± 4	110 ± 4
	3	Thiopental	? 108 ± 25	101 ± 2	103 ± 4
	4	Thiopental	84 ± 3	93 ± 3	106 ± 3

*$p < 0.02$, †$p < 0.0001$, group 1 vs groups 2, 3, 4, Hotelling t square.

TABLE 30.3. Recovery times (min, mean ± SEM)

Group	Eyelash Reflex*	Response to Commands**	Oriented
1	12.0 ± 2.6	12.1 ± 5.4	29.8 ± 2.8
2	20.6 ± 2.7†	22.7 ± 5.8†	36.4 ± 3.0†
3	6.6 ± 1.6	7.3 ± 4.0	30.7 ± 7.9
4	4.7 ± 1.6	9.7 ± 4.1	21.6 ± 7.8

†Time from termination of operation to first positive response.
*2>1>3 = 4; covariate analysis $F_{(3,85)}$ = 19.8; $p < 10^{-5}$.
**2>1>3 = 4; covariate analysis $F_{(3,85)}$ = 18.6; $p < 10^{-5}$.

controlled for the duration of anesthesia by covariate analysis of variance.

DISCUSSION

The results of this study demonstrate that rapid infusion of a large dose of alfentanil results in slower induction of anesthesia than a bolus injection of sodium thiopental; however, induction with alfentanil is associated with fewer hemodynamic alterations, particularly after paralysis with succinylcholine, laryngoscopy, and endotracheal intubation. The data also indicate that induction with alfentanil diminishes halothane anesthetic requirements for at least 40 minutes when compared to induction with sodium thiopental, and results in faster postoperative recovery. Additionally, our findings indicate that recovery after nitrous oxide–fentanyl or nitrous oxide–alfentanil anesthesia is quicker than halothane–nitrous oxide anesthesia whether the induction agent is sodium thiopental or alfentanil. The data indicate, however, that recovery after alfentanil–nitrous oxide is no faster than after fentanyl–nitrous oxide in operations of 30 minutes to 2 hours when both drugs are supplemented in multiple small boluses throughout operation. Finally, our results demonstrate that both nitrous oxide–fentanyl and nitrous oxide–alfentanil anesthesia are associated with little change in plasma catecholamines or cortisol concentrations during operation but significant increases (of catecholamines) postoperatively.

Although there are now numerous reports that document that an induction dose of alfentanil produces little or no change in arterial blood pressures, heart rate, cardiac output, and right and left ventricular filling pressures before or after paralysis, laryngoscopy, and endotracheal intubation [7–11], a few investigators have found significant hypotension and increases in ventricular filling pressures prior to laryngoscopy, and others have noted significant increases in heart rate and blood pressures at or immediately after laryngoscopy or endotracheal intubation [12–14]. On the basis of these data, some investigators have suggested that alfentanil is unreliable in providing rapid, hemodynamically event-free anesthetic induction. These differences in findings during and immediately after the induction period with alfentanil are reminiscent of some of the early reports following the introduction of fentanyl as an anesthetic in 1978, and indicate that, as with fentanyl, subtle changes in technique (premedication, rate of infusion or dose of alfentanil, pretreating muscle relaxant, paralyzing muscle relaxant) and perhaps patient selection may significantly influence hemodynamic results [15–19].

A study was conducted [12] in which alfentanil (100, 150, 200, or 250 µg/kg injected in 10 seconds) was evaluated as an anesthetic induction agent in unpremedicated ASA class I patients pretreated with d-tubocurarine, 3 mg, and paralyzed with succinylcholine for endotracheal intubation. McDonnell and coworkers [12] saw no evidence of cardiovascular depression (no hypotension or brady-cardia) after alfentanil before or after en-dotracheal intubation. Insignificant changes in arterial blood pressure and heart rate after induction with alfentanil have also been noted in ASA class I and II patients by Steen et al (unpublished data, 1983) using 100 to 150 μg/kg of alfentanil, and by Gooding (un-published data, 1983) using 125 to 175 μg/kg of alfentanil. Nauta and colleagues [7] found that patients with ASA class I or II physical status who were premedicated with atropine and pretreated with 1.5 mg of pancuronium (to minimize chest wall rigidity) developed small increases in heart rate and arterial blood pressure (from pancuronium) prior to anesthetic induction, but experienced no fur-ther hemodynamic changes after infusion of 119 μg/kg of alfentanil (over a little more than two minutes), after paralysis with suc-cinylcholine or after endotracheal intuba-tion. Using a somewhat faster alfentanil infusion (120 μg/kg/min) but otherwise sim-ilar induction technique in similar patients premedicated with secobarbital and atro-pine, Nauta et al [8] documented no signif-icant hemodynamic changes at any time throughout induction or after endotracheal intubation. These authors also found that when alfentanil was infused at 50 μg/kg/min in ASA class III and IV patients premedi-cated with lorazepam and atropine, small but significant decreases in systolic arterial blood pressure occurred in spite of lower total re-quirements of alfentanil (30 to 60 μg/kg) for unconsciousness [8]. Recently Moldenhauer and co-workers [14] noted significant hypo-tension and evidence of myocardial depres-sion (elevated ventricular filling pressures) after induction with alfentanil, 150 μg/kg in-jected over one or three minutes, in patients in ASA class II through IV premedicated with glycopyrrolate and diazepam, pre-treated with curare, and paralyzed with suc-cinylcholine. They concluded that alfentanil may not be a desirable anesthetic induction agent when combined with succinylcholine because of unpredictable, dramatic falls in arterial blood pressure. In view of the other studies cited above, the hypotension and myocardial depression observed by Molden-hauer and colleagues [14] may also be ex-plained by an interaction between alfentanil and lorazepam—also well described for fen-tanyl [15] and morphine [20] with diaze-pam—or by cardiovascular effects of alfentanil differing in patients whose phys-ical status is ASA class III and IV from that in I and II, an overdose of alfentanil, too rapid an infusion of alfentanil in patients with little cardiovascular reserve, or numerous other factors.

Hypertension and tachycardia after en-dotracheal intubation following anesthetic induction with alfentanil was not seen in this study (but was seen after induction with so-dium thiopental) and was not reported by Nauta and co-workers [7,8], de Lange et al [9–11], or Moldenhauer and colleagues [14]. Steen et al (unpublished data, 1983) saw small increases in systolic arterial blood pres-sure and Gooding (unpublished data, 1983) noted small increases in heart rate after en-dotracheal intubation after induction with al-fentanil. McDonnell et al [12] observed similar increases in arterial blood pressure and heart rate, which were unrelated to the dose of alfentanil. While we believe that nu-merous factors relating to technique and pa-tient selection may influence hemodynamics after as well as before endotracheal intuba-tion following anesthetic induction with al-fentanil, there are still insufficient data to document whether these impressions are valid in humans at the present time. In basal anesthetized, mechanically ventilated dogs, alfentanil in high doses (160 μg/kg) can re-sult in significant decreases in blood pres-sure, heart rate, and cardiac output and increases in left ventricular end-diastolic pressure [2].

In this study, arterial blood pressures and heart rate were easily maintained at or near preanesthetic values in groups 3 and 4 during operation using increments of alfentanil or fentanyl. Similar (unpublished) findings have been reported by Giesecke et al, Steen and co-workers, and Gooding. Indeed, the latter two groups of investigators suggest that alfentanil–nitrous oxide results in more stable cardiovascular dynamics than in similar patients anesthetized with concentrations of enflurane–nitrous oxide that produce approximately equal minimum alveolar concentrations.

In this study of ASA class I and II patients premedicated with diazepam and atropine, we found that 150 μg/kg of alfentanil was not always reliable in ensuring unconsciousness. Indeed, our mean requirement for anesthesia with alfentanil was 246 μg/kg. These data support the findings of McDonnell et al [12] who suggested that for alfentanil, the effective dose that causes loss of eyelid reflex in 90% of unpremedicated patients in ASA class I is probably above 250 μg/kg. Both McDonnell's and our results contrast sharply with those of Nauta et al [7]. The latter group found that ASA class I and II patients require only 119 μg/kg of alfentanil for loss of eyelid reflex when induced with an infusion rate of 50 μg/kg/hr. Using a similar alfentanil infusion rate in class III and IV patients premedicated with lorazepam, Nauta et al found that only 30 to 60 μg/kg of alfentanil was required for complete anesthesia and hemodynamically uneventful anesthetic induction. These data strongly suggest that premedication and patient selection, and perhaps other factors, have a marked effect on opioid anesthetic induction requirements and/or determination of the proper opioid induction dose. In view of these findings, we believe the use of fixed or "magic" doses for induction of anesthesia is illogical at the present time and is potentially dangerous.

Patients receiving halothane after induction with alfentanil (group 1) required significantly less halothane than those receiving sodium thiopental (group 2) and recovered more rapidly after operation. Similar findings have been reported by Steen et al in which enflurane–nitrous oxide was used after induction with alfentanil or thiopental. In the latter study the mean difference in average enflurane concentration was 0.8%.

Postoperative recovery of patients in groups 1 and 2 was slower than that of patients in groups 3 and 4 in this study. Gooding has data indicating that patients who receive enflurane–nitrous oxide after a rapid-sequence sodium thiopental induction recover more slowly than similar patients whose anesthesia is induced with alfentanil and maintained with alfentanil–nitrous oxide. These findings suggest that patients receiving higher concentrations of a potent inhalation agent recover more slowly from anesthesia than those receiving lower concentrations, even though the depth of anesthesia may be similar. The above results indicate there are potentially important practical advantages for supplementing potent induction anesthetics with short-acting opioids as has become popular in recent years. Our and Gooding's findings also indicate that recovery from nitrous oxide–opioid anesthesia with fentanyl and alfentanil is more rapid than from halothane–nitrous oxide or enflurane–nitrous oxide, irrespective of induction agent. The reason for this is undoubtedly due to the poor solubility of nitrous oxide in blood and its rapid excretion after termination of anesthesia. Whether recovery from isoflurane–nitrous oxide is also slower than from fentanyl–nitrous oxide or alfentanil–nitrous oxide is, at least to our knowledge, unknown. Furthermore, whether a 5- to 15-minute faster recovery is of any clinical importance in cost or overall patient outcome is also unknown.

That fentanyl–nitrous oxide and alfentanil–nitrous oxide did not block increases in circulating catecholamines postoperatively was not unexpected, as much larger doses of both opioids have not been capable of blocking postoperative increases in plasma concentrations of both hormones, even when administered to patients just before the end of an operation [11,19,21,22]. That both anesthetic techniques were capable of blocking increases in plasma norepinephrine and cortisol and resulted in relatively small increases in plasma epinephrine during operation was not expected because of the relatively low doses of both opioids employed in this study.

These findings suggest that the surgical procedures may not have been particularly stressful, that maintenance of unchanged hemodynamics during operation by frequent administration of alfentanil and fentanyl as described by our protocol was effective in blocking whatever mechanism it is that produces increases in plasma stress hormones, or that other unknown factors were important in maintaining both stable hemodynamics and little change in plasma concentrations of the stress hormones during this investigation. The relationship between changes in hemodynamics and plasma concentrations of epinephrine and norepinephrine has not been carefully studied. Furthermore, the value, if any, of maintaining unchanged plasma stress hormones during operation, especially when these hormones become elevated postoperatively, has not been documented.

REFERENCES

1. Niemegeers CJE, Janssen PAJ. Alfentanil (R 39209)–a particularly short-acting intravenous narcotic analgesic in rats. Drug Dev Res 1981;1:83–8.
2. de Castro J, van de Water A, Wouters L, et al. A comparative study of eight narcotics in dogs. Acta Anaesthesiol Belg 1979;30:5–99.
3. de Lange S, Stanley TH, Boscoe MJ. Alfentanil-oxygen anaesthesia for coronary artery surgery. Br J Anaesth 1981;53:1291–6.
4. Ruder HJ, Guy RW, Lipsett MB. A radioimmunoassay for cortisol in plasma and urine. J Clin Endocrinol Metab 1972;35:219–24.
5. Passon TG, Peuler JD. A simplified radiometric assay for plasma norepinephrine and epinephrine. Anal Biochem 1973;51:618–31.
6. Robertson D, Frolich JC, Can K, et al. Effects of caffeine on plasma renin activity, catecholamines and blood pressure. N Engl J Med 1978;298:181–6.
7. Nauta J, de Lange S, Koopman D, et al. Anesthetic induction with alfentanil (R 39209): a new short-acting narcotic analgesic. Anesth Analg (Cleve) 1982;61:267–72.
8. Nauta J, Stanley TH, de Lange S, et al. Anaesthetic induction with alfentanil: comparison with thiopental, midazolam, and etomidate. Can Anaesth Soc J 1983;30:53–60.
9. de Lange S, de Bruijn N, Stanley TH, et al. Alfentanil-oxygen anesthesia: comparison of continuous-infusion and frequent bolus techniques for coronary artery surgery (abstract). Anesthesiology 1981;55:A42.
10. de Lange S, Boscoe MJ, Stanley TH, et al. Antidiuretic and growth hormone responses during coronary artery surgery with sufentanil-oxygen and alfentanil-oxygen anesthesia in man. Anesth Analg (Cleve) 1982; 61:434–8.
11. de Lange S, Stanley TH, Boscoe MJ, et al. Catecholamine and cortisol responses to sufentanil-O_2 and alfentanil-O_2 anaesthesia during coronary artery surgery. Can Anaesth Soc J 1983;30:248–54.
12. McDonnell TE, Bartkowski RR, Williams JJ. ED_{50} of alfentanil for induction of anesthesia in unpremedicated young adults (abstract). Anesthesiology 1982;57:A352.
13. McLeskey CH. Alfentanil-loading dose/ continuous infusion for surgical anesthesia (abstract). Anesthesiology 1982;57:A68.
14. Moldenhauer CC, Greisemer RW, Hug CC Jr, et al. Hemodynamic changes during rapid induction of anesthesia with alfentanil. Anesth Analg (Cleve) 1983;62:245.
15. Stanley TH, Webster LR. Anesthetic requirements and cardiovascular effects of fentanyl-oxygen and fentanyl-diazepam-oxygen anesthesia in man. Anesth Analg (Cleve) 1978;57:411–16.
16. Waller JL, Hug CC, Nagle DN, et al. Hemodynamic changes during fentanyl-oxygen anesthesia for aorto-coronary bypass operations. Anesthesiology 1981;55:212–17.
17. Edde RR. Hemodynamic changes prior to and after sternotomy in patients anesthetized with high-dose fentanyl. Anesthesiology 1981;55:444–6.
18. de Lange S, Stanley TH, Boscoe M. Fentanyl-oxygen anesthesia: comparison of anesthetic requirements and cardiovascular responses in Salt Lake City, Utah and Leiden, Holland. In: Zindler M, Rugheimer E, eds. Proceedings of the Seventh World Congress of Anaesthesiology. Amsterdam: Excerpta Medica, 1980:313.
19. Stanley TH. The pharmacology if intravenous narcotic anesthetics. In: Miller RD, ed.

Anesthesia. New York: Churchill Livingstone, 1981:425–49.

20. Stanley TH, Bennett GM, Loeser EA, et
al. Cardiovascular effects of diazepam and
droperidol during morphine anesthesia.
Anesthesiology 1975;44:255–8.

21. Stanley TH, Berman L, Green O, et al.
Plasma catecholamine and cortisol re-

sponses to fentanyl-oxygen anesthesia for
coronary artery operations. Anesthesiology
1980;53:250–3.

22. Sebel PS, Bovil JG, Schellekens, et al. Hormonal effects of high-dose fentanyl anaesthesia: a study in patients undergoing cardiac surgery. Br J Anaesth 1981;53:941–7.

31 THE HEMODYNAMIC STABILITY OF SHORT-ACTING NARCOTICS

Adel Ahmed El-Etr

The popularity of large-dose, short-acting narcotics in cardiac anesthesia has been due to the remarkable cardiovascular stability seen after induction with these agents. As shown by Dr. Stanley (Chapter 30), slow induction of alfentanil is associated with lessened hemodynamic alteration, particularly after paralysis with succinylcholine, laryngoscopy, and endotracheal intubation. This stability is also seen with fentanyl induction. It is not always present, however, and in some situations hemodynamic aberrations may be seen, including significant bradycardia, hypotension, hypertension, and tachycardia. All of these adverse effects have been reported by many investigators.

Hemodynamic stability depends primarily on the induction technique whenever a large dose of short-acting narcotic is the main agent. The type of premedication also affects hemodynamic stability, as do the addition of diazepam as part of the induction technique and the rate of infusion of the drug, pretreatment with muscle relaxants, initiation of muscle paralysis, and chest wall rigidity in the absence of controlled use of muscle relaxants. Recently, convulsions [1] have been reported after very rapid injection of diazepam.

As suggested by Dr. Stanley, premedication, patient selection, and perhaps many other factors have a marked effect on anesthetic induction requirements and determination of the proper induction dose. He believes that a fixed or "magic" dose is illogical and could be potentially dangerous.

Since our main goal in using large-dose fentanyl or alfentanil is to produce hemodynamic stability, meticulous attention to induction technique can influence the end result. Changes in technique can distort the picture of hemodynamic stability and defeat the purpose of using a large-dose narcotic. The status of the patient's myocardial function is also a major consideration. In reality, hemodynamic stability is a secondary goal: our primary purpose is to prevent the development of myocardial ischemia and preserve or improve ventricular function. While hemodynamic stability is easier to measure, assess, and interpret, it does not guarantee that ischemia will not develop with or without ventricular dysfunction.

CORONARY BLOOD FLOW DURING HIGH-DOSE FENTANYL ANESTHESIA

Coronary blood flow was measured in anesthetized dogs, using radioactive microspheres, before and after the administration of fentanyl, 50 μg per kilogram of body weight [2]. No significant changes in hemodynamic variables were detected. The myocardial blood flow after 50 μg/kg of fentanyl showed progressive reduction, reaching a maximum effect at the 20-minute level. This was associated in the early studies with bradycardia, and when the dogs were given atropine there was partial reversal at 5 minutes; however, 20 minutes later, the original reduction coronary blood flow was observed. This decrease in blood flow correlated well with the decrease in myocardial oxygen demand, and there were no detectable changes in left ventricular oxygen balance.

The experience was repeated in the presence of artificially induced coronary constriction of the distal portion of the left anterior descending coronary artery. Blood flow in the areas not affected by the constriction was reduced. In the ischemic areas, there were no significant changes and coronary blood flow remained the same after fentanyl was injected. In the infarct area there was a slight increase in coronary blood flow.

In a similar unpublished study (1983) done in our institution on humans, Kleinman and Henkin used a thallium scan to evaluate coronary blood flow after the induction of anesthesia using high-dose fentanyl, 50 μg/kg. Their results show that a reduction of coronary blood flow could occur in the presence of stable hemodynamic parameters.

CONCLUSION

We are trying to achieve hemodynamic stability by meticulous attention to detail during induction. Realization of this goal provides no guarantee that there will not be changes in coronary blood flow. Whether reduction of blood flow in some of these areas of the myocardium is common or not, and whether it has any significance in relation to outcome, is not clear at the present time.

REFERENCES

1. Rao TLK, Mummaneni N, El-Etr AA. Convulsions: an unusual response to intravenous fentanyl administration. Anesth Analg (Cleve) 1982;61:1020–1.
2. Rao TLK, Jacobs HK, El-Etr AA. High-dose fentanyl and myocardial blood flow in a constricted coronary bed. Anesthesiology 1982;57:A12.

32 DOES CHOICE OF ANESTHETIC (NARCOTIC VERSUS INHALATIONAL) SIGNIFICANTLY AFFECT CARDIOVASCULAR OUTCOME AFTER CARDIOVASCULAR SURGERY?

Michael F. Roizen

The introduction, about a decade ago, of easily usable techniques for measuring cardiovascular variables [1] coincided with the rediscovery of narcotic anesthesia [2,3] and increased the popularity of performing major vascular and cardiac procedures in very ill patients. These developments led naturally to the question, Does the choice of anesthetic technique (e.g., inhalational versus narcotic) make a critical difference to outcome in those patients most susceptible to adverse perioperative events? [4–8]. Anesthetics, whether narcotic or inhalational, affect the circulation in two ways: (a) directly, as demonstrated in studies on volunteers not undergoing surgery and (b) by modifying the cardiovascular effects of surgery [9]. In turn,

both actions can be influenced by administration of adjuvant drugs and by the age, cardiovascular reserve, and disease state of the patient (e.g., chronic heart failure is accompanied by sympathetic stimulation that is depressed by anesthetic agents). Although many reports have discussed the cardiovascular effects of anesthetic agents [2–29, for example] and five studies compared outcome after narcotic versus inhalational anesthesia in humans [4–8], controversy still exists as to whether choice of anesthetic agent makes a critical difference to outcome. To answer this question, I reexamined studies in the literature and analyzed them statistically.

The studies considered in this review met

the following criteria: they were originally studies published after 1964, in English, that reported values for resting, supine subjects; they randomly allocated patients to receive a primarily inhalational or narcotic technique; and they compared the results of these techniques in patients undergoing cardiovascular surgery.

Data from four studies [4–7] met these criteria and were combined with data from another study that did not randomly allocate patients [8]. This allowed a statistical approach in which the mean values of each cardiovascular variable from each study provided single data points. Although many other studies met all criteria, only these studies examined cardiovascular effects of one type of anesthetic agent and did not compare that type with another. When data were provided in figures only, they were interpolated to derive mean values and standard deviations. Data were analyzed using analysis of variance with repeated measures, followed by the Student-Newman-Keuls test [30]. Although studies probably varied in reliability, for statistical comparison they were accorded equal weight.

CARDIOVASCULAR EFFECTS OF INHALATIONAL AGENTS

Halothane was the only volatile agent used in the comparative studies [4–8]. Induction of anesthesia with inhalational agents clearly decreased mean arterial blood pressure and cardiac index (Table 32.1). (Isoflurane was not used in the comparative studies and may not affect cardiac index [10,13].) In patients anesthetized with halothane, surgical stimulation increased heart rate and systemic vascular resistance by numerically small but significant amounts, and decreased cardiac index. Noncomparative studies examining the cardiovascular effects of inhalational agents with or without surgery have confirmed these results [10–15].

CARDIOVASCULAR EFFECTS OF NARCOTIC AGENTS

Morphine sulfate was the narcotic used in four of the five comparative studies [4–7]; fentanyl was the anesthetic used in the fifth study [8]. Induction of anesthesia with narcotic agents decreased cardiac index by a numerically small but significant amount (Table 32.2). Surgical stimulation significantly increased heart rate, mean arterial blood pressure, and systemic vascular resistance in such patients. The noncomparative studies involving narcotic anesthesia appear to confirm these results, although data for fentanyl varied more among studies than did data on morphine (16–26).

CARDIOVASCULAR OUTCOMES FOR PATIENTS ANESTHETIZED WITH INHALATIONAL AGENTS VERSUS NARCOTICS

Studying patients undergoing open heart surgery, Conahan et al [4] found that 13.1% of patients anesthetized with halothane died, while 15.1% of those anesthetized with morphine died ($p > 0.05$). Kistner et al [5] reported that changes in the ST segment indicative of ischemia occurred significantly less frequently in patients anesthetized with halothane than in those anesthetized with morphine. In a study by Wilkinson et al [6], 10 of 14 patients (71.4%) given halothane had evidence of myocardial ischemia before bypass, compared with 8 of 12 patients (66.7%) given morphine ($p > 0.05$). In a study by Moffitt et al [7], 1 of 12 patients anesthetized with halothane as the primary agent produced lactate with sternotomy, compared with 2 of 6 patients anesthetized with morphine ($p > 0.5$). Thus in the four randomized studies that examined outcome variables, only one showed a significant difference between narcotic and inhalational anesthetics.

TABLE 32.1. Cardiovascular effects of volatile agents with or without surgery in comparative studies

Reference	Agent	Dose	Adjuvant Drugs (agent/dose)	Heart Rate (beats/min)			MABP (mm Hg)			Cardiac Index (L/min/m²)			Systemic Vascular Resistance			Comments
				Pre-drug	Post-drug	Post-stim.	Pre-drug	Post-drug	Post-stim.	Pre-drug	Post-drug	Post-stim.	Pre-drug	Post-drug	Post-stim.	
Conahan et al [4]	HALO	<1.0%	50–75% N_2O, MS 1 mg/10 kg, 0.04 to 0.08/10 kg, d-tubocurarine, scopolamine	?85	68	97	120	91.6	128[a]						2210 ± 402	[a]Lower BP than MS group; outcome = 13.1% mortality; poststim. = highest postinduction to bypass
Kistner et al [5]	HALO	Mean 0.75% insp.	MS 0.1 mg/kg, scopolamine 0.4 mg, 50% N_2O, pancuronium	62	78	75	99	91	93[b]	2.9	2.6	2.4	1347	1431	1516	[b]Lower BP than MS group; stim. was sternotomy; Σ ST segments different poststim. (less in HALO group)
Wilkinson et al [6]	HALO	0.2 to 1% end-tidal	MS 0.15 mg/kg, scopolamine 0.4 mg, succinylcholine, pancuronium, 50% N_2O	63	65	66	102	74[c]	82[c]	2.8	2.5	2.2	1500	1250	1620	[c]Lower BP than MS group; 10/14 had myocardial ischemia prebypass by ST segment change or lactate production

Study		Drugs												Notes
Moffitt et al [7]	HALO <3%	Secobarbital 3 mg/kg, thiopental, MS 0.25 mg/kg, pancuronium (2 HALO groups combined—1 had MS IV, the other MS IM as premed.)	69	71	77	77	64	79[d]	2.9	2.5	2.6	1071	995	1181	[d]Lower BP than MS group; stim. was sternotomy; 1/12 had lactate production with sternotomy
Zurick et al [8]	HALO 0–5%	Thiopental, 50% N_2O, pancuronium	67	80	69	89	84[e]	83[e]	2.4	2.4	1.9	1491	1341	1623	[e]Lower BP than fentanyl patients not randomly allocated to fentanyl vs. halothane group; stim. was sternotomy; 7/12 patients received nitroglycerine after intubation

Mean	69.2	72.4	76.8*	97.4	80.9*	93.0
SD	9.2	6.4	12.1	15.9	11.8	20.2
SE	4.2	2.9	5.4	7.1	5.3	9.1

2.75	2.5*	2.77**	1352	1254	1485*s
0.24	0.08	0.29	200	187	208
0.11	0.04	0.15	100	94	104

*Significantly different from control ($p \leq 0.05$).

sSignificantly different from post-drug ($p \leq 0.05$).

MABP = mean arterial blood pressure; HALO = halothane; MS = morphine sulfate.

? = data not clear.

TABLE 32.2. Cardiovascular effects of narcotic agents with or without surgery in comparative studies

Reference	Agent	Dose	Adjuvant Drugs (agent/dose)	Heart Rate (beats/min)			MABP (mm Hg)			Cardiac Index (L/min/m²)			Systemic Vascular Resistance			Comments
				Pre-drug	Post-drug	Post-stim.	Pre-drug	Post-drug	Post-stim.	Pre-drug	Post-drug	Post-stim.	Pre-drug	Post-drug	Post-stim.	
Conahan et al [4]	MS	<2 mg/kg	50–75% N₂O, MS 1 mg/10 kg, scopolamine 0.04 to 0.08/10 kg, d-tubocurarine	?85	68	99	120	100[a]	152[a]				2832 ± 282			[a]Higher BP than HALO; Outcome = 15.1% mortality; poststim. = highest postinduction to bypass
Kistner et al [5]	MS	Mean 2.1 mg/kg	MS 0.1 mg/kg, scopolamine 0.4 mg, 50% N₂O, diazepam 5 mg, pancuronium 0.08 mg/kg	62	62	83	89	89	99[b]	2.8	2.7	2.4	1258	1300	1724	[b]Higher BP than HALO; stim. was sternotomy; Σ ST segments different poststim. (MS group had greater depression)
Wilkinson et al [6]	MS	2 mg/kg	MS 0.15 mg/kg, scopolamine 0.4 mg, diazepam, pancuronium, 50% N₂O	62	61	71	98	84[c]	116[c]	3.0	2.8	2.85	1300	1150	2150	[c]Higher BP than HALO; stim. was sternotomy; 8/12 had myocardial ischemia by ST segment change or lactate production

Reference	Drug	Dose	Other agents												Comments
Moffitt et al [7]	MS	1 mg/kg	Secobarbital 3 mg/kg, diazepam, pancuronium	64	70	81	86	62	96[d]	2.6	2.3	3.0	1386	1083	1390	[d] Higher BP than HALO; stim. was sternotomy; 2/6 had lactate production with sternotomy
Zurick et al [8]	Fentanyl	150 mg/kg	Pancuronium, succinylcholine	66	83	80	98	100[e]	97[e]	2.9	2.7	2.3	1387	1525	1725	[e] Higher BP than HALO; patients not randomly allocated to fentanyl vs. halothane groups; stim. was sternotomy; 2/10 patients were aware
Mean				68	69	82.8*s	98.2	87	112s	2.8	2.6	2.6	1333	1265	1747*s	
SD				9.8	8.8	10.1	13.3	15.6	23.8	0.17	0.22	0.34	64	196	311	
SE				4.4	3.9	4.5	6.0	7.0	10.6	0.09	0.11	0.17	32	98	156	

*Significant difference from control ($p \leq 0.05$).
sSignificant difference from post-drug ($p \leq 0.05$).
MABP = mean arterial blood pressure; HALO = halothane; MS = morphine sulfate.
? = data not clear.

IMPORTANCE OF CHOICE
OF ANESTHETIC FOR
CARDIOVASCULAR SURGERY

For some diseases, one anesthetic may have theoretical value over another. For instance, in severe aortic stenosis, afterload may be maintained more easily with fentanyl. In severe aortic insufficiency, afterload may be reduced more easily with isoflurane. Moreover, the data from nonrandomized, noncomparative studies show that anesthetic agents produce different cardiovascular effects [10–27]. Thus one might expect the choice of agent to make a difference; however, no consistent differences in cardiovascular outcome due to choice of agent have been found in the randomized comparative studies. As emphasized by Glantz [31], simply showing that one technique changed a patient's physiologic state (by producing a different blood pressure) does not mean that the technique significantly affected clinical outcome.

Focusing on these intermediate variables (process variables) rather than on more important outcome variables may lead one to believe that the choice of an anesthetic makes a clinical difference when it does not. Only if one agent is less hazardous to patients than another can it be called "better." The general impression that volatile agents produce greater decreases in blood pressure and cardiac index after induction than do narcotic agents is substantiated in the literature [3–8, 10–27]. The literature also supports the belief that narcotic analgesics, in sufficient doses, produce analgesia and hypnosis with only slight decreases in cardiac contractility and blood pressure [3,16–26]. There is also support for the belief that hemodynamic changes after strong surgical stimulation are minor with inhalational agents and only slightly greater with narcotic agents [4–9]. Frequency of arrhythmias differed only slightly between narcotics and inhalational anesthetics in our preliminary studies, even when tumors that secrete catecholamines were present [32]. This raises the question,

Why don't effects on cardiovascular outcome differ for these two types of anesthetics? Perhaps similarities occur because both types are usually combined with nitrous oxide. Nitrous oxide has cardiovascular effects of its own [3,27–29] and can modify the effects of other agents significantly. Certainly, the narcotics and inhalation agents by themselves produce different cardiovascular effects, both in vitro and in vivo.

Morphine depresses contractility of the isolated heart only in concentrations of 1×10^{-3} moles or greater. This decrease in contractility may occur after an intravenous dose of 2 mg per kilogram of body weight in children [33] or perhaps 0.5 to 1 mg/kg in very aged patients, but rarely in most patients [34]. Halothane, enflurane, and isoflurane all depress cardiac contractility in isolated heart muscle [35–37] and even more so in muscle from failing hearts [37]. Morphine slows heart rate, presumably by sympatholytic and parasympathomimetic effects (the latter by activating the vagal nerves) [9,38–40]. Morphine also reduces arteriolar resistance and increases venous capacitance in experimental animals [38,41,42], partly by releasing histamine [43] and partly by acting directly on vascular smooth muscle [44].

In humans, however, the cardiovascular effects are similar for both inhalational and narcotic techniques: small decreases in blood pressure and systemic vascular resistance with slight but usually clinically insignificant changes in heart rate and cardiac index [4–8]. With both techniques, occasionally severe decreases in blood pressure occur. When such decreases were noted after induction with narcotics, they were attributed to vagal slowing of the heart rate (in the case of fentanyl or morphine), to venous pooling of a hypovolemic blood volume [45,46], or to unknown causes. When such decreases occurred during induction with inhalational agents, they were attributed to dysrhythmias or depressed contractility [10].

The myocardial ischemia that occurs in patients given halothane is often attributed to low coronary artery filling pressure. In the comparative studies, these periods were not significantly related to onset of ischemia [4–8]. In patients anesthetized with narcotic agents, the onset of ischemia was associated with increases in rate-pressure product [4–8]. The clinical impression is that anesthesia with a narcotic and an inhalational agent provides better hemodynamic stability than does anesthesia with either type of agent alone. Our preliminary data bear this out and indicate a synergism between fentanyl and isoflurane in blocking the cardiovascular responses to surgery (Alpert R, Roizen MF, unpublished data, 1984).

It is perhaps because the clinician understands these effects so well that morbidity does not differ among anesthetic agents. Even in pharmacologic studies using animal models of ischemia, however, differences among agents have not been found. Merin et al [11] concluded, "If a high cardiac oxygen demand can be decreased without markedly interfering with oxygen supply (especially by decreasing heart rate), then the result has universally been improvement [by any anesthetic given] in the electrical, functional, and for metabolic indices of ischemia."

Perhaps the reason outcome measurements have not been found to differ between narcotic and inhalational anesthetics is that the studies done to date have not been sufficiently large to reveal such differences [4–8]. If morbid complications were predicted to be 20% for one anesthetic and 50% less for another, then, as determined by power analysis [47], the studies would have had to compare approximately 237 patients to have a confidence level of 0.05% and an 80% chance of finding such a difference. If a lower rate of complications (e.g., 15%) and a smaller difference in the rates of complications (e.g., 33%) were assumed, more patients would have to be studied to be 80% certain that no difference occurred, even at the 0.05 level. That is, approximately 764 patients would have to be compared. Obviously, low morbidity and the large number of patients who need to be studied make evaluations of outcome difficult to perform. Would any additional investigations other than outcome studies produce worthwhile results after the first one or two descriptive studies of basic cardiovascular effects had been performed?

CONCLUSION

I conclude, as did Conahan and his colleagues in 1973 [4], that no data justify the belief that any narcotic or inhalational agent is superior in its effect on outcome when used for cardiac or vascular anesthesia. The data indicate that skill and care in administration remain more critical to cardiovascular outcome than choice of anesthetic agent.

REFERENCES

1. Swan HJC, Ganz W, Forrester JS, Marcus H, Diamond G, Chonette D. Catheterization of the heart in man with use of a flow-directed balloon-tipped catheter. N Engl J Med 1970;283:447–57.
2. Bailey P, Gerbode F, Garlington L. An anesthetic technique for cardiac surgery which utilizes 100% oxygen as the only inhalant. Arch Surg 1958;76:437–40.
3. Lowenstein E, Hallowell P, Levine FH, Daggett WM, Austen WG, Laver MB. Cardiovascular response to large doses of intravenous morphine in man. N Engl J Med 1969;281:1389–93.
4. Conahan TJ, Ominsky AJ, Wollman H, Stroth RA. A prospective random comparison of halothane and morphine for open-heart anesthesia: one year's experience. Anesthesiology 1973;38:528–35.
5. Kistner JR, Miller ED, Lake CL, Ross WT. Indices of myocardial oxygenation during coronary-artery revascularization in man with morphine versus halothane anesthesia. Anesthesiology 1979;50:324–30.
6. Wilkinson PL, Hamilton WK, Moyers JR, et al. Halothane and morphine-nitrous oxide anesthesia in patients undergoing coronary artery bypass operation. Patterns of intraoperative ischemia. J Thorac Cardiovasc Surg 1981;82:372–82.

7. Moffitt EA, Sethna DH, Bussell JA, Raymond M, Matloff JM, Gray RJ. Myocardial metabolism and hemodynamic responses to halothane or morphine anesthesia for coronary artery surgery. Anesth Analg (Cleve) 1982;61:979–85.

8. Zurick AM, Urzua J, Yared J-P, Estafanous FG. Comparison of hemodynamic and hormonal effects of large single-dose fentanyl anesthesia and halothane/nitrous oxide anesthesia for coronary artery surgery. Anesth Analg (Cleve) 1982;61:521–6.

9. Roizen MF, Horrigan RW, Frazer BM. Anesthetic doses blocking adrenergic (stress) and cardiovascular responses to incision—MAC BAR. Anesthesiology 1981;54:390–8.

10. Cullen DJ, Eger EI II, Stevens WC, et al. Clinical signs of anesthesia. Anesthesiology 1972;36:21–36.

11. Merin RG, Verdouw PD, de Jong JW. Myocardial functional and metabolic responses to ischemia in swine during halothane and fentanyl anesthesia. Anesthesiology 1982;56:84–92.

12. Calverley RK, Smith NT, Prys-Roberts C, Eger EI II, Jones CW. Cardiovascular effects of enflurane anesthesia during controlled ventilation in man. Anesth Analg (Cleve) 1978;57:619–28.

13. Dolan WM, Stevens WC, Eger EI II, et al. The cardiovascular and respiratory effects of isoflurane-nitrous oxide anaesthesia. Can Anaesth Soc J 1974;21:557–68.

14. France CJ, Plumer MH, Eger EI II, Wahrenbrock EA. Ventilatory effects of isoflurane (Forane) or halothane when combined with morphine, nitrous oxide and surgery. Br J Anaesth 1974;46:117–20.

15. Eger EI II, Dolan WM, Stevens WC, Miller RD, Way WL. Surgical stimulation antagonizes the respiratory depression produced by Forane. Anesthesiology 1972;36:544–9.

16. Bailey DR, Miller ED Jr, Kaplan JA, Rogers PW. The renin-angiotensin-aldosterone system during cardiac surgery with morphine-nitrous oxide anesthesia. Anesthesiology 1975;42:538–44.

17. Rouby JJ, Eurin B, Glaser P, et al. Hemodynamic and metabolic effects of morphine in the critically ill. Circulation 1981;64:53–9.

18. Lappas DG, Buckley MJ, Laver MB, Daggett WM, Lowenstein E. Left ventricular performance and pulmonary circulation following addition of nitrous oxide to morphine during coronary-artery surgery. Anesthesiology 1975;43:61–9.

19. Wong KC, Martin WE, Hornbein TF, Freund FG, Everett J. The cardiovascular effects of morphine sulfate with oxygen and with nitrous oxide in man. Anesthesiology 1973;38:542–9.

20. Sonntag H, Larsen R, Hilfiker O, Kettler D, Brockschnieder B. Myocardial blood flow and oxygen consumption during high-dose fentanyl anesthesia in patients with coronary artery disease. Anesthesiology 1982;56:417–22.

21. Sprigge JS, Wynands JE, Whalley DG, et al. Fentanyl infusion anesthesia for aortocoronary bypass surgery: plasma levels and hemodynamic response. Anesth Analg (Cleve) 1982;61:972–8.

22. Waller JL, Hug CC Jr, Nagle DM, Craver JM. Hemodynamic changes during fentanyl-oxygen anesthesia for aortocoronary bypass operation. Anesthesiology 1981;55:212–17.

23. Lunn JK, Stanley TH, Eisele JH, Webster L, Woodward A. High-dose fentanyl anesthesia for coronary artery surgery: plasma fentanyl concentrations and influence of nitrous oxide on cardiovascular responses. Anesth Analg (Cleve) 1979;58:390–5.

24. de Lange S, Boscoe MJ, Stanley TH, de Bruijin N, Philbin DM, Coggins CH. Antidiuretic and growth hormone responses during coronary artery surgery with sufentanil-oxygen and alfentanil-oxygen anesthesia in man. Anesth Analg (Cleve) 1982;61:434–8.

25. Stoelting RK, Gibbs PS, Creasser CW, Peterson C. Hemodynamic and ventilatory responses to fentanyl, fentanyl-droperidol, and nitrous oxide in patients with acquired valvular heart disease. Anesthesiology 1975;42:319–24.

26. Stanley TH, Liu W-S. Cardiovascular effects of meperidine-N_2O anesthesia before and after pancuronium. Anesth Analg (Cleve) 1977;56:669–73.

27. Smith NT, Eger EI II, Stoelting RK, Whayne TF, Cullen DJ, Kadis LB. The

cardiovascular and sympathomimetic responses to the addition of nitrous oxide to halothane in man. Anesthesiology 1970; 32:410–21.

28. Eisele JH, Smith NT. Cardiovascular effects of 40 percent nitrous oxide in man. Anesth Analg (Cleve) 1972;51:956–63.

29. Thorburn J, Smith G, Vance JP, Brown DM. Effect of nitrous oxide on the cardiovascular system and coronary circulation of the dog. Br J Anaesth 1979;51:937–42.

30. Zar JH. Biostatistical analysis. Englewood Cliffs, NJ: Prentice-Hall, 1974:151–5.

31. Glantz SA. Primer of biostatistics. New York: McGraw-Hill, 1981:107–8.

32. Roizen MF, Horrigan RW, Koike M, et al. A prospective randomized trial of four anesthetic techniques for resection of pheochromocytoma. Anesthesiology 1982; 57:A43.

33. Dahlström B, Bolme P, Feychting H, Noack G, Paalzow L. Morphine kinetics in children. Clin Pharmacol Ther 1979;26:354–65.

34. Krishna G, Paradise RR. Effect of morphine on isolated human atrial muscle. Anesthesiology 1974;40:147–50.

35. Sugai N, Shimosato S, Etsten BE. Effect of halothane on force-velocity relations and dynamic stiffness of isolated heart muscle. Anesthesiology 1968;29:267–74.

36. Shimosato S, Sugai N, Iwatsuki N, Etsten BE. The effect of Ethrane on cardiac muscle mechanics. Anesthesiology 1969; 30:513–18.

37. Kemmotsu O, Hashimoto Y, Shimosato S. Inotropic effects of isoflurane on mechanics of contraction in isolated cat papillary muscles from normal and failing hearts. Anesthesiology 1973;39:470–7.

38. Eckenhoff JE, Oech SR. The effects of narcotics and antagonists upon respiration and circulation in man. Clin Pharmacol Ther 1960;1:483–524.

39. Marta JA, Davis HS, Eisele JH. Vagomimetic effects of morphine and Innovar® in man. Anesth Analg (Cleve) 1973;52:817–21.

40. Flaim SF, Vismara LA, Zelis R. The effects of morphine on isolated cutaneous canine vascular smooth muscle. Res Commun Chem Pathol Pharmacol 1977;16:191–4.

41. Hsu HO, Hickey RF, Forbes AR. Morphine decreases peripheral vascular resistance and increases capacitance in man. Anesthesiology 1979;50:98–102.

42. Zelis R, Mansour EJ, Capone RJ, Mason DT. The cardiovascular effects of morphine: the peripheral capacitance and resistance vessels in human subjects. J. Clin Invest 1974;54:1247–58.

43. Philbin DM, Moss J, Rosow CE, Atkins CW, Kono K, Savarese JJ. The use of H_1 and H_2 histamine blockers with morphine: a double-blind study. Anesthesiology 1980;53:S67.

44. Lowenstein E, Whiting RB, Bittar DA, Sanders CA, Powell WJ Jr. Local and neurally mediated effects of morphine on skeletal muscle vascular resistance. J Pharmacol Exp Ther 1972;180:359–67.

45. Laubie M, Schmitt H, Canellas J, Roquebert J, Demichel P. Centrally mediated bradycardia and hypotension induced by narcotic analgesics: dextromoramide and fentanyl. Eur J Pharmacol 1974;28:66–75.

46. Goldberg AH, Padget CH. Comparative effects of morphine and fentanyl on isolated heart muscle. Anesth Analg (Cleve) 1969; 48:978–82.

47. Fleiss JH. Statistical methods for rates and proportions. New York: John Wiley & Sons, 1973:178.

33 NARCOTICS VERSUS INHALATION ANESTHETICS: EFFECTS ON REGIONAL MYOCARDIAL ISCHEMIA

Sandra L. Roberts and John H. Tinker*

Comparing the cardiac effects of narcotics to those of inhalational agents is difficult, and only limited numbers of comparative studies have been published. Bland, Chir, and Lowenstein [1] studied elevation of the ST segment produced by acute occlusion of a previously normal canine coronary artery without versus with halothane. They found a significantly smaller summation of elevations with halothane. Smith et al [2] used xenon clearance to evaluate blood flow and oxygen use distal to a ligated canine anterior descending coronary artery. Halothane resulted in increased oxygen availability/consumption ratio in the areas of ischemia. In 1982 Smith et al [3] repeated their study with enflurane and obtained similar results. All three of these studies were done in dogs—an animal whose coronary circulation overlaps, and which is probably a less than op-

timal animal model of regional coronary artery disease. None of the studies mentioned examined narcotic effect on experimental ischemia in comparison to the volatile agents.

In 1982, Merin et al [4] reported a study done in pigs, whose coronary circulation is considerably more similar to humans'. They compared a relatively hypodynamic 1-MAC halothane anesthetic to a much more hyperdynamic fentanyl anesthetic. The fentanyl group had higher coronary blood flow, oxygen delivery, and myocardial oxygen demand. They then produced a 50% to 60% flow occlusion of the left anterior descending coronary artery and considered that resultant ischemia was indicated by arteriovenous oxygen differences, lactate extraction, and venoarterial potassium and hydrogen concentrations. No differences were found between the halothane and fentanyl groups, possibly because the stenoses produced were flow reductions from controls, which were

*Presented at the conference by Dr. Tinker.

very different. Use of negative overall lactate extraction as a measure of ischemia may overlook small areas of ischemia, but Merin et al did examine regional lactate extractions. Loeb et al [5] studied 20 patients with known coronary artery disease. After measuring myocardial oxygen consumption (MVO$_2$) in the awake resting state by thermodilution coronary sinus catheters, they increased MVO$_2$ by 80% by means of pacing-induced tachycardia. At that point, 17 of the 20 patients experienced angina and 14 had ST segment changes on electrocardiogram. Despite obvious regional myocardial ischemia, only three patients had negative overall myocardial lactate extraction.

COMPARISON OF VOLATILE AND NARCOTIC ANESTHESIA IN PIGS

We decided to compare, in swine, cardiac ability to perform equal amounts of external work under either volatile or narcotic anesthesia. Left ventricular external work (LVEW) divided by MVO$_2$ was considered to be myocardial oxygen utilization efficiency (Meff), after suitable unit conversion, expressed as percentage. At various mechanically determined preset workloads, we examined MVO$_2$ and Meff under halothane, enflurane, isoflurane, fentanyl (50 mg/kg bolus plus 25 mg/kg/hr bolus), and same-dose fentanyl plus propranolol.

The experimental model was a right heart bypass modified from that described originally by Sarnoff et al [6]. Inferior vena cava and superior vena cava blood flows were diverted and an indwelling right ventricular catheter was used to collect coronary blood flow (Figure 33.1). Oxygenated blood was returned to the left atrium. While holding output constant, work was adjusted by an aortic snare and/or an arteriovenous fistula to raise or lower mean arterial pressure respectively. Heart rate was held as close to 120 beats per minute as possible, with electrical pacing if necessary.

At approximately equal work levels of

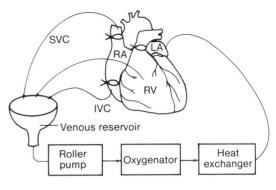

$$MVO_2 = CBF (C_{aO_2} - C_{\overline{cv}O_2})$$

FIGURE 33.1. The right heart bypass model.

1600 gm-m/min/m^2 (relatively low level cardiac work) Meff ranged from 7.71% to 11.07% for the different agents. These numbers are similar to reported values for human resting Meff. Within the low-work group, the more depressant halothane and enflurane had 10% to 11% Meff compared to 7% to 8% for the less depressant fentanyl and isoflurane (Table 33.1). With beta blockade, the Meff of fentanyl increased to 9.81%.

At higher workload levels the more depressant anesthetics probably begin to result in ventricular failure and the nondepressant anesthetics showed greater Meff. No animal exhibited frank left ventricular failure.

The oxygen consumption varied 3 to 4 cc O$_2$/min/100 gm heart between the depressant versus the nondepressant groups at low work levels (Table 33.2). None of the animals exhibited ischemia as detected by external and epicardial electrocardiographic monitoring and overall lactate extraction ratios. Catecholamine levels were slightly lower in the halothane group and higher in the propranolol-fentanyl group.

CONCLUSIONS

The study conclusions were: despite nearly identical external hemodynamics, MVO$_2$ and Meff varied substantially with different anesthetics tested; at low work levels, the more

TABLE 33.1. Myocardial oxygen utilization efficiency (percent)

Group	Workload Levels (%)		
	Low	Medium	High
Halothane (N = 9)	11.07 ± 0.62	13.50 ± 1.19	10.98 ± 1.40
Enflurane (N = 6)	10.21 ± 0.86	11.40 ± 0.71	11.38 ± 1.27
Isoflurane (N = 5)	7.71 ± 0.64	9.93 ± 1.15	11.31 ± 1.55
Fentanyl (N = 11)	7.76 ± 0.57	10.44 ± 0.79	9.88 ± 1.10
Fentanyl + propranolol (N = 6)	9.81 ± 0.56	12.28 ± 1.00	15.38 ± 0.41

TABLE 33.2. Myocardial oxygen consumption (cc O_2/100 gm ventricular weight/min)

Group	Workload Levels (%)		
	Low	Medium	High
Halothane	8.73 ± 0.65	8.79 ± 0.67	13.99 ± 2.11
Enflurane	9.07 ± 0.68	10.69 ± 1.05	16.03 ± 1.84
Isoflurane	9.71 ± 0.72	10.28 ± 0.74	13.85 ± 1.65
Fentanyl	12.70 ± 0.90	12.89 ± 0.97	18.04 ± 1.85
Fentanyl + propranolol	13.82 ± 0.87	9.49 ± 0.28	10.73 ± 0.33

depressant halothane and enflurane anesthetics were associated with better oxygen utilization efficiencies than fentanyl and isoflurane; at higher workloads the efficiency differences between anesthetics decreased; and adding propranolol to fentanyl improved the otherwise low Meff [7,8].

Hemodynamic stability is a popular goal today in cardiac anesthetic management. Does the presence of stable and identical hemodynamic states in two separate operating rooms necessarily imply identical myocardial oxygen demand? The data on Meff indicate a clinically relevant "no" answer. Increasing myocardial oxygen consumption per se was not necessarily shown to be detrimental. Pending further investigation, one could assume that this reflects increased myocardial stress. We must work hard to achieve the lowest possible MVO_2 with reasonable hemodynamics.

REFERENCES

1. Bland JL, Chir B, Lowenstein E. Halothane-induced decrease in experimental myocardial ischemia in the non-failing canine heart. Anesthesiology 1976;45:287–93.
2. Smith G, Rogers K, Thornburn J. Halothane improves the balance of oxygen supply to demand in acute experimental myocardial ischemia. Br J Anaesth 1980;52:577–83.
3. Smith G, Evans DH, Asher MJ, Bentley S. Enflurane improves the oxygen supply/demand balance in the acutely ischemic canine myocardium. Acta Anaesthesiol Scand 1982; 26:44–47.
4. Merin RG, Verdouw PD, de Jong JW. Myocardial functional and metabolic responses to ischemia in swine during halothane and fentanyl anesthesia. Anesthesiology 1982;56:84–92.
5. Loeb HS, Saudye A, Croke RP, Talano JV, Klodnychy ML, Gunnar RM. Effect of phar-

macologically induced hypertension on myocardial ischemia and coronary hemodynamics in patients with fixed coronary abstruction. Circulation 1978;57:41–6.

6. Sarnoff SJ, Brownwald E, Welch JH Jr, Case RB, Stainsby WN, Macruz R. Hemodynamic determinants of oxygen consumption of the heart with special reference to the tension time index. Am J Physiol 1958;192:148–56.

7. Tinker JH, Milde JH, Nugent M. Myocardial oxygen utilization efficiency: comparisons between four anesthetics at similar external workloads and heart rates. Submitted to Anesthesiology (in revision).

8. Tinker JH, Nugent M, Barash PG, Kay H. Cardiac O_2 use efficiency vs four anesthetics: halothane/enflurane better than fentanyl without B blockade in swine (abstract). Anesthesiology 1982;57:A18.

34 NARCOTICS AND THE CORONARY CIRCULATION

Dietrich Kettler, Otto Hilfiker, and Hans Sonntag

Morphine and other opiates have been used both to supplement balanced anesthesia and as the primary anesthetic during cardiac surgery. Since Lowenstein et al [1] introduced the practice of administering large intravenous doses of morphine during cardiac surgery, more studies have been done on the effects of large doses of newly developed synthetic narcotics such as fentanyl, sufentanil, alfentanil, and others. All reports concluded that narcotic anesthesia, especially with high doses of the newer narcotics, provided stable circulation with few side effects.

Worldwide increase in coronary artery operations has led many anesthesiologists to use narcotics for this type of surgery also. Large doses of narcotics during coronary artery bypass graft surgery were reported not only to produce stable cardiovascular dynamics, but to provide stress-free anesthesia during intubation and sternotomy. These reports are based mainly on hemodynamic, metabolic, and endocrine factors [1]. Few data are available on the influence of anesthetics, including narcotics, on myocardial blood flow, oxygenation, and metabolism. We studied the influence of various intravenous and inhalational anesthetic agents in patients with either normal or impaired cor-

onary circulation. This chapter describes the effects of morphine, fentanyl, and sufentanil on human coronary blood flow and myocardial oxygenation and compares these with effects of halothane–nitrous oxide inhalation anesthesia.

COMPARISON OF NARCOTIC VERSUS INHALATION ANESTHESIA

Measurements of myocardial blood flow (MBF) and myocardial oxygen consumption (MVO_2) have been performed in our institution during the last ten years in patients undergoing general or coronary artery surgery. Myocardial blood flow is measured by means of the argon wash-in technique [2]. In a modification of the original Kety-Schmidt technique, argon is substituted for nitrous oxide because it is less water and lipid soluble and more diffusible, and therefore allows maximum arterial and coronary sinus argon concentrations to be reached more rapidly. In contrast to nitrous oxide, argon has no anesthetic properties. During the five-minute period of MBF measurement, the patient under expiratory carbon dioxide control inhales a standard concentration of argon. Simultaneously, blood is withdrawn by motor-driven syringes from the artery and the coronary sinus and analyzed for argon content (gas chromatography).

The effects of neuroleptanalgesia (0.33 mg droperidol per kilogram of body weight followed by 7 μg/kg fentanyl) and sufentanil (0.7 μg/kg) on MFB and MVO_2 were studied in patients with normal coronary circulation undergoing general surgery. In patients scheduled for coronary artery bypass graft surgery with two- or three-vessel coronary artery disease but normal left ventricular function, the effects of 6 mg/kg morphine and 100 μg/kg fentanyl on MBF and MVO_2 were investigated after intubation and sternotomy and compared with results obtained during halothane–nitrous oxide anesthesia. In the fentanyl and halothane studies, myocardial lactate metabolism was also determined. All patients received a maintenance dose of a beta blocker (pindolol) until the day of operation.

The following scheme illustrates the stages of anesthesia and surgery when measurements were performed in the three groups.

	I	II	III
Morphine (N = 8)	Awake	10 min after infusion of 6 mg/kg morphine, after intubation	During sternotomy
High-dose fentanyl (N = 9)	Awake	10 min after infusion of 100 μg/kg fentanyl and 0.3 mg/kg etomidate, after intubation	During sternotomy
Halothane–nitrous oxide (N = 7)	Awake	After induction by mask and after intubation; mean halothane concentration 0.5 vol/% (N_2O/O_2 = 50% each)	During sternotomy, mean halothane concentration 0.9 vol/% (N_2O/O_2 = 50% each)

Patients with Normal Coronary Function

Table 34.1 presents mean values of hemodynamic and myocardial variables for awake patients after injections of droperidol followed by fentanyl (neuroleptanalgesia) and after sufentanil without droperidol. A 22% rise in heart rate ($p < 0.05$) and a 16% decrease in total peripheral resistance ($p < 0.01$) were produced by 0.33 mg/kg of dro-

TABLE 34.1. Hemodynamic and myocardial variables during neuroleptanalgesia and sufentanil analgesia in patients with normal coronary function

Variable	Neuroleptanalgesia (N = 10)			Sufentanil (N = 6)	
	Awake	Droperidol 0.33 mg/kg	+ Fentanyl 7 μg/kg	Awake	Sufentanil 0.7 μg/kg
HR (beats/min)	77	94*	79	71	64*
MAP (mm Hg)	105	91	93	92	85†
CI (L/min/m²)	3.72	3.93	3.43	3.73	3.21
SVI (ml/m²)	48	45	44	48	50
TPR (mm Hg/(ml/min/kg))	0.99	0.84†	0.98	1.09	1.08
MBF (ml/min/100 gm)	97	139†	92*	84	73*
CVR (mm Hg/(ml/min/100 gm))	0.91	0.60†	0.93	1.00	1.09
MVO_2 (ml/min/100 gm)	10.3	14.3†	9.2*	10.2	8.6

HR = heart rate; MAP = mean arterial pressure; CI = cardiac index; SVI = stroke volume index; TPR = total peripheral resistance; MBF = myocardial blood flow; CVR = coronary vascular resistance; MVO_2 = myocardial oxygen consumption (mean values).

*$p < 0.05$ versus awake.

†$p < 0.01$ versus awake.

peridol. Mean arterial pressure decreased by 15% (no significance). These hemodynamic changes were accompanied by a 43% augmentation of MBF and 39% ($p < 0.01$) of MVO_2. The succeeding injection of 7 μg/kg fentanyl completed neuroleptanalgesia and changed most of the droperidol-induced variations to the range observed during consciousness.

Injection of 0.7 μg/kg sufentanil into awake patients reduced heart rate by 10% ($p < 0.05$) and mean arterial pressure by 8% ($p < 0.01$). Myocardial blood flow decreased by 13% ($p < 0.05$) and MVO_2 by 16% (no significance).

Patients with Coronary Artery Disease

In Table 34.2 the behavior of the coronary circulation during the two narcotic techniques (morphine and fentanyl) can be compared with the effects of halothane–nitrous oxide anesthesia. Both 6 mg/kg morphine and 100 μg/kg fentanyl decreased MBF by 14% and 10% respectively ($p < 0.05$ and < 0.01). Myocardial oxygen consumption decreased under morphine by 14% ($p < 0.05$) and under fentanyl by 14% ($p < 0.01$). Halothane, 0.5%, combined with nitrous oxide, reduced MBF (29%, $p < 0.05$) and MVO_2 (29%, $p < 0.01$) to a greater extent than did morphine and fentanyl. When sternotomy (stage III) was performed under morphine and fentanyl anesthesia, MBF and MVO_2 (60%, $p < 0.05$; and 61%, $p < 0.01$) rose to values well above the conscious state. Coronary vascular resistance was unchanged under morphine, decreased considerably under high-dose fentanyl, and showed a slight increase under halothane. After fentanyl infusion (stage II), and especially during sternotomy (stage III), global lactate production by the left ventricular myocardium was detectable; however, there was considerable variation in lactate values. During stage II, five of the nine patients, and during stage III, seven of the nine patients developed dif-

TABLE 34.2. Myocardial variables during three anesthetic techniques for coronary artery bypass grafting

Variable	Morphine			High-dose Fentanyl			Halothane–Nitrous Oxide (50%)		
	I	II	III	I	II	II	I	II	III
MBF (ml/min/100 gm)	112	96*	155*	97	87†	150†	111	79*	71†
CVR (mm Hg/(ml/min/ 100 gm))	0.75	0.76	0.72	0.9	0.85†	0.56†	0.74	0.82	1.0
O_2-Sat cv (%)	33	34	35	36	36*	38*	36	38	34
MVO_2 (ml/min/100 gm)	12.3	10.6*	17.6*	11.5	9.9†	15.9†	13.7	9.4†	9.3†
Lactate (μmol/min/ 100 gm)	—	—	—	6.9	−0.9†	−1.2†	11.5	9.5	7.6

MBF = myocardial blood flow; CVR = coronary vascular resistance; O_2-Sat cv = coronary sinus oxygen saturation; MVO_2 = myocardial oxygen consumption; lactate = myocardial uptake (+) or release (−) (mean values).

I = awake.

II = after induction: Morphine, 6 mg/kg body weight; High-dose fentanyl, 100 μg/kg body weight; Halothane, 0.5% (N_2O).

III = sternotomy: Morphine = II; High-dose fentanyl = II; Halothane = 0.9% (N_2O).

*p <0.05 versus awake.

†p <0.01 among all values.

ferent degrees of myocardial lactate production. In the halothane group, lactate production was not observed at all.

Table 34.3 presents the corresponding hemodynamic variables. Morphine and fentanyl produced a mild increase in the heart rate, which further increased during sternotomy (24% and 29% respectively) compared to heart rate when conscious. Under halothane–nitrous oxide no heart rate changes were observed at any time. Arterial pressures (systemic and mean), including coronary perfusion pressure, decreased after application of the two opiates but increased considerably during sternotomy. During halothane–nitrous oxide anesthesia, arterial pressures under both concentrations were diminished by about 20% ($p < 0.01$) at stage II and 12% to 17% ($p < 0.01$) during sternotomy. Pulmonary capillary wedge pressure in all groups was slightly affected. Cardiac index decreased in a dose-dependent fashion by at most 32% ($p < 0.01$) only in the halothane group, mainly reflecting the

accompanying variations in heart rate. Stroke volume index decreased under both opiate techniques (24% and 29% respectively) and halothane–nitrous oxide (33%) as well.

EFFECTS OF ANESTHETICS ON MYOCARDIAL BLOOD FLOW AND MVO$_2$

Reports on the effects of morphine on coronary circulation in various species, first published in 1929 by Gruber and Robinson [3], attributed to morphine a coronary dilating potency. These papers neglected the relation between hemodynamic variables and coronary blood flow adjustment, however. From our experimental work [4] and data published by Patschke et al [5], a specific pharmacologic action of the synthetic opiates fentanyl (as part of neuroleptanalgesia) and piritramide could be excluded. We used a complex hemodynamic variable for calculation of MVO$_2$ after Bretschneider [6], which allows calculation of five independent oxygen-consuming processes of the heart. No

TABLE 34.3. Hemodynamic variables and blood gases during three anesthetic techniques

Variable	Morphine I	II	III	High-dose Fentanyl I	II	III	Halothane–Nitrous Oxide (50%) I	II	III
HR (beats/min)	63	68	78*	76	82†	98†	69	72	69
SAP (mm Hg)	149	128*	173*	141	124†	152†	142	108†	111†
MAP (mm Hg)	96	82*	123*	103	87†	106†	103	82†	86†
MDAP (mm Hg)	85	74*	108*	91	79†	91†	91	74†	78*
PCWP (mm Hg)	8.9	8.6	10.9*	11.2	11.8	12.8	10.3	9.7	9.3
CI (L/min/m²)	3.18	2.99	2.99	3.89	3.09	3.58	3.48	2.47†	2.35†
SVI (ml/m²)	51	45	39*	48	37†	34†	51	38†	34†
Hb (gm/dl)	13.3	12.9	13.0	14.2	13.7	13.2	15.0	14.3	14.4
Po₂ (mm Hg)	83	104	127	85	129	171	87	113	127
Pco₂ (mm Hg)	—	—	—	37	38	38	43	37	36
Arterial pH	7.36	7.39	7.38	7.39	7.38	7.37	7.35	7.42	7.42

HR = heart rate; SAP = systolic arterial pressure; MAP = mean arterial pressure; MDAP = mean diastolic arterial pressure; PCWP = pulmonary capillary wedge pressure; CI = cardiac index; SVI = stroke volume index (mean values).

Stages I, II, III: see Table 34.2.

*$p < 0.05$ versus awake.

†$p < 0.01$ between all values.

deviation was found between calculated and directly measured MVO_2 values under opiate anesthesia. Sonntag et al [7–12] demonstrated a close relationship between changes of heart rate, arterial pressure, and contractility on the one hand and MBF/ MVO_2 on the other in several clinical studies on the effects of anesthetics on human coronary circulation. Up to now, only diethyl ether has been known to produce specific anesthetic coronary vasodilation of relevant magnitude [4,13].

In the study of effects of neuroleptanalgesia [14], an anesthetic technique used frequently in Europe, droperidol produced tachycardia and a rise in MVO_2 of the same magnitude. The succeeding fentanyl injection returned both values to normal. The newer opioid sufentanil, whose analgesic potency is 7 to 10 times higher than that of fentanyl, had effects similar to fentanyl (Table 34.1) on the general and coronary circulation. The effects of morphine and fentanyl (Tables 34.2 and 34.3) in patients with coronary artery disease deserve special attention, because these patients have restricted coronary reserve and may not be able to increase MBF sufficiently during hypertensive episodes to meet the increased oxygen demand of the heart. In these patients, the importance of diastolic coronary perfusion pressure (oxygen supply) and of other hemodynamic variables (contractility, heart rate, and blood pressure: oxygen demand) becomes evident. Figure 34.1 shows only those patients of the fentanyl group who developed global left ventricular anaerobiosis. Lactate release is shown at the abscissa and is related to MVO_2 (left ordinate) and rate-pressure product (right ordinate). As indicated by the vertical connection lines, there was large individual variation of correlation between MVO_2 and rate-pressure product. The overall coefficient of correlation was 0.66. Again, the rate-pressure product proved to be an unreliable individual estimate for MVO_2.

The greatest lactate release occurred in two patients (no. 8 and no. 9) at rather moderate rate-pressure products of about 9000 and 11,000 and at moderate MVO_2 values (11.6 and 11.1 cc O_2/min/100 gm). It should be expected that sternotomy with rate-pressure products now of 15,500 and 16,600 and correspondingly increased MVO_2 values (90% and 71%) would lead to increased lactate production. The opposite effect was observed in both patients, however, in whom lactate release was considerably reduced. Two possible mechanisms may explain these findings. First, the coronary blood flow of these two patients may have been compromised in stenotic areas by a critically low coronary perfusion pressure (68 and 69 mm Hg respectively). Any increase in arterial pressures, including diastolic, would improve the oxygenation of the myocardial area supplied by the narrowed vessel despite increased global oxygen demand. Second, under surgical stress, most of the unaffected coronary vasculature may have dilated, and lactate coming from the underperfused area would be diluted in the overall increased coronary sinus blood flow. The magnitude of MBF increase observed during sternotomy does not fully explain the extent of lower lactate values, however; we cannot provide an explanation. Both effects may play a role. The difficulty of extending results from animal studies and theoretical considerations to individual patients is evident. Unfortunately, it is not yet possible to study regional blood flow and metabolism of the heart with sufficient accuracy. Measurements of human coronary blood flow obtained by measuring global blood flow must be interpreted with great caution. Larger doses of morphine and fentanyl injected into patients with two- or three-vessel coronary artery disease but normal left ventricular function caused a drop in arterial pressures accompanied by a mild increase in heart rate. Standard surgical stimulation, such as sternotomy and chest spreading, did not, however, prevent arterial hypertension and further increase in heart rate. Myocardial blood flow and MVO_2 behaved similarly. After initial diminution following drug application, sternotomy led to a

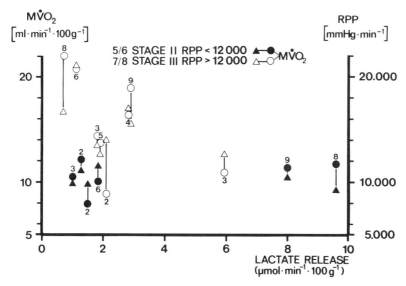

FIGURE 34.1.   Correlation between rate-pressure product (RPP, right ordinate), MV̇O₂ (left ordinate), and global myocardial lactate release (MBF × coronary sinus − arterial lactate content) during high-dose fentanyl anesthesia. Only those patients are shown who at stage II (after intubation) or stage III (during sternotomy and chest spreading) release lactate through the myocardium. Every patient can be identified by a number.

At stage II, 5 of the 6 patients had RPPs <12,000; however, patients 8 and 9 had a more than fourfold higher lactate release, indicating poor individual correlation between RPP and MV̇O₂ on the one and anaerobiosis on the other hand. Patients 8 and 9 even diminished lactate output at higher RPPs under sternotomy (III), stressing the importance of an adequate individual perfusion pressure during coronary artery disease.

At stage III, 7 of the 8 lactate-releasing patients had RPP <12,000 with poor correlation to the amount of total lactate release.

There was a large individual variation between MV̇O₂ and RPP.

relevant augmentation of MVO₂. At stage II, fentanyl without surgical manipulation depressed blood pressure and MVO₂ and caused myocardial lactate production in five of nine patients, indicating global anaerobic energy gain in the myocardium. Anaerobiosis, aggravated when sternotomy was performed, now occurred in seven of nine patients. Thus under varying hemodynamic conditions, both blood pressures below (stage II) and above (stage III) control values had a negative impact on myocardial oxygenation.

Looking at the halothane–nitrous oxide effects, the picture becomes even more confusing. In these patients arterial pressures,

heart rate, and MVO₂ were well below the values with fentanyl. No lactate production was ever observed in these patients [15]. In an editorial on a paper by Merin et al [16] dealing with the effects of fentanyl and halothane anesthesia on myocardial oxygenation, Lowenstein et al [17] discussed the possible effects of blood pressure drop on myocardial blood flow in a narrowed coronary vascular unit, comparing a "low-demand–low-pressure" state (halothane) with a "high-demand–high-pressure" state (fentanyl). Contrary to Merin et al [16], who found an equivalent depression of ischemia under both techniques, Lowenstein et al [17] calculated that fentanyl and halothane anesthesia may produce quite different degrees of ischemia in the presence of an identical degree of coronary constriction due to a greater fall of oxygen demand under halothane. Kistner et al [18] compared indirect indices of myocardial oxygenation during coronary artery bypass grafting under morphine and halothane anesthesia and found greater increases of heart rate, rate-pressure product, and tension-time index as well as a greater ST segment depression and a decreased diastolic pressure-time index/tension-time index ratio under morphine anesthesia. Our results do not support the thesis that opioids per se produce a myocardial anaerobiosis during coronary artery bypass grafting. For more than ten years we have used fentanyl in cardiac surgery in moderate doses of 10 to 20 μg/kg/hr with good results, either during neuroleptanalgesia combining fentanyl with droperidol or in conjunction with benzodiazepines (diazepam or flunitrazepam). Unpublished observations (Hilfiker O, Larsen R, Sonntag H, 1982) at our institution indicate that anesthesia for coronary artery bypass grafting with midazolam-fentanyl does not impair myocardial oxygenation. Application of analgesic doses of fentanyl during halothane or enflurane anesthesia is another way of achieving reliable and safe anesthesia during cardiovascular interventions. In our opinion, however, changing balanced anesthesia to a single anesthetic technique with sole application of enormous amounts of opioids is the wrong way to deal with the requirements of cardiovascular anesthesia. Results of various studies indicate that the opioids morphine, fentanyl, and sufentanil do not have specific dilating or constricting effects on the human coronary circulation. Myocardial blood flow under opiate action is affected by secondary hemodynamic variations (heart rate, blood pressure, wall tension) on myocardial oxygen demand.

CONCLUSION

In patients with coronary artery disease, use of a large amount of fentanyl as the sole an-

esthetic during surgical stimulation does not prevent hemodynamic reactions or augmentation of myocardial oxygen demand and the possibility of inadequate myocardial oxygenation.

REFERENCES

1. Lowenstein E, Hallowell P, Levine FH, et al. Cardiovascular response to large doses of intravenous morphine in man. N Engl J Med 1969;281:1389–93.
2. Tauchert M, Kochsiek K, Heiss HW. Measurements of coronary blood flow in man by the argon method. In: Maseri A, ed. Myocardial blood flow in man. Turin: Minerva Medica, 1970:859–64.
3. Gruber CHM, Robinson PI. Studies on the influence of morphine, papaverine and quinidine upon the heart. J Pharmacol 1926;27:429–49.
4. Kettler D. Sauerstoffbedarf und Sauerstoffversorgung des Herzens in Narkose. Anaesthesiology and Resuscitation 67. Berlin, Heidelberg, New York: Springer, 1973.
5. Patschke D, Gethmann JW, Hess W, Tarnow J, Waibel H. Hämodynamik, Koronardurchblutung und myokardialer Sauerstoffverbrauch unter hohen Fentanyl- und Piritramiddosen. Anaesthesist 1976;25:309–17.
6. Bretschneider HJ. Die hämodynamischen Determinanten des myokardialen Sauerstoffverbrauchs. In: Dengler HJ, ed. Die therapeutische Anwendung β-sympathikolytischer Stoffe. Stuttgart, New York: Schattauer, 1972:45–60.
7. Sonntag H, Schenk HD, Regensburger D, et al. Effects of Althesin (Glaxo CT 1341) on coronary blood flow and myocardial metabolism in man. Acta Anaesthesiol Scand 1973;17:218–26.
8. Sonntag H, Hellberg K, Schenk HD. Effects of thiopental (Trapanal) on coronary blood flow and myocardial metabolism in man. Acta Anaesthesiol Scand 1975;19:69–78.
9. Kettler D, Sonntag H, Donath U, Regensburger D, Schenk HD. Hämodynamik, Myokardmechanik, Sauerstoffbedarf und Sauerstoffversorgung des menschlichen Herzens unter Narkoseeinleitung mit Etomidate. Anaesthesist 1974;23:116–21.

10. Kettler D, Sonntag H. Intravenous anaesthetics: coronary blood flow and myocardial oxygen consumption (with special reference to Althesine). Acta Anaesthesiol Belg 1974;25:384–401.

11. Sonntag H. Actions of anesthetics on the coronary circulation in normal subjects and patients with ischemic heart disease. In: Prys-Roberts C, ed. Hypertension, ischemic heart disease and anesthesia. International Anesthesiology Clinics. Boston: Little, Brown & Co., 1980:111–35.

12. Hilfiker O, Larsen R, Brockschnieder B, Sonntag H. Morphin-"Anaesthesie"-Koronardurchblutung und myokardialer Sauerstoffverbrauch bei Patienten mit Koronarkrankheit. Anaesthesist 1982;31: 371–6.

13. Eberlein HJ. Koronardurchblutung und Sauerstoffversorgung des Herzens unter verschiedenen CO_2-Spannungen und Anaesthetika. Arch Kreislauf Forsch 1966; 50:18–86.

14. Sonntag H, Heiss HW, Knoll D, Regensburger D, Schenk HD, Bretschneider HJ. Über die Myokarddurchblutung und den myokardialen Sauerstoffverbrauch bei Patienten während Narkoseeinleitung mit Dehydrobenzperidol-Fentanyl und Ketamine. Z Kreislauf Forsch 1972;61:1092–1105.

15. Hilfiker O, Larsen R, Sonntag H. Myocardial blood flow and oxygen consumption during halothane-nitrous oxide anaesthesia for coronary revascularization. Br J Anaesth 1983;55:927–32.

16. Merin RG, Verdouw PD, de Jong JW. Myocardial functional and metabolic responses to ischemia in swine during halothane and fentanyl anesthesia. Anesthesiology 1982;56:84–92.

17. Lowenstein E, Hill RD, Rajagopalan B, Schneider RC. Winnie the Pooh revisited, or, the more recent adventures of Piglet. Anesthesiology 1982;56:81–3.

18. Kistner JR, Miller ED, Lake CL, Ross WT. Indices of myocardial oxygenation during coronary-artery revascularization in man with morphine versus halothane anesthesia. Anesthesiology 1979;50:324–30.

35 THE VALUE OF FENTANYL IN CARDIOVASCULAR ANESTHESIA

Paul G. Barash

Dr. Kettler's group in West Germany has contributed extensively to our understanding of coronary physiology in the clinical setting. Recently, they published a study on the coronary effects of fentanyl that I think is very controversial and gives much food for thought concerning the way we practice anesthesia. I am sure many anesthesiologists who administer fentanyl for cardiac anesthesia achieve marked hemodynamic stability without evidence of ischemia in their patients. That has been our experience, and I will describe it briefly.

THE PLACE OF FENTANYL IN INDUCTION AND MAINTENANCE OF ANESTHESIA

We have conducted clinical research using conventional hemodynamic measurements in conjunction with radionuclide techniques to assess the effects of fentanyl during induction and intubation in patients with coronary disease. In general, the observed hemodynamic profiles with a valium–nitrous oxide–enflurane sequence showed clinically significant increases in blood pressure and heart rate during laryngoscopy and intubation (15 seconds). These increases persisted for three to five minutes. The left ventricular ejection fraction, which we measure on line, decreased significantly, from a normal range of approximately 55% to 34% during intubation. That decrease in ejection fraction is more dramatic and rapid than would be seen in a stress-testing laboratory. In contrast, in the patients given 30 to 75 μg of fentanyl per kilogram of body weight, stable blood pressure, heart rate, and ejection fraction were observed.

Subsequently, we enlarged these studies to include direct measurements of coronary vascular performance. We compared two groups of patients, one treated with fentanyl, 75 μg/kg, and one that received the valium–enflurane–nitrous oxide sequence. There were no significant differences in baseline demographic data between the groups. The patients were premedicated with morphine and scopolamine, and 90 minutes later vascular catheterization, including coronary sinus catheterization, was performed under fluoroscopy. The first group received fentanyl, 75 μg/kg, with oxygen inhalation. The second group received diazepam, 0.3 mg/kg; nitrous oxide–oxygen, 3:2; and enflurane. After induction was started, the patients were given a succinylcholine infusion for muscle relaxation.

Our experience with one patient treated with fentanyl serves as an example of the typical findings in that group. Prior to intubation, this patient's coronary sinus blood flow was 122 ml/min with a myocardial oxygen consumption of 7.6 ml/min. During intubation the patient's heart rate, blood pressure, and pulmonary artery pressure remained stable. There was no loss in ejection fraction and no significant decrease in coronary blood flow or myocardial oxygen consumption. In contrast, in a patient treated with the diazepam-enflurane sequence, blood pressure and heart rate increased significantly, while ejection fraction decreased precipitously, from 52% to 37%, during 15-second intubation. Coronary sinus blood flow increased by 70%, while myocardial oxygen consumption almost doubled.

Neither group of patients showed signs of lactate production. Our study could detect only global changes in left ventricular and coronary performance; regional ventricular dysfunction could not be assessed.

CONCLUSION

How can we account for the differences in our results and Dr. Kettler's? First, Kettler's group used a combination of drugs, etomidate and fentanyl; we used fentanyl-oxygen technique. Second, they intubated patients at a fentanyl dose of 10 μg/kg plus 0.3 mg/kg etomidate; we intubated at 75 μg/kg fentanyl. Third, we did not carry our data collection through to sternotomy; they did.

Despite these differences, I believe Dr. Kettler's group and ours are in certain agreement about the place of fentanyl. I view it as an excellent induction agent for these patients. After induction, one then has to match the anesthetic depth to the surgical stimulus; we add enflurane. Finally, although the findings of our respective studies differ, I think we also concur that fentanyl has established its place in maintenance of anesthesia.

Part V DISCUSSION

DR. EDMOND I. EGER II: Dr. Barash, I was impressed with Dr. Roizen's comment that it is more important to consider the skills and desires of the anesthetists than the anesthetics we choose. I noticed that in the cases where you saw increases in blood pressure and pulse rate, you had administered enflurane at only one-third MAC. The hemodynamic problems may have had nothing to do with your choice of anesthetic. Regardless of the drug you select, be it fentanyl or alfentanil, the issue is adequate suppression of the cardiovascular response to stress. Perhaps more anesthetic rather than less would have been desirable in this case, or perhaps propranolol would have been more appropriate. A combination of fentanyl and enflurane might also have helped to diminish these cardiovascular effects.

DR. PAUL G. BARASH: Actually, we have used enflurane at concentrations below one-third MAC, but we were accused of doing our intubations in awake patients so we decided to increase the dose. The problem here is of using inhalation anesthesia in patients with coronary artery disease. It is very difficult in the operating room to administer inhalation agents in higher concentrations without causing blood pressure to drop. We did a series of studies in which we used 60 mm Hg as our lowest allowable mean blood pressure. This gave us even lower diastolic pressures, and I don't think many people would accept levels much below that. Our patients were receiving relatively high doses of beta blockers, averaging about 177 mg per day, and they were given their last dose of the beta blocker with their premedication.

These patients were also given nitrous oxide. I don't want to argue with you about MAC, but as I recall, the MAC for enflurane with nitrous oxide in this age group is about 0.65 or 0.7 mg/kg, so with nitrous oxide we were almost at 1 MAC. As a matter of fact, we were concerned about whether we were giving these patients too much enflurane, so I'm glad to hear you say you think they were not receiving enough.

DR. EGER: My thought was not that they were given too much or too little as an anesthetizing dose, but that they received too little to suppress the stress response. The fact that the patients received what would seem to be an adequate dose of propranolol does not mean they were given enough medication to block the stress response. You were still seeing stress-related cardiovascular effects such as tachycardia and hypotension.

DR. EDWARD LOWENSTEIN: Can I ask you, Dr. Eger, what you would have done differently to ensure that the stress response would in fact be blocked?

DR. EGER: I think I might have given fentanyl along with the enflurane. I might also have given more propranolol.

DR. JOHN H. TINKER: I'd like to comment on another aspect of Dr. Barash's study, the relationship between heart rate and ejection fraction. A paper published in *Circulation* in 1983 described changes in ejection fraction in patients receiving ventricular pacing. When contractions were increased, in increments of 10, from 50 to 100 beats per minute, the ejection fractions dropped from 58% to 47%. Dr. Barash has also shown a dramatic rate dependency for ejection fraction, which decreased to 37% in his patients. His patients who were given fentanyl had a nice, slow heart rate that may well have been responsible for their higher and more satisfying ejection fractions.

DR. BARASH: I agree with the study in *Circulation*—I think that a declining ejection fraction is certainly an index of ventricular function. Cardiac performance is profoundly altered, which is surely deleterious. I'm not sure if it is due to blood pressure or heart rate, though heart rate probably plays a role. We were unable to show lactate production, so I couldn't say whether the effect is injurious in terms of myocardial oxygen balance or pumping function.

DR. LOWENSTEIN: Dr. Stanley, your average alfentanil dose for inducing sleep was 250 µg/kg, I believe. Others at this symposium have stated that 150 µg/kg is a large dose. How do you explain this difference?

DR. THEODORE H. STANLEY: It is explained by the premedication we used, by our patients' age and degree of cardiovascular dysfunction, and by the many other factors that alter anesthetic requirements. Each patient is different, and there are no magic doses for alfentanil just as there are none for enflurane, halothane, isoflurane, or any other compound we use in anesthesia.

DR. ELI M. BROWN: Dr. Barash, you said you tested patients at doses ranging from 30 to 75 µg/kg of fentanyl. Since you showed us only results for the

75-μg/kg dose, should we assume that there was no marked difference at the lower doses?

DR. BARASH: The reason we showed our results at 75 μg/kg was that this was the only dose at which our patients had the coronary sinus catheter in place. Our patients who were given 30 and 50 μg/kg, using exactly the same protocol with the exception of the coronary sinus determinations, showed the same cardiovascular stability. In other words, the ejection fraction was preserved during intubation at both the 30- and 50-μg/kg fentanyl doses. The only difference we observed was an 8% increase in blood pressure during intubation at the 30-μg/kg dose. We saw no change in heart rate.

DR. BROWN: So you feel we can use the smaller doses, then?

DR. BARASH: Yes, for induction. Following induction you then must decide whether you want to use an infusion, go to an inhalation agent, or whatever.

DR. LOWENSTEIN: Are you saying that a ceiling effect may in fact be a change in concentration?

DR. BARASH: Yes.

DR. DHUN SETHNA: I have two comments regarding coronary sinus blood flow and myocardial lactate extraction studies. Dr. Tinker pointed out that coronary artery disease is a regional disorder and coronary sinus lactate measurements reflect the final common effluent from the left ventricle, that is, it is a global measurement. In patients like those Dr. Barash studied and those I reported with Dr. Moffitt, the absence of lactate extraction in coronary sinus blood does not necessarily mean that there was no regional ischemia. One must be very cautious in one's interpretation when there is a negative finding on this test.

DR. BARASH: I agree. For example, there could be regional abnormalities in vessel walls that our radionuclide technique would not be able to detect. I think some of Dr. El-Etr's work is fascinating, and if it is borne out, it might have some very important implications for our practice.

DR. SETHNA: You are right. With procedures such as regional wall motion studies using radionuclide techniques, we should be able to detect regional abnormalities.

DR. MICHAEL F. ROIZEN: It appears that the transesophageal echocardiograph can also detect myocardial wall motion. This procedure has had an initially high success rate in predicting future myocardial dysfunction, and I would hope we will be able to use it to prevent these problems as well.

DR. TINKER: I would like to emphasize that the reason we can detect these abnormal areas is because the rest of the myocardium clearly compensates for an ischemic region and uses more lactate.

DR. SETHNA: In this context, the study of Dr. Gertz and associates from San Francisco (*Circulation* 1980;63:1273) is relevant. Using a radiolabeled tracer method, they showed that myocardial lactate metabolism is heterogeneous at rest in patients with coronary artery disease; a significant amount of lactate can be released by the myocardium at a time when chemical analysis of arterial–coronary sinus blood indicates global extraction.

Furthermore, the presentations at these sessions have made it clear that myocardial ischemia can still be present even when there are no excessive changes in heart rate or blood pressure. The reason may be that heart rate and blood pressure measurements fail to consider an important determinant of myocardial oxygen consumption, that is, myocardial contractility. Surgical stimuli that increase heart rate and blood pressure would also affect myocardial contractility. For example, my studies with Dr. Moffitt have shown that digoxin produces a significant increase in myocardial oxygen consumption with no accompanying changes in heart rate or blood pressure. Digoxin increases myocardial contractility, but this change is not reflected in the heart rate or blood pressure.

In another study we observed that in six patients receiving morphine anesthesia, while very moderate increases in heart rate and blood pressure occurred after sternotomy, two of the patients produced lactate. Heart rate and blood pressure, then, are poor indicators of myocardial oxygen consumption. I think the belief that a rate-pressure product that is not very high precludes myocardial ischemia is misleading.

DR. LOWENSTEIN: Dr. Kettler, you have some opinions about the rate-pressure product that are based upon a fair amount of data. Do you agree with what Dr. Sethna has just stated?

DR. DIETRICH KETTLER: Yes. Dr. Sethna has just described something I think most of us agree with:

the rate-pressure product is a poor measure of ischemia.

DR. CARL E. ROSOW: Dr. Roizen's provocative presentation raised a question in my mind about the prevalence in much of our research of the type II statistical error. I'm referring to the absence of statements describing the degree to which a study can actually detect the differences it purports to detect. For example, it would have been virtually impossible for him to have found any difference in outcome between halothane versus narcotic anesthesia, given the variance in the studies he reviewed. It would require some huge number of patients to show a difference between two drugs or two modes of treatment. I wonder if anyone on the panel agrees that in future comparative studies we should perhaps begin to demand a statement of statistical power.

DR. ROIZEN: This is an important point. Comparative studies of outcome are difficult to do. We are not as successful as we would like to be in detecting things such as the myocardial infarction rate. Still, if you find that 71% of the patients in a study have myocardial ischemia, you don't need a large number of cases to conclude that this differs from the norm.

DR. LOWENSTEIN: Studies of anesthetic outcome must include death, but the mortality rate in pa-
tients undergoing cardiac surgery is so dependent upon what occurs directly to the heart in surgery that perhaps these patients are poor models for evaluating anesthetic technique past the beginning of bypass. Dr. Roizen, how suitable do you think the cardiac surgical population is for a study assessing the effects of anesthesia?

DR. ROIZEN: I think patients undergoing vascular surgery would be much better subjects for this kind of evaluation. The disease is just as severe, but no intervention involving the heart is taking place.

DR. LOWENSTEIN: Dr. Kettler, you mentioned that diethyl ether is the only anesthetic with coronary vasodilating properties. I understand, though, that some strong evidence will be available soon that isoflurane is in fact a profound coronary vasodilator. What are your feelings about that?

DR. KETTLER: I am familiar with the results of the study Dr. Reiz performed in Umea, Sweden, that showed coronary dilatation accompanied by myocardial lactate production in a group of patients anesthetized with isoflurane. He used a technique involving continuous thermodilution in the coronary sinus by Swan-Ganz catheter. We have made these determinations in just one patient, employing the argon inert gas technique, so it's too early for us to offer an opinion.

VI USE OF OPIOIDS IN CARDIOVASCULAR ANESTHESIA

36 OPIOIDS AND CORONARY ARTERY SURGERY

F. G. Estafanous and A. M. Zurick

The debate continues as to whether the preferred anesthetic agents for patients with coronary artery disease are opioids or inhalational agents. All are in agreement, however, that the management of anesthesia in these patients should ensure a positive balance between myocardial oxygen supply and demand. Among the advantages claimed for opioid anesthesia are decreased heart rate, maintained blood pressure (perfusion pressure), absence of responses to sympathetic stimulation during stressful situations, particularly during endotracheal intubation, and lack of myocardial depression or increase in pulmonary capillary wedge pressure. These advantages, together with the development of many new synthetic opioids that are very potent, have fewer side effects, and have variable durations of action, explain why opioid anesthesia has become very popular in the last decade.

Morphine can be considered the prototype narcotic anesthetic. It was used in the late nineteenth century combined with scopolamine as a complete anesthetic. It was abandoned, however, because of the number of deaths associated with its use. In the late 1960s Hasbrouck [1] and Lowenstein et al [2,3] reintroduced large doses of morphine as a good anesthetic for the severely ill and

for patients undergoing heart surgery for valve replacement. They demonstrated that such usage in patients with aortic valve disease was followed by an increase in cardiac index, stroke index, and central venous pressure and a decrease in systemic vascular resistance. Since then, large-dose morphine anesthesia has attained great popularity and is widely used.

Nevertheless, as early as 1972, Dalton [4] alerted us that patients with coronary artery disease (CAD), anesthetized with large doses of morphine, developed tachycardia, hypertension, and electrocardiographic signs of ischemia. Stoelting and Gibbs in 1973 [5] demonstrated that the addition of nitrous oxide to morphine anesthesia caused significant bradycardia and decreased mean arterial pressure, cardiac index, and systemic vascular resistance in patients with either valve or coronary artery disease. They also reported, in the same study, that hypertension was a frequent complication during endotracheal intubation and at the time of the skin incision.

Conahan et al demonstrated in 67 patients undergoing heart valve replacement that large doses of morphine, 2 mg per kilogram of body weight, caused severe hypertension during induction in 10% of the patients.

Later, intraoperatively, systemic vascular resistance increased and there was severe hypertension that required control of blood pressure in 50% of the patients [6].

The popularity of morphine anesthesia did not fade, however. Many anesthesiologists used large doses of morphine for patients with valve disease as well as coronary heart disease who underwent open heart surgery. Meanwhile, conflicting reports continued with regard to the hemodynamic effects of morphine anesthesia.

Lappas et al [7] in 1975 reported that in patients with CAD, the use of 2 mg/kg of morphine to which succinylcholine was added before endotracheal intubation did not cause any significant change in hemodynamic values. They later reported that the addition of 5% nitrous oxide to morphine anesthesia significantly decreased mean arterial pressure, cardiac index, and left ventricular stroke work index and increased pulmonary capillary wedge pressure [8].

In 1979 Kistner et al demonstrated that morphine, 2.1 mg/kg, and pancuronium bromide, 0.08 mg/kg, when administered to patients with CAD, caused significant increases in blood pressure and heart rate as well as relative myocardial ischemia evidenced by ST segment depression in lead V and concomitant significant decrease in diastolic pressure-time index/tension-time index before cardiopulmonary bypass [9].

Meanwhile, the other side effects of large-dose morphine anesthesia became more apparent, including venodilation with increased intravascular volume and increased fluid requirement during surgery [10], high frequency of intraoperative awareness unless other amnesics were used, histamine release and allergic-like response, and prolonged postoperative amnesia and respiratory depression that required mechanical support.

All these prompted the examination of other narcotic analgesics as the main anesthetic for patients with CAD.

FENTANYL ANESTHESIA AND PATIENTS WITH CAD

Fentanyl, long known as a narcotic, has been used as a component of neuroleptic anesthesia for the last two decades. In 1978 Stanley and colleagues introduced it as a complete anesthetic for patients undergoing mitral valve replacement [11] as well as coronary artery surgery [12], and claimed that its use was accompanied by maximum hemodynamic stability.

Fentanyl is supposed to be a better anesthetic than morphine. It is 50 times as potent as morphine. Due to the inverse relationship between the potency of opioids and their metabolic and cardiovascular toxicity [13], it is assumed to be safer. Fentanyl has a negative chronotropic effect [14] and it reduces the neurologic, endocrine, and metabolic responses to surgical stress [15].

Initially, Stanley had reported that doses of fentanyl as low as 20 μg/kg provided adequate anesthesia and did not increase either the heart rate or blood pressure during endotracheal intubation; and with a total dose of up to 40 to 60 μg/kg there were no significant hemodynamic changes before cardiopulmonary bypass. Late in 1980, however, de Lange, Stanley, and Boscoe [16] reported that the amount of fentanyl required to depress cardiovascular reflexes was higher when the same protocol was repeated in a different population. Also in 1980, Barash et al [17] reported that with doses of 75 μg/kg plus 100% oxygen there was no significant change in ventricular function.

Such repeated reports promoted fentanyl as the main anesthetic agent providing hemodynamic stability for patients with CAD; however, under no circumstances can this statement be unqualified. Further clinical studies with fentanyl anesthesia for patients with CAD demonstrated that hemodynamic changes with fentanyl anesthesia do occur, although less frequently than those observed with morphine or inhalational anesthetics. As with morphine, the addition of nitrous oxide to fentanyl anesthesia resulted in ventricular depression. Also, Lunn et al [18] found that the use of 60% nitrous oxide together with fentanyl, 70 μg/kg, resulted in tachycardia, decreased cardiac output, and increased systemic vascular resistance.

In 1980 Lappas et al [19] used fentanyl, 75 μg/kg, and diazepam for induction of anesthesia, and pointed out that this did not block the sympathetic cardiovascular reflexes. Waller et al [20] used 50 μg/kg fentanyl without significant hemodynamic changes, but after administration of pancuronium bromide there was significant tachycardia and hypertension. Also Zurick et al [21] reported that even with the use of very large doses of fentanyl, 100 to 150 μg/kg, for induction, together with pancuronium bromide, there was an increase in the heart rate without changes in blood pressure. A good reason for the conflicting reports was the different designs of the studies, mainly the doses used, points of measurement in relation to endotracheal intubation, type of muscle relaxant used, and timing of drug administration. It is clear from reviewing this literature, however, that the hemodynamic changes that accompany fentanyl anesthesia are minimal.

Currently, our anesthesia technique for patients undergoing coronary artery bypass surgery is as follows. Beta-blocker therapy is continued until the morning of surgery. Premedication consists of morphine, 0.15 mg/kg; scopolamine, 0.4 mg, and long-acting nitroglycerine, a 10-cm patch. For induction of anesthesia we use fentanyl, 40 to 60 μg/kg, and either pancuronium bromide or a combination of two-thirds metocurine, one-third pancuronium. One-fourth of the muscle relaxant is administered prior to the fentanyl and the rest of the intubating dose is given simultaneously during fentanyl administration. For maintenance of anesthesia we use either increments of fentanyl, 5 to 10 μg/kg, or an inhalational agent, depending on the patient's hemodynamic status.

We have found that this technique is flexible and provides the best hemodynamic stability for normotensive, hypertensive, or hypotensive patients. Occasionally, β-adrenergic blockers and/or vasodilators are required to adjust episodes of hypertension and/or tachycardia. The prevalence of hypotension with this technique is very low.

SUFENTANIL ANESTHESIA AND PATIENTS WITH CAD

Recently, sufentanil was recommended as a better alternative than fentanyl for opioid anesthesia in patients with CAD. Initial animal and human studies demonstrated that sufentanil anesthesia minimized intraoperative hypertension and tachycardia [22,23] reduced myocardial oxygen consumption [24], and produced shorter postoperative respiratory depression [25].

Sufentanil is a potent synthetic opioid, structurally related to fentanyl, five to ten times more potent, and with a safety margin 90 times that of fentanyl [26]. It has a faster onset and shorter duration of action. Sufentanil is highly specific to opioid receptors and produces electroencephalographic (EEG) signs of anesthesia with relatively small doses; therefore, possibly it does not interfere with other receptors as much as with cardiovascular receptors.

Initial studies of sufentanil anesthesia in patients with CAD using pancuronium bromide as a muscle relaxant demonstrated a high frequency of tachycardia and hypertension, 28% and 47% respectively [27]. In later studies, as droperidol was added, the frequency of hypertension was insignificant and the incidence of tachycardia dropped to 7.4% [28].

In 1982 de Lange et al [29] used sufentanil and succinylcholine for induction, followed by pancuronium bromide for muscle relaxation. They compared changes in hemodynamic variables with this technique to those with fentanyl. Tachycardia and hypertension occurred less than with fentanyl anesthesia; however, 6% to 20% of patients anesthetized with sufentanil developed a rise in blood pressure, mainly prior to cardiopulmonary bypass, that required management [29].

Independently, Sebel and Bovill [30] also studied sufentanil anesthesia, 15 μg/kg, with pancuronium bromide, 0.8 mg/kg, in the same types of patients and reported that overall there were no significant cardiovascular changes after induction of anesthesia. Sixteen of 40 patients (40%) developed an increase in blood pressure immediately after skin incision [30], however, which was controlled in 12 of them by additional doses of sufentanil.

During 1981–1982, our group studied and compared sufentanil versus halothane anesthesia for patients with CAD [31]. We also studied and compared the effects of different muscle relaxants and different doses of sufentanil [32]. We selected patients without severe left ventricular impairment, valvular dysfunction, hypertension, or diabetes, or with a major systemic disease. Beta-blocker therapy was continued until the time of surgery, and all received the premedication mentioned with our fentanyl technique.

The following hemodynamic variables were monitored and measured: heart rate, mean arterial blood pressure, cardiac output, pulmonary capillary wedge pressure, calculated systemic vascular resistance, and cardiac index. Measurements were taken before induction (baseline measurement), one minute prior to intubation, one minute after intubation, one minute prior to incision, one minute after incision, one minute after sternotomy, and immediately before cannulation.

We also reported awakening time (time from the end of surgery until the patient became responsive to verbal stimuli); duration of postoperative respiratory depression (time from the end of surgery until the patient was able to maintain adequate ventilation to be extubated, defined as ability to generate an inspiratory pressure rate of -20 cm H_2O and

tidal volume above 1000 ml); and the incidence of recall and global evaluation by both the patient and the anesthesiologist as to the quality of anesthesia and recovery.

EVALUATION OF SUFENTANIL-PANCURONIUM VERSUS HALOTHANE IN PATIENTS WITH CAD UNDERGOING CORONARY ARTERY SURGERY

We compared sufentanil anesthesia to halothane anesthesia using pancuronium bromide as a muscle relaxant in both groups. We used relatively large doses of both sufentanil and halothane. Sufentanil was administered at the rate of 5 μg/kg/min with a total dose of 15 to 20 μg/kg for the surgical procedure and pancuronium bromide, total dose of 0.12 to 0.15 μg/kg, for induction.

The results of this study demonstrated that with sufentanil, anesthesia was adequate without incidence of recall. The patients evaluated anesthesia as satisfactory. Administration of 1.5 to 2 mg of pancuronium bromide prior to the administration of sufentanil and the administration of the balance of the muscle relaxant concomitantly with sufentanil prevented muscle rigidity in all patients. With the use of such large doses of sufentanil, return to consciousness and postoperative respiratory depression were rather prolonged compared with results following halothane anesthesia (Table 36.1).

TABLE 36.1.   Time to return to consciousness

Agents	Minimum	Maximum	Median
Halothane-pancuronium	0.9	4.5	2.7
Sufentanil-pancuronium	1.0	8.9	3.5
Sufentanil-metocurine	0.3	4.0	2.3
Sufentanil-metocurine (EEG)	0.3	5.5	2.6

Hemodynamic Changes

The hemodynamic changes that accompanied sufentanil anesthesia and pancuronium bromide were rather mixed. Basically, the cardiac output and pulmonary capillary wedge pressure were maintained; if any change occurred, it was an increase in cardiac output and decrease in wedge presure. This was a definite advantage over halothane anesthesia, which was accompanied by a significant increase in wedge pressure after intubation and by decreased cardiac output, significantly so after sternotomy.

Contrary to previous reports and studies, we found a significant increase in the heart rate at all points of measurement. Nine of 17 patients had episodes of tachycardia (above 110 beats per minute) that required treatment regardless of continuation of beta-blocker therapy. There was also a high incidence of hypertension whereby patients developed a rise in blood pressure (20% above baseline values) that required control with peripheral vasodilators (Table 36.2).

The increases in heart rate and blood pressure were rather disturbing in patients with CAD, as these changes can shift the balance between myocardial oxygen supply and demand to the negative side. We postulated that such undesirable changes in heart rate and blood pressure may well be due to the use of large doses of pancuronium bromide. Indeed, we used a total dose of 0.12 to 0.15 mg/kg, versus 0.08 mg/kg used by Sebel and the initial use of succinylcholine in de Lange's study. These results prompted our next two studies, using a different muscle relaxant and smaller doses of sufentanil in one of them.

EVALUATION OF SUFENTANIL-PANCURONIUM VERSUS SUFENTANIL-METOCURINE IN PATIENTS WITH CAD UNDERGOING CORONARY ARTERY SURGERY

In this study, we followed the same protocol and used the same dose of sufentanil, but substituted pancuronium bromide with 0.35 to 0.5 mg/kg doses of metocurine.

The incidence of tachycardia and hypertension was much higher when pancuronium bromide was used [32]. The differences in heart rate and blood pressure between the groups were not only statistically significant but clinically desirable at all points of measurement. The indications for either vasodilators or beta blockers to control the rises in heart rate and blood pressure were infrequent (Table 36.2). It became apparent that the difference in the occurrence of hypertension and tachycardia between the study groups was related to the differences in the pharmacologic properties of the muscle relaxants. Pancuronium bromide has vagolytic, sympathomimetic, and direct myocardial stimulant effects; it can increase both heart rate and blood pressure in doses that produce muscle relaxation [33–35]. Such effects usually are not apparent with halothane, which is a myocardial depressant, or with morphine, which produces venodilation and occasionally hypotension. Increases in heart rate and blood pressure were observed when pancuronium bromide was used with fentanyl [20,21] anesthesia, but not to the extent or frequency observed when it was combined with sufentanil.

TABLE 36.2. Occurrence of hypertension and tachycardia that required treatment

Agents	Patients Studied	Hyper-tension Requiring Treatment	Tachy-cardia Requiring Treatment
Halothane-pancuronium	12	12	4
Sufentanil-pancuronium	17	16	9
Sufentanil-metocurine	15	8	1
Sufentanil-metocurine (EEG)	15	9	1

The exaggerated effect of pancuronium bromide on heart rate and blood pressure when used with sufentanil can be explained on the basis of the high potency and high specificity of sufentanil to opioid receptors. Due to this high specificity, very small doses can produce EEG signs of anesthesia and may not interfere with the cardiovascular receptors or reflexes. Therefore, when sufentanil was combined with pancuronium bromide, the cardiovascular effects of the latter were augmented.

The combination of sufentanil-metocurine was accompanied by minimum hemodynamic changes. Unlike pancuronium bromide, metocurine does not block the muscarine receptors or produce tachycardia. Also, it does not have sympathetic or direct myocardial stimulant effects [36,37].

This study demonstrated that selection of muscle relaxant is a critical determinant of the suitability of using sufentanil anesthesia for patients with coronary artery disease. It also emphasized the advantages of sufentanil, namely, that it does not cause myocardial depression and it sustains cardiac output and blood pressure with minimum occurrence of tachycardia or hypotension.

SUFENTANIL REQUIREMENTS FOR ANESTHESIA AS DETERMINED BY THE ELECTROENCEPHALOGRAM

We performed this study to determine: (a) the smallest dose of sufentanil that can produce EEG signs of anesthesia (low-frequency wave forms with little or no frequency response in the processed EEG); (b) the effect of such small doses on hemodynamic variables at the same time points of measurement used in our previous two studies; and (c) the relationship between the total dose of sufentanil administered and the time to return to consciousness and the duration of postoperative respiratory

depression. For monitoring we used the Neurometrics monitor, which displays a computer-processed EEG. The clinical status was correlated with the EEG pattern as described by Smith et al [38].

Cortical depression was observed in doses as low as 2.6 to 3.7 µg/kg. Changes in EEG patterns took place in less than 30 seconds (stage 4) and the EEG became profoundly depressed in a mean time of 72 seconds. Sufentanil, although it is a very short-acting opioid, produced long-acting central nervous system depression (anesthesia lightening starting on or about 97 ± 47 minutes in 50% of the patients). The remainder of the patients stayed in clinical stage 4 until the end of surgery (three to four hours). There was no epileptiform activity in any patient.

The results of this study demonstrated that a small dose of sufentanil can produce effective anesthesia (2.6 µg/kg). A total dose of ± 10 µg sufentanil was adequate for a surgical procedure that lasted three hours, compared with the 25 µg/kg we had used in our previous studies. With such small doses, the awakening time and the time to extubation were very much reduced (Table 36.3). Early recovery from the effects of anesthesia is desirable, as it allows easy evaluation of the patient's neurologic status as well as shortening the need for mechanical support of

TABLE 36.3. Time to extubation

Agents	Minimum	Maximum	Median
Halothane-pancuronium	6.9	30.1	11.0
Sufentanil-pancuronium	9.7	33.1	16.5
Sufentanil-metocurine	6.4	21.9	15.0
Sufentanil-metocurine (EEG)	8.7	20.4	12.5

ventilation. These are two major advantages with respect to the workload in intensive care recovery units and the cost of the patients' stay in such units.

CONCLUSIONS

Sufentanil is a potentially good anesthetic for patients with coronary artery disease for a number of reasons. Its use did not cause myocardial depression; both the cardiac output and pulmonary capillary wedge pressure were maintained. When sufentanil was combined with a muscle relaxant that does not have significant cardiovascular effects (metocurine), the frequency of tachycardia and hypertension was minimal. Sufentanil doses of 2.6 to 3.0 μg/kg were adequate for induction of anesthesia, and a total dose of 10 to 12 μg/kg produced adequate anesthesia for procedures lasting three to four hours, with short duration of postoperative respiratory depression. Most patients were extubated within 16.5 hours. With proper timing in the administration of muscle relaxants, the occurrence of chest wall rigidity was negligible. Patients compared sufentanil very favorably to halothane, and there were no instances of recall. Finally, vasoactive drugs and beta blockers were only occasionally needed to adjust the hemodynamics.

I must emphasize that our studies were performed in patients with only mild to moderately impaired ventricular function and without hypertension or accompanying valve lesions. The results could have been different in other categories of patients. Clearly, it has to be stated that more clinical experience is needed with sufentanil anesthesia, particularly in different categories of patients and with the new family of muscle relaxants.

Finally, results obtained from experimental studies and controlled protocols may not be easy to duplicate in clinical practice. In a clinical setup the hemodynamic changes are the sum of the effects of the preexisting hemodynamic condition, preoperative therapy, preoperative medication, muscle relaxants used, anesthetic agent used, and, obviously, the method of administration and techniques of the individual anesthesiologist.

REFERENCES

1. Hasbrouck JD. Morphine anesthesia for open-heart surgery. Ann Thorac Surg 1970;10:364–9.
2. Lowenstein E, Hallowell P, Levine FH, et al. Cardiovascular response to large doses of intravenous morphine in man. N Engl J Med 1969;281:1389–93.
3. Lowenstein E. Morphine "anesthesia"—a perspective. Anesthesiology 1971;35:563–5.
4. Dalton B. Anaesthesia and coronary heart disease. J Ir Coll Phys Surg 1972;2:36–40.
5. Stoelting RK, Gibbs PS. Hemodynamic effects of morphine and morphine-nitrous oxide in valvular heart disease and coronary-artery disease. Anesthesiology 1973;38:45–52.
6. Conahan TJ III, Ominsky AJ, Wollman H, et al. A prospective random comparison of halothane and morphine for open-heart anesthesia: one year's experience. Anesthesiology 1973;38:528–35.
7. Lappas DG, Geha D, Fischer JE, et al. Filling pressures of the heart and pulmonary circulation of the patient with coronary-artery disease after large intravenous doses of morphine. Anesthesiology 1975;42:153–9.
8. Lappas DG, Buckley MJ, Laver MB, et al. Left ventricular performance and pulmonary circulation following addition of nitrous oxide to morphine during coronary-artery surgery. Anesthesiology 1975;43:61–9.
9. Kistner JR, Miller ED, Lake CL, et al. Indices of myocardial oxygenation during coronary-artery revascularization in man with morphine versus halothane anesthesia. Anesthesiology 1979;50:324–30.
10. Stanley TH, Gray NH, Stanford W, Armstrong R. The effects of high-dose morphine on fluid and blood requirements in open heart operations. Anesthesiology 1973;38:536.

11. Stanley TH, Webster LR. Anesthetic requirements and cardiovascular effects of fentanyl-oxygen and fentanyl-diazepam-oxygen anesthesia in man. Anesth Analg (Cleve) 1978;57:411.

12. Stanley TH, Philbin DM, Coggins CH. Fentanyl-oxygen anesthesia for coronary artery surgery: cardiovascular and antidiuretic hormone responses. Can Anaesth Soc J 1979;26:168.

13. de Castro J, van de Water A, Wouters L, Xhonneux R, Reneman R, Kay B. Comparative study of cardiovascular, neurological and metabolic side-effects of eight narcotics in dogs. Acta Anaesthesiol Belg 1979;30:5.

14. Vusse GJ, van der Belle H, van Gerven W, Kruger R, Reneman RS. Acute effect of fentanyl on haemodynamics and myocardial carbohydrate utilization and phosphate release during ischaemia. Br J Anaesth 1979;51:927.

15. Hall GM. Analgesia and the metabolic response to surgery. Stress-free anaesthesia. International Congress Symposium series no. 3. London: Royal Society of Medicine, 1978:22.

16. de Lange S, Stanley TH, Boscoe MJ. Fentanyl-oxygen anesthesia: comparison of anesthetic requirements and cardiovascular responses in Salt Lake City, Utah and Leiden, Holland. Abstracts of the Seventh World Congress of Anaesthesiology, Hamburg. Amsterdam: Excerpta Medica, 1980:313.

17. Barash P, Kopriva C, Giles R, et al. Global ventricular function and intubation: radionuclear profiles (abstract). Anesthesiology 1980;53:S109.

18. Lunn JK, Stanley TH, Eisele JH, Webster L, Woodward A. High-dose fentanyl anaesthesia for coronary artery surgery: plasma fentanyl concentrations and influence of nitrous oxide on cardiovascular responses. Anesth Analg (Cleve) 1979;58:390.

19. Lappas DG, Fahmy NR, Slater EE, et al. Catecholamines, renin and cardiovascular responses to fentanyl-diazepam anesthesia. Anesthesiology 1980;53:S14.

20. Waller J, Hug CC Jr, Nagle DM, et al. Hemodynamic changes during fentanyl oxygen anesthesia for aorto-coronary bypass operations. Anesthesiology 1981;55:212–17.

21. Zurick AM, Urzua J, Yared JP, et al. Comparison of hemodynamic and hormonal effects of large single-dose fentanyl anesthesia and halothane/nitrous oxide anesthesia for coronary artery surgery. Anesth Analg (Cleve) 1981;60:521–5.

22. de Castro J. Practical applications and limitations of analgesic anaesthesia. Acta Anaesthesiol Belg 1976;27:107–1218.

23. van de Wall J, Lauwers PL, Andriaensen H. Double-blind comparison of fentanyl and sufentanil in anaesthesia. Acta Anaesthesiol Belg 1976;27:129–35.

24. Hempelmann G, Seitz V, Piepenbrock S, et al. Vergleichende Untersuchungen zu kardialen und vaskulären Effekten des neuens Analgetikums Sufentanil (R 30730) und Fentanyl. Prakt Anaesth 1978;13:429–37.

25. Kay B, Rolly G. Duration of analgesic supplements to anaesthesia: a double-blind comparison between morphine, fentanyl and sufentanil. Acta Anaesthesiol Belg 1977;28:25–32.

26. de Castro J, van de Water A, Wouters L, et al. Comparative study of cardiovascular, neurological and metabolic side effects of eight narcotics in dogs. Acta Anaesthesiol Belg 1979;30:5–99.

27. Dubois-Primo J, Dewachter B, Massaut J. Analgesic anaesthesia with fentanyl and sufentanil in coronary surgery. A double-blind study. Acta Anaesthesiol Belg 1979;2:113–26.

28. Dubois-Primo J. Double-blind study comparing fentanyl and sufentanil in 150 patients. Symposium fentanyl-sufentanil. Beerse, March 31-April 1, 1977.

29. de Lange S, Boscoe MJ, Stanley TH, Pace N. Comparison of sufentanil-O_2 and fentanyl-O_2 for coronary artery surgery. Anesthesiology 1982;56:112–18.

30. Sebel PS, Bovill JG. Cardiovascular effects of sufentanil anesthesia. Anesth Analg (Cleve) 1982;61:115–19.

31. Khoury GF, Estafanous FG, Samonte AF, et al. Evaluation of sufentanil-O_2 versus halothane-N_2O_2 anesthesia for coronary artery surgery. Anesthesiology 1982;57:A290.

32. Khoury GF, Estafanous FG, Zurick AM, et al. Sufentanil/pancuronium versus sufentanil/metocurine anesthesia for coronary artery surgery. Anesthesiology 1982;57:A47.

33. Kelman GR, Kennedy BR. Cardiovascular effects of pancuronium in man. Br J Anaesth 1971;43:335–8.

34. Segarra Domenech J, Carlos Garcia R, Rodriquez Sasiain JM, Quintana Loyola A, Santafe Oroz J. Pancuronium bromide: an indirect sympathomimetic agent. Br J Anaesth 1976;48:1143–8.

35. Duke PC, Fung H, Gartner J. The myocardial effects of pancuronium. Can Anaesth Soc J 1975;22(6):680–6.

36. Zaidan J, Philbin DM, Antonio R, Savarese J. Hemodynamic effects of metocurine in patients with coronary artery disease receiving propranolol. Anesth Analg (Cleve) 1977;56:255–9.

37. Zaidan JR, Kaplan JA. Cardiovascular effects of metocurine in patients with aortic stenosis. Anesthesiology 1982;56:395–7.

38. Smith NT, Demetrescu M. The EEG during high-dose fentanyl anesthesia. Anesthesiology 1980;53:S7.

37 CONSIDERATIONS ON THE USE OF OPIOIDS IN CARDIOVASCULAR SURGERY

Theodore H. Stanley and Joost van der Maaten

Before the first patient was ever given large doses of fentanyl anesthesia in Salt Lake City, somewhere between 150 and 200 dogs were anesthetized with doses ranging from 2 to 5 mg per kilogram of body weight. In these studies numerous other drugs were often used, many kinds of muscle relaxants evaluated, and many adjuvants to fentanyl studied. On the basis of this work, certain impressions were formed that resulted in the original technique described in our first paper on fentanyl anesthesia and in many of our subsequent articles.

As our human and animal experience grew, the technique we used became subtly refined. On the basis of numerous years of experience with patients undergoing surgery for cardiac disease, the approach we take is that muscle relaxants should be used rationally and with a great deal of caution, especially when one is dealing with opioids. This chapter shares some of the conclusions we have reached based on our work with narcotic anesthetics in cardiovascular surgery.

HEMODYNAMIC EFFECTS OF THE MUSCLE RELAXANTS

One of the strong impressions we still retain is that muscle relaxants, as Dr. Estafanous indicates (Chapter 36), can have an effect on hemodynamics during narcotic anesthesia. One of the early alfentanil studies demonstrated this fact. In that study, 1.5 mg of pancuronium was used as a pretreatment drug to prevent muscle rigidity. Three minutes after administration of a 1.5 mg/70 kg dose, small increases in systolic blood pressure and heart rate were observed.

We have always used succinylcholine for laryngoscopy and endotracheal intubation because of the relative absence of hemodynamic effects associated with the drug after premedication with atropine or other belladonna preparations 60 to 90 minutes prior to induction of anesthesia. Our studies in dogs suggested that a belladonna premedication was also important in minimizing the sometimes impressive vagal effects (decrease in heart rate) of an anesthetic dose of virtually any narcotic.

In the early human studies, succinylcholine was used not only to enable rapid paralysis, but to allow patients to recover rapidly from paralysis. This approach was adopted to see if, in fact, the patients were anesthetized. At the time that approach was begun, we talked to the patients before and throughout the surgical procedure to reevaluate whether they were anesthetized. Often we found that after what we had considered an adequate induction dose of fentanyl, patients would recover and respond to verbal command. Additional doses of fentanyl were required to ensure that patients became nonresponsive again and remained so throughout the operation.

Muscle relaxation was our original rationale for using these agents. Subsequently we used relaxants in our studies and our clinical practice for their hemodynamic effects as well. This required careful attention to choice of agent and dosage. When patients have attained satisfactory hemodynamic status after induction of anesthesia, the relaxant should not alter that status. Therefore a large dose of pancuronium as a bolus for endotracheal intubation would be inappropriate. Metubine would be a better choice because it is an agent that causes minimal hemodynamic alterations after induction; pancuronium in small increments is another alternative.

Of course, after smooth anesthetic induction, especially in a hypertensive patient or one with a high heart rate, it makes no sense to use 0.1 mg/kg of pancuronium for muscle relaxation for laryngoscopy and intubation. Similarly, this approach makes little sense after endotracheal intubation. On the other hand, in a patient who is hypertensive even before induction of anesthesia, one can use d-tubocurarine for its ganglionic blocking and sympatholytic actions without being concerned about hypertension or, usually, tachycardia.

DOSAGE OF THE OPIOIDS AND MUSCLE RELAXANTS

Another important point to consider is dosage. The right dose of a narcotic opioid is extremely important, as Dr. Estafanous points out (Chapter 36), but it is difficult to predict. Certainly there is no definable "magic" dose that is effective in every patient. Determinations of the median or 90% effective dose are useful for understanding relative potency, but they should not be relied upon in administering induction or even maintenance doses of opioids. Inhalation anesthesia is not conducted by producing minimum alveolar concentrations of 1 MAC or 1.5 MAC or 1.32 MAC—an anesthetic is given to achieve a desired effect, and there is no reason to use narcotics in any other way.

There is no magic dose for fentanyl, just as there is none for the muscle relaxants. Because we give to effect, clinical skill is as relevant to our practice today as it has always been. New agents may make it easier and safer to give to effect, but we still must observe the patient and monitor the drug's effect to determine adequacy of anesthesia. A skilled anesthesiologist can block hemodynamic responses to endotracheal intubation with an inhalation anesthetic as well as with fentanyl. The only difference is that it requires a little more skill with an inhalation agent.

Regardless of how one uses opioids, I believe it is important to establish what the induction dosage requirement is. The "sleep dose" varies with premedication, disease, cardiac output, and probably a host of other factors. By giving a large, fixed magic dose, one can never tell what the induction dose is, and therefore it is difficult to predict how much additional drug is needed.

CONCLUSION

Our experience with the narcotic opioids has led us to believe that several considerations are of primary importance when these agents are used in cardiovascular surgery. A cautious approach is warranted, with careful attention to choice of muscle relaxant and its dosage and to the induction dose of opioid. Because these agents are administered until the desired effect occurs, achieving the proper dose depends on the clinical proficiency of the anesthesiologist. Clinical skill remains central to effective practice.

38 OPIOID ANESTHESIA FOR VALVE REPLACEMENT SURGERY: EXPERIENCE WITH FENTANYL, SUFENTANIL, AND ALFENTANIL

James G. Bovill, Patrick J. Warren, Harry B. van Wezel, and Martine H. Hoeneveld

The use of high doses of opioids to produce anesthesia for patients undergoing cardiac surgery is extremely popular. This technique originated with the observation in 1969 by Lowenstein and colleagues [1] that morphine, 0.5 to 3 mg per kilogram of body weight, given to patients with severe aortic valve disease, produced surgical anesthesia with minimal hemodynamic disturbances. Indeed, induction of anesthesia with morphine often improved the cardiovascular status of these patients, possibly due to the accompanying reduction in vascular resistance and cardiac workload.

Subsequent to this report, morphine anesthesia gained widespread acceptance among cardiac anesthesiologists. Within a few years, however, it became apparent that the use of morphine in high doses was not always trouble free. Several significant complications were reported, including hypotension possibly related to venodilation and histamine release, hypertension during or after sternotomy, and increased intraoperative and postoperative blood and fluid requirements [2,3]. These problems became accentuated when the technique was used to produce anesthesia for patients undergoing coronary artery surgery. Whereas the patients who had valve replacement surgery were often in poor physical state as a result of long-standing cardiac failure and extensive myocardial damage, those who underwent coronary artery surgery were often relatively healthy without a history of chronic cardiac disease. In this group of patients it was found that much larger doses of morphine—sometimes 10 to 12 mg/kg—were required to produce anesthesia.

In an attempt to overcome these problems, Stanley and Webster [4] began using fentanyl in a dose of 50 to 75 µg/kg as an alternative opioid anesthetic. In patients with mitral valve disease they found that, with the exception of 15% to 18% decreases in blood pressure and heart rate, fentanyl had no other significant influence on hemodynamics. Subsequently, fentanyl in doses up to 150 μg/kg has been extensively evaluated and in the 1980s is probably the most widely used opioid in cardiac anesthesia.

Recently, two new fentanyl derivatives, sufentanil and alfentanil, have become available for clinical investigation. Sufentanil is approximately ten times as potent as fentanyl and in animal experiments has an extremely high safety margin, the ratio of median effective to median lethal dose (ED_{50}/LD_{50}) being 25,200 [5]. The equivalent ratios for morphine and fentanyl are 67 and 270 respectively. The elimination half-life of sufentanil (164 minutes) is shorter than that of fentanyl [6]. Alfentanil is one-third to one-fifth less potent than fentanyl [7] and has a very short elimination half-life of only 95 minutes [8–10]. Both of these new opioids have been successfully used to produce anesthesia for patients undergoing cardiac surgery, with hemodynamic stability comparable to that of fentanyl [11–14].

All these published reports have involved almost exclusively patients with coronary artery disease undergoing coronary artery revascularization. The problems these patients present to the anesthesiologist are often very different from those that occur when anesthetizing patients with severe aortic or mitral valve disease. In the latter group, the clinical manifestations of the valvular disease are frequently the result of a chronic disease process such as rheumatic carditis, which may have severely compromised myocardial function. In addition, the mechanical abnormalities associated with disruption of valve function can impose severe volume or pressure loads on the ventricle, resulting in additional interference with cardiac function. These patients are often extremely sensitive to alterations in myocardial contractility, cardiac rhythms, or changes in vascular resistance. It is therefore important to choose an anesthetic technique that will cause minimal disturbances to these variables.

Our initial experience using high-dose opioid anesthesia with fentanyl and the newer drugs, sufentanil and alfentanil, for patients undergoing valve replacement has been favorable and is reported here.

METHODS

Sixty patients undergoing elective surgery for either aortic or mitral valve replacement were studied. They were allocated randomly to three groups of 20 patients, each group receiving fentanyl, sufentanil, or alfentanil for anesthesia. Eight patients in both the sufentanil and alfentanil groups and seven patients in the fentanyl group underwent mitral valve surgery. The remaining patients underwent aortic valve surgery. Patients in the three groups were comparable with respect to age and weight. The overall mean ($\pm$ SEM) age was 61 $\pm$ 2.7 years and the mean ($\pm$ SEM) weight was 69 $\pm$ 2.6 kg.

Technique of Anesthesia

All patients were given oral lorazepam, 3 to 5 mg, 1.5 hours before surgery. On arrival in the operating room, electrocardiographic electrodes were applied and a radial artery cannula and two peripheral infusion cannulas were inserted percutaneously under local analgesia. A flow-directed pulmonary artery catheter was inserted.

After preoxygenation, pancuronium, 2 mg, was given intravenously, followed one minute later by the induction dose of the appropriate drug administered over a two- to four-minute period. The preinduction dose of pancuronium was given for two reasons: to prevent opioid-induced muscle rigidity and to minimize the bradycardia that high doses of opioids can produce. The induction doses of the three drugs were as follows:

Fentanyl, 75 μg/kg
Sufentanil, 15 μg/kg
Alfentanil, 125 μg/kg

When the patient became unresponsive to verbal commands, additional pancuronium, 6 mg, was given in divided doses.

Three minutes after the induction dose had been given, the patient's trachea was intubated and the lungs ventilated with an oxygen-air mixture (FIO_2 = 0.5). Ventilation was adjusted to achieve an end-tidal carbon dioxide concentration of 4.5% to 5.0%. Because of the short duration of action of alfentanil, patients in this group received a continuous infusion, 0.5 mg/kg/hr, to maintain surgical anesthesia. Patients in the other groups were given additional doses of either fentanyl, 25 µg/kg, or sufentanil, 5 µg/kg, immediately before the skin incision.

During anesthesia and surgery, the electrocardiogram and arterial, right atrial, and pulmonary arterial pressures were continuously recorded. Pulmonary artery capillary wedge pressure and cardiac output (thermodilution) were measured intermittently. Heart rate was determined from the electrocardiogram. When atrial fibrillation was present, heart rate and pressure data at each measurement point were derived from the paper recording and were taken as the average value over at least one minute of recording.

Statistical Analysis

Data were analyzed using two-way analysis of variance. Where indicated, a modified t test was used to identify significant differences between or within groups, using critical values of p calculated according to the method of Bonferroni [15]; $p < 0.05$ was considered significant.

RESULTS

The preinduction (control) hemodynamic variables and the changes from the control value after induction of anesthesia, endotracheal intubation, skin incision, and sternotomy are given in Table 38.1 (aortic valve replacement) and Table 38.2 (mitral valve replacement). Control values were not statistically different among the three anesthetic groups although there were some significant differences between patients with aortic and mitral valve disease. Mean pulmonary artery pressure in patients with mitral valve disease was significantly higher ($p < 0.05$) than in those with aortic disease in the fentanyl and alfentanil but not in the sufentanil group. Control pulmonary capillary wedge pressure was also higher in those having mitral valve replacement who received fentanyl. In the sufentanil group the control values for systemic vascular resistance were significantly higher for mitral valve replacement. Pulmonary vascular resistance preinduction was also higher in patients having mitral valve surgery in the fentanyl and alfentanil groups but not in those receiving sufentanil.

Changes during Anesthesia and Surgery

With the exception of mean arterial blood pressure (MABP) and systemic vascular resistance (SVR), there were no significant changes from control hemodynamic variables in any of the groups at induction, intubation, or skin incision, or after sternotomy.

In patients undergoing mitral valve replacement there was no significant change in MABP or SVR at any time in the alfentanil group. Mean arterial pressure decreased by an average of 24.5 mm Hg ($p < 0.01$) after induction of anesthesia in patients given sufentanil and was still less than control value at skin incision. Systemic vascular resistance also decreased after induction of anesthesia in this group, although the change from control was not statistically significant. In the fentanyl group, MABP and SVR increased significantly above control after sternotomy.

Among patients having aortic valve replacement, MABP was significantly higher than control in the fentanyl group at two minutes after sternotomy and in all groups

TABLE 38.1. Control hemodynamic values and changes from control in three groups of patients undergoing aortic valve surgery anesthetized with fentanyl (F; N = 13), sufentanil (S; N = 12), or alfentanil (A; N = 12)*

Determination		Control Value	Maximum Change from Control at:				
			Induction	Intubation	Incision	Sternotomy +2 min	Sternotomy +5 min
MABP (mm Hg)	F	86.1 ± 3.79	−6.5 ± 2.83	−1.2 ± 2.60	6.6 ± 2.95	12.3 ± 2.85‡	17.4 ± 3.81‡
	S	85.6 ± 4.46	−5.8 ± 3.82	−3.8 ± 2.56	4.3 ± 2.72	6.4 ± 3.15	8.6 ± 3.17†
	A	81.8 ± 4.81	−6.0 ± 3.97	−1.2 ± 3.90	3.7 ± 3.25	6.1 ± 4.02	9.3 ± 4.55†
HR (beats/min)	F	77.0 ± 2.98	−2.0 ± 2.07	−1.4 ± 2.51	−4.9 ± 2.95	−1.4 ± 3.15	+2.8 ± 3.83
	S	76.3 ± 3.86	2.3 ± 3.94	2.9 ± 5.25	−1.5 ± 4.64	2.9 ± 5.72	7.4 ± 6.00
	A	74.1 ± 3.49	2.5 ± 1.83	3.3 ± 2.42	5.0 ± 2.77	6.2 ± 2.84	8.9 ± 3.32
RAP (mm Hg)	F	2.6 ± 0.81	0.2 ± 0.55	−0.6 ± 0.56	−0.5 ± 0.64	0.0 ± 0.78	−0.2 ± 0.73
	S	2.2 ± 1.16	1.2 ± 1.12	−0.2 ± 0.87	0.4 ± 0.88	0.3 ± 0.85	0.1 ± 0.90
	A	0.9 ± 0.85	0.7 ± 0.65	1.4 ± 0.52	1.0 ± 0.35	0.3 ± 0.45	0.2 ± 0.36
PAP (mm Hg)	F	14.8 ± 2.28	−0.4 ± 0.65	1.0 ± 0.91	0.8 ± 1.04	1.6 ± 1.34	2.1 ± 1.62
	S	20.3 ± 2.79	−1.9 ± 1.66	−2.1 ± 1.79	−2.8 ± 1.72	−2.1 ± 1.95	−1.8 ± 2.09
	A	17.1 ± 1.71	−1.1 ± 0.77	1.3 ± 1.13	−0.3 ± 1.32	0.2 ± 1.55	1.0 ± 1.38
PCWP (mm Hg)	F	8.2 ± 1.75	−0.4 ± 0.76	0.0 ± 0.84	1.3 ± 0.56	1.8 ± 1.30	1.7 ± 1.26
	S	9.8 ± 1.43	−0.6 ± 1.03	0.0 ± 1.09	−0.3 ± 1.54	0.25 ± 1.57	−0.4 ± 1.41
	A	9.9 ± 1.56	−2.3 ± 1.02	−1.6 ± 1.27	−2.3 ± 1.36	−1.1 ± 1.40	−1.2 ± 1.27
CI (L/min/m²)	F	3.1 ± 0.22	−0.3 ± 0.13	−0.2 ± 0.21	−0.3 ± 0.22	−0.3 ± 0.23	−0.0 ± 0.18
	S	3.4 ± 0.22	−0.3 ± 0.21	−0.2 ± 0.24	−0.3 ± 0.14	−0.2 ± 0.13	−0.1 ± 0.14
	A	2.8 ± 0.16	−0.3 ± 0.18	−0.0 ± 0.17	0.0 ± 0.12	0.0 ± 0.14	−0.1 ± 0.18
SI (ml/beat/m²)	F	39.5 ± 2.28	−3.0 ± 1.96	−1.8 ± 2.94	0.1 ± 3.09	−2.3 ± 3.15	−0.4 ± 2.53
	S	45.3 ± 3.26	−5.1 ± 2.11	−3.0 ± 2.47	−1.8 ± 3.37	−2.8 ± 3.77	−5.0 ± 3.22
	A	39.1 ± 2.61	−4.9 ± 2.14	−2.0 ± 1.92	−3.5 ± 2.10	−3.2 ± 1.85	−3.0 ± 2.08
SVR (dyne-sec/ cm⁻⁵)	F	1224 ± 110.2	8 ± 65.4	26 ± 84.3	231 ± 85.7†	353 ± 103.8‡	299 ± 95.4‡
	S	1126 ± 82.1	−4 ± 60.7	0 ± 94.0	148 ± 78.3	130 ± 76.2	194 ± 80.1†
	A	1312 ± 85.6	−27 ± 48.7	−18 ± 37.3	107 ± 52.1	93 ± 41.5	118 ± 72.0

LVSWI (gm-m/ m²/beat)	F	41.6 ± 3.24	-5.7 ± 2.77	2.4 ± 4.16	3.1 ± 4.46	6.8 ± 3.44
	S	48.1 ± 5.21	-5.9 ± 2.53	-1.6 ± 2.81	-2.3 ± 2.52	-2.0 ± 2.65
	A	40.4 ± 5.37	-6.5 ± 3.64	-3.5 ± 2.74	-1.1 ± 3.22	0.1 ± 3.36
PVR (dyne-sec/ cm⁻⁵)	F	97.3 ± 10.19	14.6 ± 7.02	21.3 ± 17.07	8.5 ± 10.29	10.3 ± 10.12 17.5 ± 11.40
	S	167.5 ± 44.94	-12.0 ± 19.39	-29.3 ± 23.26	-32.1 ± 17.18	-48.9 ± 25.16 -23.8 ± 20.01
	A	110.4 ± 12.73	33.0 ± 14.28	49.8 ± 13.03	53.4 ± 16.78	25.5 ± 12.87 35.8 ± 10.46

*Values are mean ± SEM.

†$p <0.05$ comparison against control value.

‡$p <0.01$ comparison against control value.

MABP = mean arterial blood pressure; HR = heart rate; RAP = right atrial pressure; PAP = pulmonary artery pressure; PCWP = pulmonary capillary wedge pressure; CI = cardiac index; SI = stroke volume index; SVR = systemic vascular resistance; LVSWI = left ventricular stroke work index; PVR = pulmonary vascular resistance.

TABLE 38.2. Control hemodynamic values and changes from control in three groups of patients undergoing mitral valve surgery anesthetized with fentanyl (F; $N = 7$), sufentanil (S; $N = 8$), or alfentanil (A; $N = 8$)*

Determination		Control Value	Maximum Change from Control at:				
			Induction	Intubation	Incision	Sternotomy +2 min	Sternotomy +5 min
MABP (mm Hg)	F	97.2 ± 5.08	−7.4 ± 3.65	−7.3 ± 3.88	4.6 ± 4.41	8.9 ± 3.30†	15.5 ± 5.60‡
	S	96.1 ± 4.12	−24.5 ± 3.64‡	−19.7 ± 4.70‡	−9.1 ± 2.68†	−2.2 ± 2.34	2.0 ± 3.20
	A	86.2 ± 4.24	−7.8 ± 3.74	3.1 ± 4.93	3.8 ± 3.54	5.1 ± 3.66	6.6 ± 4.22
HR (beats/min)	F	70.6 ± 5.93	4.6 ± 4.73	7.3 ± 5.01	15.1 ± 6.56	10.4 ± 5.39	3.4 ± 3.72
	S	83.6 ± 4.89	−2.3 ± 3.23	−8.7 ± 2.67	−7.8 ± 5.44	−4.5 ± 3.46	3.1 ± 4.40
	A	71.3 ± 5.01	4.9 ± 4.30	15.1 ± 6.74	11.1 ± 7.48	14.4 ± 7.20	17.5 ± 7.71
RAP (mm Hg)	F	5.0 ± 2.99	0.8 ± 0.71	0.7 ± 0.90	0.3 ± 0.71	−0.2 ± 1.09	−0.2 ± 0.87
	S	2.2 ± 0.61	−0.7 ± 0.52	−0.6 ± 0.47	−0.4 ± 0.45	−1.2 ± 0.42	−0.6 ± 0.53
	A	3.8 ± 1.10	−0.1 ± 0.50	0.6 ± 0.63	−0.6 ± 0.71	−0.6 ± 0.88	−0.8 ± 0.65
PAP (mm Hg)	F	27.0 ± 3.93	−1.9 ± 2.51	−2.9 ± 2.73	2.2 ± 4.30	−0.8 ± 3.64	0.2 ± 4.42
	S	21.5 ± 2.73	0.7 ± 0.68	−1.8 ± 1.08	−2.5 ± 1.41	−2.3 ± 1.66	−1.6 ± 1.47
	A	23.8 ± 2.50	0.7 ± 3.30	3.6 ± 3.34	−0.9 ± 2.63	−1.0 ± 2.79	1.9 ± 2.86
PCWP (mm Hg)	F	15.7 ± 2.61	−0.2 ± 1.01	0.3 ± 2.13	1.5 ± 3.06	−0.4 ± 2.93	−0.5 ± 2.74
	S	14.3 ± 1.76	10.0 ± 11.78	8.4 ± 11.99	8.5 ± 10.10	8.4 ± 10.16	8.8 ± 10.13
	A	11.5 ± 2.38	3.0 ± 1.29	4.6 ± 1.52	3.3 ± 1.31	3.3 ± 1.20	4.8 ± 1.40
CI (L/min/m²)	F	2.8 ± 0.31	−0.3 ± 0.13	−0.3 ± 0.15	0.1 ± 0.25	0.1 ± 0.22	−0.1 ± 0.19
	S	3.0 ± 0.32	−0.5 ± 0.20	−0.5 ± 0.16	−0.6 ± 0.11	−0.4 ± 0.21	−0.4 ± 0.21
	A	2.8 ± 0.25	−0.5 ± 0.14	−0.3 ± 0.25	−0.4 ± 0.20	−0.3 ± 0.18	−0.1 ± 0.26
SI (ml/beat/m²)	F	39.5 ± 2.28	−4.9 ± 2.01	−6.5 ± 2.29	−6.6 ± 2.18	−4.1 ± 2.67	−4.6 ± 3.42
	S	45.3 ± 3.26	−6.3 ± 3.09	−3.1 ± 1.93	−3.0 ± 2.47	−4.2 ± 1.76	−3.7 ± 3.45
	A	39.1 ± 2.61	−8.6 ± 2.76	−9.7 ± 4.13	−9.4 ± 3.91	−9.1 ± 3.45	−7.6 ± 4.34
SVR (dyne-sec/ cm⁻⁵)	F	1566 ± 114.6	97 ± 133.1	73 ± 102.3	262 ± 260.6	312 ± 267.1	560 ± 273.0‡
	S	1655 ± 166.7	−251 ± 129.4	−178 ± 146.6	168 ± 98.5	310 ± 113.5	299 ± 154.5
	A	1441 ± 144.6	99 ± 88.1	198 ± 177.2	319 ± 89.0	239 ± 87.1	169 ± 127.7

LVSWI (gm-m/ m²/beat)	F	43.9 ± 5.17	−9.5 ± 2.52	−8.6 ± 3.24	−6.5 ± 3.93	0.1 ± 4.36	2.69 ± 4.53
	S	38.8 ± 5.74	−20.8 ± 7.88	−14.5 ± 8.35	−12.1 ± 6.66	−10.3 ± 6.87	−8.6 ± 8.21
	A	40.6 ± 5.23	−13.5 ± 3.37	−10.0 ± 5.07	−9.0 ± 5.31	−8.8 ± 4.72	−7.2 ± 5.70
PVR (dyne-sec/ cm⁻⁵)	F	200.0 ± 39.81	−9.7 ± 15.02	−25.3 ± 19.41	−3.5 ± 27.26	−6.5 ± 45.90	30.9 ± 54.61
	S	159.1 ± 29.62	37.9 ± 32.92	7.4 ± 15.78	8.4 ± 23.63	−2.9 ± 20.90	2.3 ± 19.29
	A	213.7 ± 39.26	−39.9 ± 30.27	−19.3 ± 39.49	−45.9 ± 41.56	−61.9 ± 36.71	−50.8 ± 35.27

*Values are mean ± SEM.

†$p < 0.05$ comparison against control values.

‡$p < 0.01$ comparison against control values.

Abbreviations are the same as in Table 38.1.

at five minutes after sternotomy. The SVR was also increased at these times in the fentanyl and sufentanil groups, but the increase in the alfentanil group did not reach statistical significance.

Two patients in the sufentanil group and one from both the alfentanil and fentanyl groups developed significant hypotension (systolic blood pressure below 80 mm Hg). This was associated with 40% to 60% reduction in right atrial and pulmonary capillary wedge pressure and 25% to 50% decrease in cardiac output. Two of these patients—one in the sufentanil group and one in the fentanyl group—had mitral stenosis. Of the remaining two, one (alfentanil group) had aortic stenosis and one (sufentanil group) had aortic incompetence and stenosis. In all four patients the hypotension was transient and blood pressure returned to acceptable values during endotracheal intubation without the need for specific interventions. With these exceptions, no complications were experienced prior to cardiopulmonary bypass in any of the groups.

DISCUSSION

The results of this study confirm that both fentanyl and its newer derivatives, sufentanil and alfentanil, are capable of producing satisfactory anesthesia for patients undergoing cardiac surgery for valve replacement. In this respect, our results are comparable to those previously reported when these drugs were used in patients with coronary artery disease. De Lange et al [14], in a study comparing sufentanil and fentanyl anesthesia for coronary artery surgery, concluded that sufentanil may be a more suitable drug than fentanyl for this type of surgery because of its ability to control poststernotomy hypertension. In another study during coronary artery surgery [13] there was a 40% incidence of poststernotomy hypertension, which responded to additional sufentanil in 90% of patients.

Alfentanil has also been evaluated in patients undergoing coronary artery surgery. When alfentanil was given by repeated boluses, a very high incidence of hypertension occurred [11], presumably due to inadequate drug concentrations during periods of stress (e.g., sternal spread). When alfentanil is given by continuous infusion, the incidence of hypertension after sternotomy is low [12].

Poststernotomy hypertension associated with increases in systemic vascular resistance was observed in this study. The increase in MABP and SVR was highest in the patients receiving fentanyl. Indeed, in the group of patients undergoing mitral valve surgery, only those given fentanyl showed significant increases in these variables after sternotomy. Although this apparent inability of fentanyl to prevent poststernotomy hypertension may be a result of the pharmacologic properties of the drug, it is perhaps more likely that we were not comparing equally potent doses of the agents studied. If one accepts a potency ratio between fentanyl and sufentanil of 1:10, then the dose of sufentanil used in this study (20 µg/kg) is equivalent to 200 µg/kg fentanyl, that is, two times the dose we actually used. This difference can also explain the greater decrease in MABP during induction of anesthesia with sufentanil in patients with mitral valve disease. The more stable hemodynamics in the alfentanil group probably resulted from the use of a continuous infusion and maintenance of persistently high plasma (and brain) drug concentrations. In another study using infusions of alfentanil at rates similar to those used here, plasma alfentanil concentrations between 1.1 and 2.1 µg/ml were measured (Bovill JG, Sebel PS, unpublished observations, 1981). These concentrations are considerably higher than the probable threshold level required to produce surgical anesthesia [16].

The short elimination half-life of alfentanil makes it feasible to maintain these high plasma and brain concentrations during the most stressful periods of surgery, which in cardiac procedures is almost always the prebypass period. By reducing the infusion rate during the less stimulating periods of surgery, for example, after cardiopulmonary bypass, it should be possible, where desired, to have a patient be awake and capable of spontaneous ventilation within a few hours from the end of surgery. No attempt was made in this study to limit the total dose of alfentanil or to measure recovery times. De Lange et al [11] reported return of consciousness on average 1.4 hours after the end of surgery in a group of patients given doses of alfentanil comparable to those we used. The average time until patients fulfilled their criteria for extubation was four hours. Although it may be possible to minimize the incidence of poststernotomy hypertension considerably by giving large (150 to 200 μg/kg) doses of fentanyl, this is likely to result in many patients needing mechanical ventilation for longer than 24 hours. This would be unacceptable as a routine practice in most cardiac surgical centers.

CONCLUSION

Satisfactory anesthesia for patients undergoing valve surgery can be achieved with fentanyl, sufentanil, or alfentanil. In our study, hemodynamic stability was good and most of the observed differences among the drugs could be explained by noncomparability of doses. Our findings confirm the statement in a recent editorial by Lowenstein and Philbin [17] that "the similarities between opiates are greater than the differences."

REFERENCES

1. Lowenstein E, Hallowell P, Levine FH, Daggett WM, Austen WG, Laver MB. Cardiovascular response to large doses of intravenous morphine in man. N Engl J Med 1969;281:1389–93.
2. Lowenstein E. Morphine anesthesia: a perspective. Anesthesiology 1971;35:563–5.
3. Stanley TH, Gray NH, Stanford W, Armstrong R. The effects of high-dose morphine on fluid and blood requirements in open-

heart surgery. Anesthesiology 1973;38:536–41.
4. Stanley TH, Webster LR. Anesthetic requirements and cardiovascular effects of fentanyl-oxygen and fentanyl-diazepam-oxygen anesthesia in man. Anesth Analg (Cleve) 1978;54:411–6.
5. Niemegeers CJE, Schellekens KHL, van Bever WFM, Janssen PAJ. Sufentanil, a very potent and extremely safe morphine-like compound in mice, rats and dogs. Arzneim Forsch 1976;26:1551–6.
6. Bovill JG, Sebel PS, Blackburn CL, Heykants J. Kinetics of alfentanil and sufentanil: a comparison. Anesthesiology 1981; 55:A174.
7. Kay B. Postoperative pain relief. Use of an on-demand analgesia computer (ODAC) and a comparison of the rate of use of fentanyl and alfentanil. Anaesthesia 1981; 35:949–51.
8. Bovill JG, Sebel PS, Blackburn CL, Heykants J. The pharmacokinetics of alfentanil (R 39209): a new opioid analgesic. Anesthesiology 1982;57:439–43.
9. Bower S, Hull CJ. Comparative pharmacokinetics of fentanyl and alfentanil. Br J Anaesth 1982;54:871–7.
10. Camu F, Gepts E, Rucquoi M, Heykants J. Pharmacokinetics of alfentanil in man. Anesth Analg (Cleve) 1982;61:657–61.
11. de Lange S, Stanley TH, Boscoe MJ. Alfentanil-oxygen anaesthesia for coronary artery surgery. Br J Anaesth 1981;53:1291–6.
12. Sebel PS, Bovill JG, van der Haven A. Cardiovascular effects of alfentanil anaesthesia. Br J Anaesth 1982;54:1185–90.
13. Sebel PS, Bovill JG. Cardiovascular effects of sufentanil anaesthesia. Anesth Analg (Cleve) 1982;61:115–19.
14. de Lange S, Boscoe MJ, Stanley TH, Pace N. Comparison of sufentanil-O₂ and fentanyl-O₂ for coronary artery surgery. Anesthesiology 1982;56:112–18.
15. Wallenstein S, Zucker CL, Fleiss JL. Some statistical methods useful in circulation research. Circ Res 1980;47:1–9.
16. Stanski DR, Hug CC Jr. Alfentanil—a kinetically predictable narcotic analgesic. Anesthesiology 1982;57:435–8.
17. Lowenstein E, Philbin DM. Narcotic "anesthesia" in the eighties. Anesthesiology 1981;55:195–7.

39 THE VALUE OF OPIOIDS IN VALVE REPLACEMENT PROCEDURES

Stephen J. Thomas

Dr. Bovill and colleagues very nicely demonstrated in the preceding chapter that "industrial-strength" narcotics provide hemodynamic stability in patients with either mitral or aortic valvular heart disease who undergo open heart surgery. It seems to matter little whether that narcotic is fentanyl, sufentanil, or alfentanil. The only trace of hemodynamic disturbance occurred in the fentanyl group, where mean arterial pressure increased during sternotomy. With this exception, all of the hemodynamic values remained similar to control. Similar cardiovascular stability has been demonstrated in patients with coronary artery disease [1–3], but this is one of the first reports using this technique in patients with valvular disease. The ultimate role of sufentanil is yet to be determined, since in its hemodynamic effects and duration of action it is very similar to fentanyl. Alfentanil, however, because of its shorter duration of action and its suitability for infusion techniques, may prove extremely useful. The mean time to extubation in Bovill's alfentanil group was only four hours, shorter than that reported with fentanyl or sufentanil.

A few comments seem pertinent concerning the design of the study. The first is that, in common with most other studies evaluating the effects of anesthetics in patients with valve disease, all patients are lumped into one large category regardless of specific valvular lesion. This disregards the physiologic differences between stenotic and regurgitant lesions. Patients with aortic or mitral stenosis usually prefer (in the hemodynamic sense) maintenance of heart rate without either bradycardia or tachycardia. Maintenance of adequate systemic blood pressure is equally important, especially in patients with aortic stenosis. Vasodilators have little to offer this group with the possible exception of patients with severe pulmonary hypertension and right ventricular failure secondary to mitral stenosis. In contrast, modest tachycardia is often beneficial in patients with valvular regurgitation, and forward cardiac flow is almost always improved by afterload reduction. The second comment concerns the choice of muscle relaxant. Since tachycardia may be detrimental in patients with stenotic lesions, metocurine or succinylcholine might be preferable. It would appear that this is more a theoretical objection than a real one, since tachycardia did not occur in this study.

The last aspect of Dr. Bovill's study that deserves comment is the severity of valvular disease present in these patients. The mean cardiac index was greater than 3.0 L/min/m^2, while mean pulmonary artery, right atrial, and pulmonary capillary wedge pressures were all within the normal range. Our intuitive feeling was that the patients who come to valve surgery in New York present a different hemodynamic picture than their cohorts in Amsterdam.

To see if Dr. Bovill's technique was equally effective for the "sicker" denizens of New York, we used a similar protocol with a few notable exceptions. For admission to the study, the mean pulmonary artery pressure had to be above 30 mm Hg. In addition, we used only fentanyl; the other two narcotics were unavailable. We reduced the fentanyl dose because of our uncertainty about the results in these patients; because in Stanley's original report [4] patients became unconscious at 11 µg/kg and the total dose needed for the entire procedure was 50 to 75 µg/kg; and because of two recent cases at our institution where profound hypotension followed 50 µg/kg of fentanyl in patients undergoing mitral valve replacement. Because of the limited number of patients in our series, we too are guilty of lumping the various valve lesions together. We will rectify the situation when more data are available.

METHODS

Eight patients (six women and two men) with mean pulmonary artery pressures of approximately 30 mm Hg were selected at random. Our patients averaged 60 ± 2 years, 68 ± 6 kg, with a body surface area of 1.71 ± 0.09 m^2. There were five mitral valve operations (three mitral valve replacements, two open mitral commissurotomies), two aortic valve replacements, and one combined aortic and mitral valve replacement with a coronary artery bypass graft.

Premedication consisted of morphine, 0.1 mg/kg, and scopolamine, 0.04 mg, in six patients. The other two patients received an additional 2 to 4 mg of lorazepam.

Vascular cannulas, including a 14-gauge intravenous catheter, a 20-gauge intraarterial catheter, and a pulmonary artery catheter, were inserted using local anesthesia. Anesthesia was induced with fentanyl, 25 µg/kg, combined with pancuronium, 0.1 mg/kg, administered intravenously over two minutes. Sixty to 90 seconds after the injection was completed the trachea was intubated. During the next 20 minutes, while the skin was prepared and draped and a urinary catheter inserted, an additional 25 µg/kg of fentanyl was administered. Measurements of heart rate, cardiac output (thermodilution), and radial, pulmonary artery, pulmonary capillary wedge, and right atrial pressures were made six times: 1—during oxygen breathing after vascular cannulation but before induction; 2—one minute after the induction drugs were given but before intubation; 3—two minutes after intubation; 4—immediately prior to incision; 5—two minutes after incision; and 6—two minutes after sternotomy. Cardiac and stroke work index, systemic and pulmonary vascular resistance index, and left ventricular stroke work index were calculated using appropriate formulas. Student's t test was used for statistical analysis.

RESULTS

Both measured and calculated variables for the study are shown in Table 39.1. While heart rate and mean arterial pressure were similar to those in Dr. Bovill's study, our patients had higher pulmonary artery, pulmonary capillary wedge, and right atrial pressures, lower cardiac and stroke work indexes, and higher pulmonary and systemic resistance indexes. Pressures tended to fall minimally in the absence of surgical stimulation (periods 2 and 4) and to rise somewhat with intubation (period 3) and sternotomy (period 6). The change in pulmonary artery pressure was significant for periods 2, 4, and

TABLE 39.1. Hemodynamic values with fentanyl administration to patients with valvular heart disease

Period	HR	MAP	PA	PCWP	RAP	CI	SI	SVRI	PVRI	LVSWI
1	82 ± 8	93 ± 3	53 ± 7	30 ± 2	14 ± 1	1.97 ± 0.19	26 ± 4	3419 ± 343	1038 ± 312	22 ± 3
2	89 ± 9	85 ± 5	48 ± 7*	30 ± 2	14 ± 2	2.14 ± 0.23	27 ± 5	2814 ± 252*	774 ± 237*	21 ± 5
3	90 ± 5	93 ± 7	53 ± 6	34 ± 2*	14 ± 2	2.23 ± 0.27	26 ± 4	2918 ± 112	782 ± 219*	23 ± 6
4	82 ± 6	89 ± 8	46 ± 7*	31 ± 3	12 ± 1	1.93 ± 0.22	25 ± 4	3275 ± 246	762 ± 340	22 ± 7
5	87 ± 7	89 ± 9	47 ± 8*	28 ± 2	12 ± 1	2.00 ± 0.32	25 ± 5	3185 ± 244	871 ± 396	25 ± 10
6	86 ± 8	92 ± 10	51 ± 8	30 ± 4	12 ± 1	2.05 ± 0.27	25 ± 4	3487 ± 237	509 ± 139	28 ± 8

HR = heart rate; MAP = mean arterial pressure; PA = mean pulmonary artery pressure; PCWP = pulmonary capillary wedge pressure; RAP = right atrial pressure; CI = cardiac index; SI = stroke index; SVRI = systemic vascular resistance index; PVRI = pulmonary vascular resistance index; LVSWI = left ventricular stroke work index.

*$p < 0.05$ compared to control (period 1).

5 compared to control, as was pulmonary capillary wedge pressure for period 3. These changes were of minimal clinical importance. Although there were no significant blood pressure changes during the study, one patient with aortic valve disease was eliminated from the study after the fifth measurement period because of a mean arterial pressure above 120 mm Hg. In addition, two other patients with aortic valve disease developed sustained hypertension after the last measurement period and required treatment with vasodilators. There was an initial drop in systemic vascular resistance after the initial fentanyl administration, with values gradually returning toward control. Pulmonary vascular resistance showed a similar initial decrease but then fell again in the last measurement period. This latter finding may be spurious since in two patients the wedge pressure could not be obtained during these measurement periods, and therefore pulmonary vascular resistance was not calculated. Stroke index was unchanged throughout the study.

No patient had any memory of the operative procedure.

DISCUSSION

Our protocol was based on that designed by Dr. Bovill. Hemodynamically, the New Yorkers behaved similarly to the European cohort despite the great disparity in initial cardiovascular state. Induction and intubation were achieved without major hemodynamic perturbation, and the only alteration of note was the development of hypertension in three patients. This may not have been ameliorated by higher doses of fentanyl since Bovill's patients had a mean arterial pressure of 109 mm Hg after a total dose of 100 μg/kg of fentanyl. This observation may be in keeping with similar experiences reported in patients with coronary artery disease. It is of interest that the hypertension seen in our patients occurred only with aortic valve disease, but our sample is much too small to allow any meaningful conclusions.

Although there were no significant changes in heart rate, there was wide variation among patients. Heart rate increased 5 to 25 beats per minute. It is not known whether this is due to the vagolytic or sympathetic stimulating properties of pancuronium, the previous use of drugs such as digitalis, or the severity of the valvular disease. It will be worthwhile in future studies to see if these changes in heart rate can be controlled better with the use of alternative muscle relaxants.

CONCLUSION

We have demonstrated that fentanyl is an excellent induction and initial maintenance agent in patients with severe valvular disease associated with pulmonary artery pressures greater than 30 mm Hg. Our sample was very small and must be enlarged before meaningful clinical conclusions can be drawn. This will also allow us to respond to our initial comment and see if the responses differ in patients with stenotic versus regurgitant valvular lesions.

REFERENCES

1. de Lange S, Boscoe MJ, Stanley TH, et al. Comparison of sufentanil-O_2 and fentanyl-O_2 for coronary artery surgery. Anesthesiology 1982;56:112.
2. Lunn JK, Stanley TH, Eisele JH, et al. High-dose fentanyl anesthesia for coronary artery surgery: plasma fentanyl concentrations and influence of nitrous oxide on cardiovascular responses. Anesth Analg (Cleve) 1979;59:390.
3. Quintin L, Whalley DG, Wynands JE, et al. Oxygen high-dose fentanyl-droperidol anesthesia for aortocoronary bypass surgery. Anesth Analg (Cleve) 1981;60:412.
4. Stanley TH, Webster LR. Anesthetic requirements and cardiovascular effects of fentanyl-oxygen and fentanyl-diazepam-oxygen anesthesia in man. Anesth Analg (Cleve) 1978;57:411.

40 NARCOTIC REQUIREMENTS FOR INTRAVENOUS ANESTHESIA IN CORONARY ARTERY SURGERY

J. Earl Wynands

The title of this chapter suggests that narcotics may be complete anesthetics, and how individual opiates must be used and in what dosages to produce complete anesthesia. Complete anesthesia is defined as unconsciousness, analgesia, absence of awareness, and suppression of an adrenergic response to noxious stimuli. Previous experience with morphine for open heart surgery has suggested that it may not be a complete anesthetic, and we have studied intravenous fentanyl to that end.

ANESTHETIC INDEXES

The minimum alveolar concentration (MAC) of an inhalation anesthetic has been defined as the minimum end-tidal alveolar anes-thetic concentration that inhibits movement in response to a noxious stimulus in 50% of subjects. It has proved to be a remarkably accurate and easily measurable index of anesthetic potency, and is used to define therapeutic indexes and quantify anesthetic effects of various volatile anesthetics [1]. The concept of MAC has been extended to MAC BAR, defined as the minimum end-tidal alveolar anesthetic concentration that inhibits adrenergic response to a noxious stimulus in 50% of individuals [2]. Thus a more quantifiable physiologic value can be used to measure responses. The question arises whether a minimal intraarterial concentration (MIC BAR) of an opiate such as fentanyl, given intravenously to achieve anesthesia, can be similarly defined.

FENTANYL ANESTHESIA

Fentanyl-oxygen anesthesia has become an established anesthetic technique for various cardiac and other surgical procedures. While it has the advantages of ease of administra-

The greater part of this chapter is a duplication of the article entitled "Narcotic requirements for intravenous anesthesia" published in *Anesthesia and Analgesia* 1984;63:(2)101–105 and printed here with the permission of the publisher.

tion, satisfactory anesthesia, and modification of hormonal stress responses [3,4], it produces prolonged respiratory depression and may not completely eliminate hemodynamic instability [5,6]. The therapeutic and threshold narcotic analgesic concentrations of fentanyl have not been clearly defined [7]. The MIC BAR (therapeutic concentration) would be the intraarterial plasma fentanyl concentration (PFC) that would prevent an adrenergic response to noxious stimuli in 50% of patients in the prebypass period.

To determine if a MIC BAR for fentanyl could be identified, we studied 43 patients undergoing aortocoronary bypass surgery (ACBP) with fentanyl anesthesia [8]. Five groups of comparable patients premedicated with diazepam, morphine, and scopolamine were anesthetized with different loading doses and infusions of fentanyl that were designed to produce a different PFC in each group. Their adrenergic response to intubation, skin incision, sternotomy, and dissection about the root of the aorta was correlated with PFC.

Adrenergic Response

It is conventionally accepted that noxious stimuli in the presence of light or inadequate anesthesia will lead to an increase in blood pressure and pulse rate that is mediated through the release of endogenous catecholamines. In this study, an adrenergic response was considered to be a 20% increase in systolic blood pressure above control. Heart rate was not used because all the patients were given pancuronium as a muscle relaxant and most were taking beta-blocking drugs that may alter the tachycardic response to noxious stimuli. When an adrenergic response was encountered, it was correlated with the PFC, which was inferred from a plasma fentanyl concentration-time curve constructed for each patient.

Plasma Fentanyl Concentrations

Figure 40.1 shows the approximate PFC at the time of each anesthetic or surgical event

studied in all patients, and indicates which patients became hypertensive at that time. When patients became hypertensive, they were treated with a volatile agent and removed from subsequent events in the study. One patient, with a PFC of 12.3 ng/ml, became hypertensive at intubation. Eight of 42 patients became hypertensive at skin incision with a PFC between 9.4 and 32.8 ng/ml. Seven of 34 patients became hypertensive at sternotomy, and the PFCs ranged from 8.7 to 18.3 ng/ml. Fifteen of 27 patients developed hypertension at aortic dissection, and the range of PFCs varied from 9.1 to 27 ng/ml. Of the 43 patients studied, only 4 with PFCs above 20 ng/ml developed hypertension before cardiopulmonary bypass. Two of these patients became hypertensive at aortic dissection while four with a PFC above 20 ng/ml did not. At the same time, 13 of 21 patients with a PFC below 20 ng/ml became hypertensive. The difference in the incidence of hypertension at aortic dissection in patients with PFC above and below 20 ng/ml is not statistically significant. There was no significant difference in the number of patients who became hypertensive at skin incision as compared to sternotomy, but significantly more patients became hypertensive at aortic dissection as compared to either skin incision or sternotomy.

The PFC of patients who became hypertensive versus those who did not at each event studied is shown in Table 40.1. There was no significant difference in the PFC of patients who becamse hypertensive at each event. There was a significant difference in the PFC of patients who became hypertensive (13 ± 1.2) compared to those who did not (18.2 ± 1.6) at sternotomy.

CORRELATION OF PLASMA FENTANYL CONCENTRATION AND ADRENERGIC RESPONSE

The range of PFC at each stress period was expected to be large, as the fentanyl anesthesia protocols were so designed. The unexpected finding was the wide range of PFCs

FIGURE 40.1. The plasma fentanyl concentration and number of patients having a hypertensive response at each event studied is shown. *From Wynands [8]. By permission of the publisher of Anesthesia and Analgesia.*

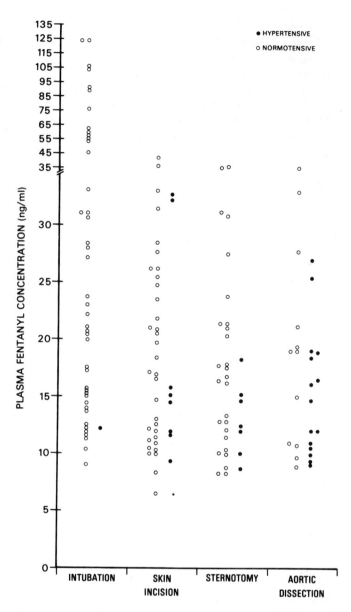

TABLE 40.1. Plasma fentanyl concentrations in patients who did and did not develop hypertension (mean ± SEM)

Response	Intubation	Skin Incision	Sternotomy	Aortic Dissection
Hypertensive response	12.3 (1)	17.9 ± 3.2 (8)	13 ± 1.2 (7)	15.4 ± 1.5 (15)
Nonhypertensive response	38.37 ± 5.1 (42)	19.2 ± 1.5 (34)	18.2 ± 1.6 (27)	19.1 ± 2.5 (12)

From Wynands [8]. By permission of the publisher of *Anesthesia and Analgesia*.

over which patients developed a hypertensive response at a given stress period, for example, 9 to 33 ng/ml at skin incision. This could not be explained. The demographic data for patients who became hypertensive was comparable to those for patients who did not. Factors that are known to affect the MAC of inhaled anesthetics and might be expected to affect the MIC BAR of intravenous narcotics, such as pH, arterial oxygen, and carbon dioxide tension [1], were controlled. Premedication will reduce MAC [1] and presumably MIC BAR. These patients were all given the same premedication at approximately the same time prior to induction of anesthesia, so that variability in premedication was an unlikely cause for the wide range of PFCs over which hypertension was encountered. There appeared to be a trend that patients with a PFC above 20 ng/ml were less likely to become hypertensive than those with lower plasma concentrations. Only four patients in the series with a PFC above 20 ng/ml became hypertensive. This is in agreement with Moldenhauer and Hug [9], who found that in six patients with a PFC of 20 ng/ml, only one had a slight hypertensive response during ACBP. In our study, however, there was no statistically significant difference in the incidence of hypertension at aortic dissection between patients whose PFC was greater than 20 ng/ml (2 of 6) and those with a PFC below 20 ng/ml (13 of 21).

Two facts suggest that fentanyl is not a complete anesthetic: a PFC of 30 ng/ml did not abolish an adrenergic response at skin incision, and Murphy and Hug [10] have found that there is a ceiling effect to which the MAC of enflurane can be reduced, which is a PFC of 30 ng/ml.

Minimum Intraarterial Concentration That Inhibits Adrenergic Response

A MIC BAR could not be established from the study because of great variability in the PFC of patients who became hypertensive,

and because steady-state concentrations of fentanyl were not always achieved. At aortic dissection, where the majority (15 of 27) of patients were hypertensive, only 2 of 6 (33%) became hypertensive when the PFC exceeded 20 ng/ml. We have a personal prejudice that if a MIC BAR does exist, it will be found to be about 18 ng/ml, which is based on the low adrenergic response rate above 20 ng/ml. The fact that there were patients who had an adrenergic response with a PFC above 30 ng/ml suggests that the slope of MIC BAR is relatively horizontal and may not reach a zero response. In comparison, the slope for MAC is fairly vertical, and zero and 100% responses are encountered on either side of the 50% response rate.

Adverse Effects

PFCs in excess of 20 ng/ml were achieved at aortic dissection in patients given a 75-μg/kg loading dose followed by a 0.75-μg/kg/min infusion. A 100-μg/kg loading dose and a 0.35-μg/kg/min infusion would also produce a PFC in excess of 20 ng/ml. Patients with a PFC in excess of 20 ng/ml at steady state required prolonged periods of postoperative artificial ventilation and received significantly more vasoconstricting drugs postoperatively compared with patients given 75 μg/kg fentanyl as a loading dose and volatile anesthetics as indicated [11].

ADVANTAGES AND RECOMMENDATIONS

The advantages of fentanyl anesthesia such as relative hemodynamic stability, ease of administration, smooth induction, and modification of hormonal stress response [3–5] make it advantageous for cardiac surgery. We support the belief that 30 to 40 μg/kg fentanyl given as a loading dose will produce smooth induction in the majority of patients [12]. Only 1 patient of the 43 studied became hypertensive at induction, and this patient had a PFC of 12.3 ng/ml. Five patients with lower PFCs did not become hypertensive at this period. As a loading dose, 30 μg/kg should produce a PFC of about 10 to 15 ng/ml at intubation (8 to 10 minutes) and a smooth induction sequence. When signs of inadequate anesthesia occur, a subanesthetic concentration of a volatile anesthetic is usually effective in restoring hemodynamic stability.

CONCLUSION

Predictions as to the dose of other narcotics required to produce anesthesia may be made knowing the potency, lipid solubility, volume of distribution, clearance, and β elimination half-life relative to fentanyl [7]. On the basis of our experience with fentanyl and other reports [13,14] that narcotics do not reliably block sympathetic response to noxious stimuli in patients with coronary artery disease, we suspect that new narcotics may exhibit the same inability to block totally the adrenergic response to noxious stimuli in the dose ranges that do not produce unacceptable morbidity.

REFERENCES

1. Quasha AL, Eger EI II, Tinker JH. Determination and application of MAC. Anesthesiology 1980;53:315–34.
2. Roizen MF, Horrigan RW, Frazer BM. Anesthetic doses blocking adrenergic (stress) and cardiovascular responses in incision-MAC BAR. Anesthesiology 1981;54:390–8.
3. Lunn JK, Stanley TH, Eisele JH, Webster L, Woodward A. High-dose fentanyl anesthesia for coronary artery surgery: plasma fentanyl concentrations and influence of nitrous oxide on cardiovascular responses. Anesth Analg (Cleve) 1979;58:390–5.
4. Stanley TH, Berman L, Green O, Robertson D. Plasma catecholamine and cortisol responses to fentanyl-oxygen anesthesia for coronary-artery operations. Anesthesiology 1980;53:250–3.
5. Waller JL, Hug CC Jr, Nagle DM, Craver JM. Hemodynamic changes during fentanyl-oxygen anesthesia for aortocoronary bypass operation. Anesthesiology 1981;55:212–17.
6. Quintin L, Whalley DG, Wynands JE, Morin JE, Mayer R. Oxygen–high-dose fentanyl-droperidol anesthesia for aortocoronary bypass surgery. Anesth Analg (Cleve) 1981;60:412–16.
7. Stanski DF, Hug CC Jr. Alfentanil—a kinetically predictable narcotic analgesic. Anesthesiology 1982;57:435–8.
8. Wynands JE, Wong P, Townsend GE, Sprigge JS, Whalley DG. Narcotic requirements for intravenous anesthesia. Anesth Analg (NY) 1984;63:101–5.
9. Moldenhauer CC, Hug CC Jr. Continuous infusion of fentanyl for cardiac surgery (abstract). Anesth Analg (Cleve) 1982;61:206.
10. Murphy MR, Hug CC Jr. The anesthetic potency of fentanyl in terms of its reduction of enflurane MAC. Anesthesiology 1982;57:485–8.
11. Wynands JE, Townsend GE, Wong P, Whalley DG, Srikant CB, Patel YC. Blood pressure response and plasma fentanyl concentrations during high- and very high-dose fentanyl anesthesia for coronary artery surgery. Anesth Analg (NY) 1983;62:661–5.
12. Barash PG, Giles R, Marx P, Berger H, Zaret B. Intubation: is low dose fentanyl really effective? (abstract). Anesth Analg (Cleve) 1982;61:168.
13. Sonntag H, Larsen R, Hilfiker O, Kettler D, Brockschnieder B. Myocardial blood flow and oxygen consumption during high-dose fentanyl anesthesia in patients with coronary artery disease. Anesthesiology 1982;56:417–22.
14. Lowenstein E. Morphine "anesthesia"—a perspective. Anesthesiology 1971;35:563–4.

41 THE LIMITATIONS OF FENTANYL FOR CARDIOVASCULAR SURGERY

Joel A. Kaplan

Dr. Wynands is one of the pioneers in the field of anesthesia for patients with coronary disease. In the preceding chapter he tries to do what many of the speakers at this symposium have recommended be done, namely, compare the pharmacokinetics of the opioids with their pharmacodynamics. This is extremely important and is not necessarily easy to do. I congratulate him for attempting it.

I agree with Dr. Wynands that in his study he has not identified the minimum intraarterial concentration at which the adrenergic response is inhibited in 50% of patients, the MIC BAR$_{50}$. The 18 ng/ml figure that he picked is probably a little low; work from other institutions shows that it may be in the 20 to 30 ng/ml range. In addition, we do not have the more important number, the MIC BAR$_{95}$. What level do we need to suppress responses in most of our patients, not just 50%? This is especially important in patients with coronary artery disease and good left ventricular function, and/or hypertension.

VARIATIONS IN RESPONSES

There is great variability in both plasma fentanyl levels and thresholds in this study. Pre-vious work by Hug et al [1] used fentanyl infusions with a different technique and achieved much more predictable and stable blood levels. Wynands gave a loading dose of 30 to 75 µg per kilogram of body weight over two to five minutes, at a rate of 1 mg/min, then he started the infusion. Hug et al used a double-infusion technique, which is a very important difference and could explain why their blood levels were stable and predictable. They gave 50 µg/kg, but over 20 minutes by infusion, and at the same time they started the maintenance infusion of 0.3 µg/kg/min. The total fentanyl doses were lower than with the bolus and infusion technique Wynands used, and they had fairly predictable blood levels of 20 ng/ml.

There was also great variability in the threshold responses of patients in this study. The hemodynamic responses in these types of patients are often unpredictable and frequently were labile. In addition, a number of these patients were taking antihypertensive medications including nitrates, beta blockers, and diuretics. It is interesting that of the patients who became hypertensive in this study, a much higher percentage were taking nitroglycerine and diuretics. The implications of antihypertensive therapy, not only on kinetics but on cardiac output and liver blood flow, are still totally unknown.

POSSIBLE CONTRAINDICATIONS TO HIGH-DOSE NARCOTIC ANESTHESIA

I still have some serious concerns about high-dose narcotic anesthesia for patients with coronary artery disease. One concern is the heart itself, which is the organ we are trying to protect. The work of Sonntag et al [2] is very important, since it shows that when things get out of control—as they do with any anesthetic, including fentanyl-oxygen—lactate production occurs together with myocardial ischemia. In other studies using acute infarction models in dogs, fentanyl led to more arrhythmias and more myocardial cell death then did halothane.

Dr. Lowenstein mentioned the goals of fentanyl-oxygen anesthesia. I do not think we have attained any of those goals so far. Circulatory stability is not guaranteed; we still have hypertension. It might be guaranteed if it was a fentanyl-nitroglycerine anesthetic, but not a fentanyl anesthetic by itself. We have not prevented all the stress responses; catecholamines are elevated during bypass. We have not avoided the big increases in fluid that were needed with morphine; Wynands found that these patients need vasopressors and large amounts of fluids. Finally, fentanyl is not a short-acting drug when given in the large doses that we are using today.

Two other areas of concern where more work is needed are awareness and seizures. Moldenhauer [3] found six reports of awareness in the literature, even one with a patient receiving benzodiazepines. I have seen a few

such cases myself, and I believe this is still a serious problem.

Harp et al showed that when they gave animals fentanyl, doses of 200 to 400 μg/kg produced seizures. Janssen has said that codeine and meperidine produce convulsions. I think it is fairly clear that fentanyl can also produce convulsive activity. Why are we not seeing this more in patients? I think it is due to the lower doses being used and the fact that most of our patients are receiving benzodiazepines. If these seizures are coming from the same area where the benzodiazepines work, this may be what is preventing them in some cases.

CONCLUSION

Why are we trying to do total anesthesia with a drug that I believe is only a partial anesthetic? There is a ceiling effect with all narcotics. Production of amnesia and muscle relaxation, as well as control of cardiovascular responses, are best done with other drugs.

REFERENCES

1. Hug CC Jr, Moldenhauer CC. Pharmacokinetics and dynamics of fentanyl infusions in cardiac surgical patients. Anesthesiology 1982;57:A45.
2. Sonntag H, Larsen R, Hilfiker O, et al. Myocardial blood flow and oxygen consumption during high-dose fentanyl anesthesia in patients with coronary artery disease. Anesthesiology 1982;56:417–22.
3. Moldehauer CC. New narcotics. In: Kaplan JA, ed. Cardiac anesthesia. Vol. II. Cardiovascular pharmacology. New York: Grune & Stratton, 1983:31–78.

Part VI DISCUSSION

DR. JOEL A. KAPLAN: Dr. Philbin has stated in a number of recent presentations that our stress response measurements do not necessarily correlate with hemodynamic changes, at least during cardiac surgery. Could you comment on that, Dr. Roizen?

DR. MICHAEL F. ROIZEN: We have seen excellent correlation between changes in blood pressure and changes in plasma norepinephrine levels when we used a narcotic anesthetic such as morphine or fentanyl alone or with nitrous oxide. When we added other drugs, such as hypnotic adjuvants or inhalation agents, to the anesthetic regimen, however, the correlation was not as strong.

Another question that has come up several times concerns the desirability of blocking the stress response perioperatively. My view is that it is desirable for cardiovascular operations but not for procedures involving the central nervous system. I think we'll be hearing a lot more about that question in the next couple of years.

DR. J. G. REVES: We have been trying to determine whether the stress response is important during extracorporeal perfusion. In one of our studies (*AM J Cardiol* 1984;53:722–8) we looked at whether the elevations in epinephrine and norepinephrine that occur during bypass can be correlated with postoperative cardiac function, myocardial damage, lactate release during reperfusion, and a number of other metabolic measurements. We found that there was no association between rises in catecholamines, which are particularly high during cardiac reperfusion, and myocardial function in the postoperative period. I agree with an earlier statement that surgery and myocardial preservation techniques are the major events affecting a patient's outcome. Our data show that, compared with these factors, the rises in catecholamines probably are not very important in contributing to myocardial damage during reperfusion of the postischemic heart.

DR. JAMES G. BOVILL: I'd like to comment on the catecholamine response during bypass. Everyone gets nervous when norepinephrine levels reach 1000 pg/ml or so, but we have to put this in some sort of perspective. Our biochemist recently completed a study, using himself and healthy volunteers, in which he measured catecholamines in a resting control state and then repeated the mea-

surement after walking up one flight of stairs. He found catecholamine levels three to four times those reported in most coronary patients during bypass. So I think the level we see during perfusion, although it certainly is statistically significant, may not be particularly relevant to the patient.

DR. FAWZY G. ESTAFANOUS: Over the past ten years we have exhausted ourselves talking about the stress response and hormonal changes during cardiopulmonary bypass. I don't know how much of this is applicable to the practicing anesthesiologist or how much we can benefit by adjusting our anesthetic techniques. Some 200 variables that occur during cardiopulmonary bypass can affect the outcome, and among the least of these are hypothermia, hemodilution, high blood pressure, low blood pressure, reflexes from the heart, reflexes from the great vessels, and so forth. Yet we sit here trying to correlate everything from induction of anesthesia to the changes that occur during bypass with our selection of an anesthetic agent. I really think the time has come for us to stop talking about this topic.

DR. PAUL G. BARASH: We recently completed a study in which we looked at norepinephrine and epinephrine uptake at the myocardial level in patients undergoing coronary artery bypass surgery. We found no correlation between the catecholamines and anything we could measure, and we observed very wide variations among our patients. Like Dr. Estafanous, I have serious questions about all this information we're collecting on the stress response and catecholamines, and what it really means in our research and our practice.

DR. JOAN W. FLACKE: I want to get back to the adrenergic response here for a minute. In our work with catecholamines—and we have extensive experience in measuring them—we have found, as has Dr. Roizen, an excellent correlation between plasma catechol levels and the changes in blood pressure and heart rate caused by surgical stimuli. This correlation is modified by the drugs we use and by secondary reflex responses; but if the cardiovascular changes are watched for carefully over a period of several minutes surrounding the time the plasma sample is taken, they are there.

Addressing Dr. Bovill's comments, we too have measured catecholamine levels in normal volunteers and have found them to be very low. We found, though, that nine out of ten people will show very little change in norepinephrine and epinephrine levels after exercise; however, the tenth person will. So perhaps your colleague who walked up the stairs should have himself evaluated further.

DR. ESTAFANOUS: Still, while these data may be useful for research purposes, we have no clinical data on cardiopulmonary bypass that can be applied in our clinical practice. I don't know of any standard value for catecholamines or hormones during bypass that we can apply for even 10% to 20% of our patients.

DR. PAUL F. WHITE: Dr. Roizen indicated that in the presence of 70% nitrous oxide he was able to define a MAC BAR equivalent for fentanyl. We have completed studies with continuous infusions of alfentanil (in the presence of 70% nitrous oxide and metocurine) in patients undergoing either superficial or more stressful intraabdominal procedures. For the superficial procedures, an alfentanil concentration of 100 to 200 ng/ml was usually adequate to suppress hemodynamic responses. For patients undergoing intraabdominal procedures, however, steady-state alfentanil levels of 200 to 500 ng/ml in combination with 70% nitrous oxide and muscle relaxants were unable consistently to block blood pressure responses to manipulations of the abdominal aorta.

DR. DONALD STANSKI: I'm a little disappointed, Dr. Kaplan, regarding the negative nature of your critique of Dr. Wynands's work, and I think some of it is inappropriate. His method of administering the drug was perfectly reasonable in terms of kinetic principles, and I don't think the differences in bolus dose between what he used and what Drs. Moldenhauer and Hug employ could explain the difference in blood levels he found. Ten to 15 minutes into an infusion following a bolus and a loading dose, there should be good equilibrium between brain and blood levels of the anesthetic. Even if these levels are not maintained throughout the full 30 to 60 minutes before perfusion is begun, blood levels should fairly accurately reflect the level in the brain.

Dr. Wynands's study is the first in which a decent-sized group was used to examine the therapeutic and threshold effects of fentanyl in cardiopulmonary bypass. The changes Dr. Moldenhauer and Dr. Hug found may be related to their smaller patient populations. What Dr. Wynands has done is impressive and elegant, and it finally begins to confirm the prediction by Drs. Hug and

Moldenhauer that use of a sole narcotic may not provide a maximal therapeutic response.

DR. KAPLAN: I think you misinterpreted some of what I said. I certainly agree that Dr. Wynands's work was elegant. It was very different from the work done by Dr. Moldenhauer, though, and I would be interested in Dr. Moldenhauer's comments.

DR. J. EARL WYNANDS: I agree with basically everything I've heard and am not disturbed by Dr. Kaplan's remarks—some of them were valid. Unfortunately for our studies, many patients with coronary artery disease are receiving drugs such as nitroglycerine or propranolol, and I think we have to consider the effects of these agents before drawing any conclusions from our findings. As for the stability of blood levels in our patients, we have a great deal more data than I could show in the time I was allotted.

DR. THEODORE H. STANLEY: In the first study we published on the use of fentanyl for coronary artery surgery, the blood levels measured at the time of sternotomy were usually greater than 40 ng/ml, while during cardiopulmonary bypass the mean plasma values ranged between 23 and 30 ng/ml. This is consistent with Dr. Wynands's findings, and perhaps it offers an explanation why there were relatively few unstabilizing hemodynamic events.

DR. BARASH: I have a question for Dr. Kaplan about recall during anesthesia. Obviously, this is probably not a desirable occurrence, but I think there has been an implication recently that narcotic anesthesia is associated with recall while inhalation anesthesia is not. Yet the literature contains numerous reports of recall during inhalation anesthesia. And if we go back to ether, the paleolithic anesthetic, there was a very popular technique early in open heart surgery in which patients were actually told they would remember the operation—it was felt that they could be maintained at a more hemodynamically stable state. So I think, Dr. Kaplan, that when we talk about recall we are speaking about an adverse effect that can occur not only with the narcotic anesthetics, but with all anesthetic agents. It can occur in cases where, for other reasons, we cannot anesthetize a patient to an adequate depth.

DR. KAPLAN: I'm not sure there is a question there, but I agree with the comment. Without question, there have been cases of recall under inhalation anesthesia. Cardiac and obstetric surgery are the two classic instances, since patients are kept at extremely light levels of anesthesia. Using an inhalation anesthetic will not avoid that possibility, but I think there's a much greater chance of it happening with a narcotic.

DR. CRAIG MOLDENHAUER: My comments are directed to Dr. Kaplan regarding his concern over fentanyl-induced seizures. We have looked in several ways at the electroencephalogram (EEG) after large doses of fentanyl, and we have not seen seizures. Recognizing the results obtained in animals, however, we designed a study to produce extremely high plasma fentanyl levels or high sustained fentanyl levels in patients to see if seizures would occur.

We recorded 8 leads of the raw (not computer-processed) EEG in eight patients with good left ventricular function. We started with a fentanyl dose of 50 μg/kg, administered in 20 seconds, to repeat the work of others and to convince ourselves it was safe. We then increased the dosage to 150 μg/kg, given over one or several minutes. At this point, some patients received up to 250 cc of fentanyl in a minute, which produced plasma fentanyl concentrations as high as 1800 ng/ml. We then monitored the EEG to look for seizures and to track the decline in plasma levels.

Our results were entirely consistent with what Dr. Sebel and Dr. Bovill found, including the sharp waves. We showed Dr. Wauquier our EEG results, and he thought some of our sharp wave activity was probably artifactual in that there seemed to be no anatomic focus to it.

When we gave fentanyl, 150 mg/kg, incrementally, we produced plasma levels in the range of 200 to 600 ng/ml that were sustained for about 12 minutes. Again, we saw very typical fentanyl EEG patterns with slow, high-amplitude delta waves and artifactual sharp waves, but nothing to indicate seizure activity.

DR. N. TY SMITH: We tape-record our EEGs and examine them very carefully during playback. We certainly have not seen any seizures, but then we haven't given the large doses Dr. Moldenhauer is talking about. Perhaps, though, as I suggested earlier, we are not seeing seizures because we are not recording the EEG in the right area—subcortically deep in the amygdala, for example. So even though we have not documented seizure activity in our patients, we can't say it does not exist in the deeper areas of the brain.

DR. AMIRA SAFWAT: I just reported the case of a patient who developed grand mal seizures after being given 200 μg of fentanyl over a five-minute interval. The patient was 80 years old.

DR. CARL C. HUG, JR.: What we need to bring this discussion into perspective is some kind of end point, and that is one thing we don't have. We've all been looking at hemodynamics, but as Dr. Kaplan mentioned, one of our major concerns as anesthesiologists is patient awareness during anesthesia. We need a means of examining this parameter, and some of us are starting to look at the EEG as the potential monitor for anesthetic depth.

I have a word of caution to offer in that regard. Dr. Wauquier and I have some data from dogs in which all the EEG changes occurred at alfentanil concentrations that none of us would consider adequate for anything. I would like Dr. Bovill and Dr. Sebel to reflect back with me on the EEG changes they reported. All occurred at induction, and even though we know that with the dose they used blood levels of fentanyl certainly were falling, and presumably brain levels were as well, there was no further change in the EEG. Dr. Wauquier and I know that we produced stable levels in our dogs, and we varied the actual concentrations over a considerable range without observing any changes in the EEG. My concern is that the EEG, as a monitor of anesthetic depth and a predictor of awareness, may not be able to give us meaningful data at the levels of anesthesia we are reaching. Dr. Bovill, do you have any reaction to that thought based on the EEG changes you reported?

DR. BOVILL: We recently completed a study that attempted to compare blood levels of alfentanil, particularly during recovery, with EEG changes, and I think our findings are similar to what you saw in the dogs. At higher blood levels we found no changes in the EEG, but at some point as the blood level drops it's as if a switch is being thrown. I've seen this occur in several patients where, within a two-minute period, they switched from an apparently deep EEG level to a reading that indicated a state of alertness. But certainly, there was no good correlation between EEG and blood levels that we could find.

DR. SIMON DE LANGE: I would like to make a comment about titrating to effect. We found in a recent study that there was good correlation between the induction dose of alfentanil used for coronary artery surgery and the total dose of alfentanil given as an infusion. In many of the studies presented at this conference, however, induction was achieved by giving a large bolus dose of narcotic with a muscle relaxant. With this technique a valuable indication of the patient's needs is lost. By titrating opioids initially to produce unconsciousness, I think we gain a good indication of further requirements for the drug during anesthesia.

DR. STEPHEN J. THOMAS: I'd like to reply to that. Is unconsciousness enough of a basis to begin titrating? Is it enough to provide hemodynamic stability? Once the patient is unconscious, what other levels do you assess in terms of titrating to effect?

DR. DE LANGE: We found, for example, that we needed a slightly higher dose of alfentanil for intubation. But both doses, for induction and for intubation, correlated well with the total dose of alfentanil needed for the procedure. Nothing else we examined, such as duration of anesthesia or the patient's age or weight, correlated well with this total dose.

DR. RONALD D. MILLER: I think everyone here is concerned with measuring an effect. I'm not a narcotic pharmacologist, but I would like to ask whether the animals we use, the rat and the dog, are valid models in which to study the convulsant effects of a narcotic when the data are then to be applied to human beings.

DR. BOVILL: I have no experience with rats. Dogs have received considerably larger doses of fentanyl than we give to our patients and there has been no evidence of convulsions. But I agree that it's very difficult, and probably erroneous, to try to extrapolate from one species to another.

DR. MILLER: The reason I asked the question is that this type of comparison is certainly not true for morphine. I don't know about fentanyl or other anesthetics, but with morphine it is very dangerous to extrapolate the EEG effects from dog to man.

DR. KAPLAN: Obviously we all recognize that point. It has been shown in cats, in dogs, and in rats. Maybe we have not yet found the species that's analogous to man. It certainly has been shown that convulsions can occur in patients, though, and we just heard Dr. Safwat describe another case. I think we need to be more cautious than to dismiss Dr. Rao's cases as flukes. I'm afraid we could be trying to ignore them simply because we don't want to acknowledge the problem.

DR. SMITH: To examine the effects of thiopental on patients with porphyria, one first needs to have a patient with porphyria. To show whether fentanyl can produce convulsions in man, perhaps we should select that very small group of patients who are predisposed to convulsions.

DR. HUG: I think Dr. Smith is absolutely correct. But in addition to his point, we do have to recognize that very high doses of narcotics kill. They kill all species that I'm aware of, including rodents and dogs, although, fortunately, I haven't heard of this happening in human beings during anesthesia. Even if we support ventilation, they kill by convulsions and hemodynamic instability. This is a dose-related effect, and I think Dr. de Castro's work with the fentanyl analogs has shown that. Whether the dog is relatively more or less sensitive than man is certainly a valid question, but, qualitatively at least, the dog seems to match human beings in the nature of the response.

DR. MILLER: My concern is that dogs convulse at nonanesthetic doses of morphine.

DR. SMITH: I'd like to bring this discussion into perspective by referring to some of our earlier studies with inhalation agents. With enflurane, for example, 6 of 12 unpremedicated volunteers experienced frank seizures, and all twelve subjects experienced epileptiform activity. Postanesthetically, the EEG showed only slowing of the alpha frequency, which then returned to normal after two days. In addition, the few postanesthetic psychologic changes that we observed represented an improvement rather than a decline. Although halothane produced no seizures, postanesthetically the EEG demonstrated a slowing similar to that seen with enflurane. In half of these subjects there was de novo sharp wave activity, which we did not see with enflurane. This sharp wave activity is similar to that seen occasionally with fentanyl. In the subjects receiving halothane, there were postanesthetic psychologic disturbances suggesting depression.

Other inhalation agents, such as ether and fluroxene, produced seizures in normal volunteers. We use these agents frequently without recording the EEG. These anecdotal reports about an occasional seizure with fentanyl are very interesting, but their frequency with fentanyl seems to be nowhere near what we see in well-controlled studies with most of the inhalation agents. The EEG patterns observed with enflurane, for example, represent classic epileptic or epileptiform activity. Those with fentanyl in humans have not, thus far. I worry that many of the reports of so-called seizures with fentanyl actually represent marked rigidity. We have seen such rigidity with large doses of alfentanil if no muscle relaxant is administered. The electromyographic artifact present during rigidity could be misinterpreted as EEG convulsant activity. I would need to see EEG seizure activity during complete paralysis before I believed these reports.

DR. ESTAFANOUS: We agree with you, Dr. Smith, that any of these effects can happen to anyone. The main goal, then, is individualization of anesthesia.

DR. M. M. GHONEIM: I'd like to get back to the issue of awareness. This is something that involves learning and memory functions, and I would suggest that monitoring the EEG is not going to be of much help in studying this problem. I think we have to borrow from the techniques used by psychologists in order to measure these functions.

Another point is the different effects narcotic and inhalation anesthetics have on memory. I have no information about large doses of narcotics, but there is no doubt that inhalation agents in anesthetic and certain subanesthetic concentrations have strong effects on memory function, while narcotics in the modest doses we can give to volunteers have virtually none.

DR. LEROY VANDAM: I'd like to conclude this discussion on a historical note. If we look back to the first use of nitrous oxide anesthesia, the student who was having his tooth removed screamed out in pain. Later on, he admitted he could not remember the tooth being extracted. When Edward Gilbert Abbott was anesthetized by William Thomas Green Morton, and the demonstration was described as being "no humbug," Abbott recalled a sensation as if a hoe had been drawn across his face. And John Snow wrote that in all of his use of ether anesthesia, his patients, with only three exceptions, were completely unaware of the operation. These three were patients in whom anesthesia had been discontinued when the surgeon decided that he had to place a few more sutures.

So there has been awareness in anesthesia all along. Whether or not it has been harmful turns out to be a very interesting question.

VII ADJUVANTS TO OPIOID ANESTHESIA

42 INTERACTION OF BENZODIAZEPINES AND NARCOTICS

J. G. Reves

Narcotics are not total anesthetic drugs, and one potentially major problem with their use in anesthesia is awareness. This deficit brings into play the use of benzodiazepines as adjuvants. The benzodiazepines have several effects, the one most useful in conjunction with narcotic anesthesia being that they produce amnesia. For this reason, benzodiazepines are commonly given in combination with or as adjuvants to narcotic anesthesia. An interesting issue arises, namely, the interactions, or possible interactions, that can occur between narcotics and benzodiazepines. Obviously, many are possible; for example, hemodynamic, analgesic, respiratory, and hypnotic. This chapter discusses the hemodynamic interaction.

CHARACTERISTICS OF THE INTERACTION

When benzodiazepines and narcotics are combined, the result is frequently a surprise—usually more decreases in blood pressure and cardiac output than were intended. The following are some data about benzodiazepines when used alone in hypnotic doses, that is, doses that put people to sleep. Samuelson et al [1] showed that midazolam, 0.2 mg per kilogram of body weight, and diazepam, 0.5 mg/kg, produce almost no change in hemodynamic measurements: heart rate is unchanged; pulmonary capillary wedge pressure may decrease slightly but not significantly; cardiac index is absolutely unaltered. With midazolam there may be a slight but clinically insignificant decrease in blood pressure; with diazepam there is no change in hemodynamics [1]. We have seen what happens when fentanyl is given in hypnotic doses: no change occurs in heart rate, wedge pressure, cardiac index, or blood pressure [2–5]. The results are the same when either narcotics or benzodiazepines are given alone—there is little or no change in hemodynamics.

Tomicheck and associates [6] looked at the interaction of diazepam and fentanyl. They studied four groups of patients in whom the first, a control group, received no diazepam. The others were given increasing doses of the drug—0.125, 0.25, and 0.5 mg/kg—before they were all given fentanyl. Fentanyl was administered in increments up to 50 µg/kg. Regardless of the dose of diazepam, it and fentanyl in combination caused significant decreases in mean arterial pressure and systemic vascular resistance (Figure 42.1).

CAUSES OF THE INTERACTION

I think it is important to try to learn what causes this interaction. Some evidence from Tomicheck et al [6] suggests that it might result from a reduction in sympathetic tone, which can be measured indirectly by looking at circulating catecholamines. Perhaps the mechanism involves a direct effect on smooth muscle that also dictates the vascular tone. Events may be taking place in the venous circulation that we cannot measure very effectively; parasympathetic activity might also

be involved. There may be central mechanisms that we do not understand. There are many potential causes for the interaction between narcotics and benzodiazepines. We have investigated the possibility that myocardial contractility is involved; in other words, the two drugs may exert direct effects on the inotropic state of the heart.

The inotropic effects of fentanyl and diazepam were investigated in rats using an isolated heart preparation (Langendorf method) [7]. We measured left ventricular contractility from the heart paced at a rate of 300 beats per minute. We used isovolumetric contractions to measure the maximum rate of rise of left ventricular pressure (dP/dt_{max}) and calculated the amount of drug required to produce 50% depression in dP/dt, or in left ventricular contractility, with

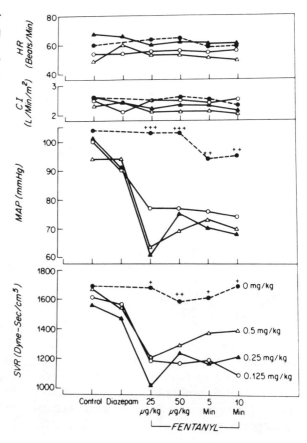

FIGURE 42.1. Hemodynamic data for groups given 0, 0.125, 0.25, and 0.5 mg/kg of diazepam and 25 and 50 μg/kg of fentanyl. Significant intergroup difference designated by + ($p < 0.05$), + + ($p < 0.01$), or + + + ($p < 0.001$). From Tomicheck [6]. By permission.

both diazepam and fentanyl; this methodology was used previously to examine the interaction of halothane and nifedipine [8]. We calculated the relative potency of depression with both fentanyl and diazepam. Equipotent depressive doses were then given in three increments to cause depression of 20% to 80% so that we could calculate again a median effective dose with an equipotent combination of the drugs. Then we performed isobolographic analysis to characterize the interaction between the drugs. In terms of direct effect of the two agents on contractility, the isobolographic analysis showed a purely additive response [7,9] (Figure 42.2).

CONCLUSION

We looked at only one aspect of the interaction between fentanyl and diazepam—the direct inotropic effects—and found that they are purely additive. It is probably necessary to look elsewhere to explain the supraadditive effects on blood pressure and cardiac output that have been found in humans.

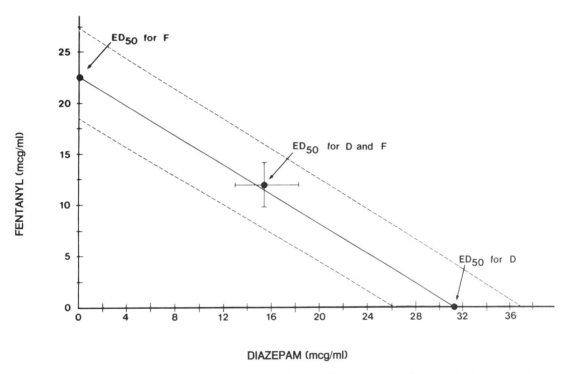

FIGURE 42.2. Isobologram for the interaction of the negative inotropic effects of fentanyl and diazepam at ED_{50} level (50% decrease from control in dP/dt_{max}. ED_{50} values for fentanyl and diazepam alone are plotted on the ordinate and abscissa, respectively. ED_{50} for an equipotent combination of fentanyl and diazepam is plotted in the dose field. The ED_{50} additive line was generated by connecting the ED_{50} for fentanyl with that for diazepam (*solid line*). All ED_{50} points are plotted with SD. The dotted lines connect the end points of 67% confidence limits for fentanyl and diazepam. Note that the combined drug value falls along the additive line, indicating that the combined effects of fentanyl and diazepam are additive. Had the point been above and to the right of the additive line, the interaction would be infraadditive, and if it were to the left and under the additive line, it would be a supraadditive effect. Note that the combination of fentanyl and diazepam has an additive negative inotropic effect at ED_{50}. *From Reves et al [9]. By permission.*

REFERENCES

1. Samuelson PN, Reves JG, Kouchoukos NT, Smith LR, Dole KM. Hemodynamic responses to anesthetic induction with midazolam or diazepam in patients with ischemic heart disease. Anesth Analg (Cleve) 1981;60:802–9.
2. Stanley TH, Webster LR. Anesthetic requirements and cardiovascular effects of fentanyl-oxygen and fentanyl-diazepam-oxygen anesthesia in man. Anesth Analg (Cleve) 1978;57:411–16.
3. Lunn JK, Stanley TH, Eisele JH, Webster L, Woodward A. High-dose fentanyl anesthesia for coronary artery surgery: plasma fentanyl concentrations and influence of nitrous oxide on cardiovascular responses. Anesth Analg (Cleve) 1979;58:390–5.
4. Waller JL, Hug CC Jr, Nagle DM, Craver JM. Hemodynamic changes during fentanyl-oxygen anesthesia for aortocoronary bypass operation. Anesthesiology 1981;55:212–17.
5. Sebel PS, Bovill JG, Boekhorst RAA, Rog N. Cardiovascular effects of high-dose fentanyl anaesthesia. Acta Anaesthesiol Scand 1982;26:308–15.
6. Tomicheck RC, Rosow CE, Philbin DM, Moss J, Teplick RS, Schneider RC. Diazepam-fentanyl interaction—hemodynamic and hormonal effects in coronary artery surgery. Anesth Analg (NY) 1983;62:881–4.
7. Reves JG, Kissin I, Fournier S. Additive negative inotropic effect of a combination of diazepam and fentanyl (abstract). Anesthesiology 1983;59:A326.
8. Marshall AG, Kissin I, Reves JG, Bradley EL Jr, Blackstone EH. Interaction between negative inotropic effects of halothane and nifedipine in the isolated rat heart. J Cardiovasc Pharmacol 1983;5:592–7.
9. Reves JG, Kissin I, Fournier SE, Smith LR. Additive negative inotropic effect of a combination of diazepam and fentanyl. Anesth Analg (NY) 1984;63:97–100.

43 BENZODIAZEPINES AS SUPPLEMENTS TO OPIOID ANESTHESIA

M. M. Ghoneim

The benzodiazepines in therapeutic doses have little if any direct effect on the heart and blood vessels. Their effects on the cardiovascular system are caused by a central site of action. A central depression of parasympathetic and sympathetic outflows may be mediated by the potentiating effect of benzodiazepines on γ-aminobutyric acid (GABA)-ergic activity. The cardiovascular effects vary as function of the dose and the central state of the organism [1].

The drugs may lower arterial blood pressure and either increase or fail to affect the heart rate. The cardiac output and stroke volume may be reduced. An increase, a decrease, and no effect on peripheral vascular resistance have been reported. Diazepam has been reported to decrease left ventricular end-diastolic pressure, rate of systolic pressure increase (dP/dt), and myocardial oxygen consumption [1].

It seems that in healthy patients or those with compensated heart disease, these drugs used in doses to induce anesthesia (e.g., 0.2 to 0.3 mg diazepam) produce clinically acceptable cardiovascular depression. This may not be the case, however, in hypovolemic patients or those taking large doses of beta blockers, in whom compensatory increases in contractility, heart rate, and central blood volume mobilization may not occur.

The addition of diazepam to large doses of opioids results in cardiovascular depression [2,3]. Although there are statistically significant changes in various cardiovascular variables associated with the addition of diazepam, many of the changes are small and perhaps of limited clinical significance [4].

ADVANTAGES OF USING BENZODIAZEPINES FOR ANESTHESIA

Benzodiazepines are useful drugs to facilitate sleep the night before surgery and to reduce anxiety and produce amnesia on the day of surgery. During the operation itself, pure opioid or opioid–nitrous oxide anesthesia has several drawbacks that may be counteracted by the addition of benzodiazepines.

The fact that occasionally patients under pure opioid anesthesia may be aware of certain events during anesthesia and surgery and be able to recall them postoperatively is well recognized [5,6]. Benzodiazepines produce

253

specific memory impairment [7], which should prevent this from happening, according to the dose used. The effects of benzodiazepines on memory can probably be supplemented by scopolamine and/or nitrous oxide.

Clinical signs of anesthesia are unreliable. Patients anesthetized with opioids and even with added nitrous oxide may suddenly move or open their eyes, if they are not paralyzed, with no warning from observations of blood pressure, heart rate, pupillary size, skin moisture, and so on. Even with large doses, there seems to be a ceiling to the effectiveness of these drugs as anesthetics [8]. Long-acting sedative-hypnotics such as the benzodiazepines would decrease the incidence of such embarrassing incidents. Benzodiazepines potentiate the activity of other centrally depressant agents.

Hypertension may occur during certain surgical manipulations. Sometimes treatment with more opioids is ineffective. A benzodiazepine may succeed, particularly when the rise in blood pressure is due to light anesthesia.

Addition of a benzodiazepine to opioids and nitrous oxide can provide an optimal balance between anesthesia and antinociception with minimal side effects during and after balanced anesthesia. Tammisto et al [9] and Aromaa et al [10] attempted to estimate the optimal balance between the actions of the drugs used in this type of anesthesia by studying their effects on consciousness (eyelid reflex), superficial nociception (pinching in inguinal skin fold), respiration, and circulation. Their results were that supplementing N$_2$O with fentanyl alone (2 or 3 µg/kg) produced unnecessarily pronounced respiratory depression without providing adequate anesthetic effect. Supplementing N$_2$O with thiopental or diazepam alone did not offer adequate antinociception. They therefore concluded that an optimal balance between anesthesia and antinociception with minimal side effects during and after balanced general anesthesia requires reinforce-

ment of nitrous oxide anesthesia not only with fentanyl but with hypnotic sedatives.

Benzodiazepines attenuate centrally mediated autonomic nervous and endocrine responses to emotions and to excessive afferent stimuli. The antinociceptive properties of benzodiazepines may be due to their actions on the GABAergic system, increasing GABA levels in the central nervous system. Recently Whitwam [11] has shown that intrathecal midazolam reversibly blocks somatosympathetic reflexes evoked by noxious stimulation.

Central actions of opioids and benzodiazepines have several convergent effects. Increasing GABA levels in the brain enhances opioid analgesia, and GABA itself has analgesic properties that do not depend on an opioid system. There is also a relationship between benzodiazepines and endogenous opioid mechanisms. Acute benzodiazepine treatment is associated with a naloxone-reversible release of striatal enkephalin, and some of the behavioral effects of benzodiazepines are reversed by opiate antagonists. Also, patients being maintained with methadone express a preference for concurrent use of diazepam, claiming that it boosts the effects derived from methadone [12].

Opioids commonly produce muscle rigidity when used in relatively large doses. Benzodiazepines can inhibit this effect. Unfortunately, the dose necessary to abolish the rigidity is large. The median effective dose of diazepam that inhibits the Straub tail in mice is 1.25 mg/kg [13].

The anticonvulsant action of benzodiazepines may be useful when large doses of opioids, particularly meperidine, are administered. Both meperidine and its main metabolite, particularly the latter, can produce convulsions.

CONCLUSION

Benzodiazepines have virtually no direct actions on organs and tissues outside the brain and spinal cord [1]. They have a very wide safety margin. In spite of their widespread use, proof is still lacking for a lethal outcome after overdosage in the absence of other drugs. Benzodiazepines are useful supplements to opioid and balanced anesthesia.

REFERENCES

1. Haefely W, Pieri L, Polc P, Schaffner R. General pharmacology and neuropharmacology of benzodiazepine derivatives. In: Hoffmeister F, Stille G, eds. Handbook of experimental pharmacology. Vol. 55, part II. New York: Springer-Verlag, 1981:13–201.
2. Stanley TH, Bennett GM, Loeser EA, Kawamura R, Sentker CR. Cardiovascular effects of diazepam and droperidol during morphine anesthesia. Anesthesiology 1976;44:255–8.
3. Stanley TH, Webster LR. Anesthetic requirements and cardiovascular effects of fentanyl-oxygen and fentanyl-diazepam-oxygen anesthesia in man. Anesth Analg (Cleve) 1978;57:411–16.
4. Lappas DG, Fahmy NR, Moss J, Slater EE. Effects of fentanyl-diazepam anesthesia on hemodynamics, plasma catecholamines and renin activity in critically ill patients. Anesthesiology 1981;55:A250.
5. Hilgenberg JC. Intraoperative awareness during high-dose fentanyl-oxygen anesthesia. Anesthesiology 1981;54:341–4.
6. Mummaneni N, Rao TLK, Montoya A. Awareness and recall with high-dose fentanyl-oxygen anesthesia. Anesth Analg (Cleve) 1980;59:948–9.
7. Ghoneim MM, Mewaldt SP. Effects of diazepam and scopolamine on storage, retrieval and organizational processes in memory. Psychopharmacology (Berlin) 1975;44:257–62.
8. Murphy MR, Hug CC Jr. The anesthetic potency of fentanyl in terms of its reduction of enflurane MAC. Anesthesiology 1982;57:485–8.
9. Tammisto T, Aromaa U, Korttila K. The role of thiopental and fentanyl in the production of balanced anaesthesia. Acta Anaesthesiol Scand 1980;24:31–5.
10. Aromaa U, Korttila K, Tammisto T. The role of diazepam and fentanyl in the production of balanced anaesthesia. Acta Anaesthesiol Scand 1980;24:36–40.
11. Whitwam JG. Benzodiazepine receptors. Anaesthesia 1983;38:93–5.
12. Cooper SJ. Minireview: benzodiazepine-opiate antagonist interaction to feeding and drinking behavior. Life Sci 1983;32:1043–51.
13. Niemegeers CJE, Lewi PJ. The anticonvulsant properties of anxiolytic agents. In: Fielding S, Lal H, eds. Industrial pharmacology. Vol 3. New York: Futura Publishing Co., 1979:141–58.

44 NITROUS OXIDE AS AN ADJUVANT TO NARCOTIC ANESTHESIA

Ira Michaels, J. Richard Trout, and Paul G. Barash*

Incomplete analgesia and amnesia may require supplementation to a narcotic-based anesthetic [1,2]. Nitrous oxide is commonly administered to potentiate the analgesic effects of narcotic anesthetics. The literature concerning the cardiovascular effects of nitrous oxide–narcotic interaction is contradictory. In certain clinical settings, nitrous oxide is reputed to exert significant hemodynamic effects. Numerous studies have reported that nitrous oxide depresses cardiovascular performance in patients anesthetized with a high-dose narcotic technique [3–7]. A recent investigation has shown no cardiac depression associated with nitrous oxide administration to patients undergoing open heart surgery who had good preoperative left ventricular (LV) function [8]. Variables that reportedly alter cardiovascular function during a N_2O–narcotic technique include poor LV function, surgical stimulation, and cardiac lesion [8–10]. Since a reduced inspired oxygen fraction (FIO_2) rather than the addition of nitrous oxide may be the cause of some of the previously reported changes, we designed a prospective randomized study to

examine the possible hemodynamic consequences of 70% nitrous oxide inhalation in patients anesthetized with sufentanil. To compare the differential effects of nitrous oxide with a reduced FIO_2 ($= 0.3$), we contrasted the cardiovascular effects of 70% nitrous oxide–oxygen, 70% nitrogen–oxygen, and 100% oxygen inhalation in patients anesthetized with sufentanil, 20 μg per kilogram of body weight.

METHODS

Twenty patients (mean age 57 ± 3 years) undergoing elective open heart surgery were evaluated. Eleven had good LV function, while nine had poor function. Poor LV function defined on the basis of cardiac catheterization data included LV ejection fraction of less than 40%, pulmonary capillary wedge pressure over 15 mm Hg, and/or significant regional wall abnormalities. Of the 20 patients, 14 underwent coronary revascularization, 4 underwent valve replacement, and 2 had combined coronary revascularization and valve replacement. Informed consent was obtained in accordance with the Human In-

---

*Presented at the conference by Dr. Barash.

vestigation Committees approved protocol. Induction of anesthesia was accomplished with intravenous oxygen-sufentanil, 20 μg/kg, and pancuronium, 0.1 mg/kg, for muscle relaxation (Figure 44.1).

The study consisted of two phases. *Phase I:* 10 minutes after intubation, during steady-state conditions, control hemodynamic measurements were made while the patient breathed 100% oxygen. Based upon hospital unit number, the patients were then randomized to alternating sequences of a 15-minute period of 70% nitrogen-oxygen inhalation followed by a 15-minute period of 70% nitrous oxide–oxygen or the reverse. At the end of each 15-minute period, hemodynamic measurements were recorded. *Phase II:* 10 minutes after sternotomy, under steady-state conditions with the patient breathing 100% oxygen, phase II control hemodynamic measurements were made. This was again followed by periods of nitrous oxide–oxygen and nitrogen-oxygen administration with the reverse sequence of that used in phase I. An additional set of measurements with 100% oxygen concluded phase II of the study. Six of the 20 patients required additional therapy for hypertension (systolic pressure >160 mm Hg) before the initiation of either phase I or phase II. Therapy consisted of sufentanil, 5 to 10 mg/kg, or sodium nitroprusside <1 μg/kg/min. Where additional therapy was required, steady-state hemodynamic conditions were achieved before control measurements were recorded. No therapy was initiated during the actual study period.

A hemodynamic tracking profile included the following measurements made at end-exhalation: heart rate, arterial blood pressure, right atrial pressure, pulmonary artery and capillary wedge pressure, and thermodilution cardiac output [11]. Statistical analysis was performed using analysis of variance and the General Linear Models techniques. Adjusted means plus or minus grouped SEM were reported for the appropriate subgroup interaction and $p<0.05$ was considered statistically significant.

RESULTS

The pertinent positive findings of this study were associated with changes in systemic blood pressure (Table 44.1). During phase I, changing from 100% oxygen to 70% nitrous oxide resulted in a 23% decrease in systolic blood pressure. Changing from 100% oxygen to 70% oxygen (30% nitrogen) was associated with an 8% decrease in systolic pressure. In phase II, nitrous oxide exerted a more profound vasodilator action. The systolic pressure decreased 21% with the addition of nitrous oxide, while stroke volume index decreased 19%.

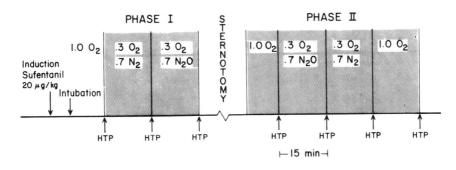

HTP = Hemodynamic Tracking Profile

FIGURE 44.1. Protocol for the study (N = 20).

TABLE 44.1.   Changes in hemodynamic variables with nitrous oxide anesthesia

Determination	O_2	N_2O	N_2	O_2
Phase I (N = 20): Preincision				
HR (beats/min)	68 ± 1	60 ± 1*†	66 ± 1	
SBP (mm Hg)	130 ± 2	105 ± 2*†	120 ± 2*	
$\overline{BP}$ (mm Hg)	86 ± 2	70 ± 2*†	80 ± 2*	
PCWP (mm Hg)	14 ± 1	12 ± 1	13 ± 1	
CI (L/min/m²)	2.9 ± 0.1	2.5 ± 0.1*†	2.9 ± 0.1	
SVI (cc/beat/m²)	44 ± 1	43 ± 1	45 ± 1	
SVRI (RU/m²)	27 ± 1	25 ± 1	26 ± 1	
		*p <0.05 compared to O_2		
		†p <0.05 N_2 vs N_2		
Phase II (N = 20): Poststernotomy				
HR (beats/min)	66 ± 1	63 ± 1*†	68 ± 1‡	65 ± 1
SBP (mm Hg)	137 ± 2	109 ± 2*†‡	127 ± 2*	128 ± 2
$\overline{BP}$ (mm Hg)	90 ± 2	72 ± 2*†‡	82 ± 2*	83 ± 2
$\overline{PCWP}$ (mm Hg)	13 ± 1	12 ± 1‡	13 ± 1‡	11 ± 1
CI (L/min/m²)	2.7 ± 0.1	2.6 ± 0.1‡	2.6 ± 0.1	2.3 ± 0.1*
SVI (cc/beat/m²)	42 ± 1	41 ± 1†‡	39 ± 1*	36 ± 1*
SVRI (RU/m²)	33 ± 1	27 ± 1*†‡	31 ± 1	34 ± 1
		*p <0.05 vs first O_2		
		†p <0.05 N_2 vs N_2O		
		‡p <0.05 vs second O_2		

HR = heart rate; SBP = systolic blood pressure; $\overline{BP}$ = mean blood pressure; $\overline{PCWP}$ = mean pulmonary capillary wedge pressure; CI = cardiac index; SVI = stroke volume index; SVRI = systemic vascular resistance index; RU = resistance units.

Associated with changes in phase I, cardiac index decreased by 14% with nitrous oxide administration; however, the heart rate showed a significant decrease of 12% with nitrous oxide as compared to oxygen. Thus stroke volume index remained constant. When this is taken into account, there were no signs of cardiac depression as evidenced by the relationship of stroke volume index and pulmonary capillary wedge pressure. In phase II, similar relationships of stroke volume index or cardiac index and wedge pressure were seen.

The presence or absence of a cardiac lesion (coronary artery or valvular disease) and good or diminished LV function did not further influence the effects of nitrous oxide as compared to nitrogen (Figure 44.2).

DISCUSSION

This randomized prospective study suggests that nitrous oxide does not consistently exert deleterious effects on cardiovascular performance in patients anesthetized with sufentanil. In contrast, Stoelting et al [6] reported a decrease in mean arterial blood pressures and cardiac index after nitrous oxide administration in patients undergoing open heart surgery (coronary artery or valve replacement) anesthetized with fentanyl. Wong et al [12] reported similar results in normal volunteers who received intravenous morphine, 2 mg/kg. Eisele et al [13] also reported cardiovascular dysfunction after 40% nitrous oxide administration to patients with coronary artery disease and poor LV function.

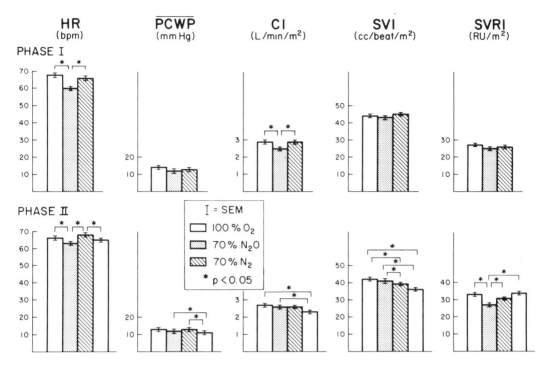

FIGURE 44.2. Data obtained for selected variables (for abbreviations, see Table 44.1).

Balasaraswathi et al documented that nitrous oxide depresses LV function in patients with poor LV reserve [8]. After nitrous oxide administration to patients with well-preserved LV function, however, no cardiovascular depression was reported.

In a clinical setting, it may be difficult to observe the effects of nitrous oxide on regional LV function. Thus Philbin et al [14], using a canine model with implanted ultrasonic crystals, noted reversible abnormalities in regional wall motion associated with 66% nitrous oxide inhalation. Moffitt et al [15], however, using direct measurements of coronary blood flow in humans with coronary artery disease, observed no signs of ischemia as judged by lactate production. The hemodynamic patterns in their patients following 50% nitrous oxide were similar to those reported in the present series.

In comparison to our previous investigation in a group of patients under a similar protocol, sufentanil, 20 μg/kg, has similar

hemodynamic actions as fentanyl, 100 μg/kg [16]. There is a suggestion that nitrous oxide–sufentanil has a more profound effect than nitrous oxide–fentanyl on systolic pressure during surgical stimulation.

Logistic considerations did not allow an additional measurement period at FIO_2 = 1.0 at the conclusion of phase I. The results of phase I and phase II were very similar during nitrous oxide and nitrogen inhalation measurements. Since the periods of nitrous oxide and nitrogen were randomized, the time from infusion of sufentanil to the measurement is not a factor. Decreased analgesia with 100% oxygen inhalation is probably not the reason for the increase in blood pressure seen during control measurements. On a theoretical basis, both 100% oxygen and 70% nitrogen were administered at similar levels of "anesthesia." Furthermore, the addition of nitrous oxide to fentanyl anesthetic does not appear to change anesthetic depth as measured by electroencephalography [17].

On the basis of our observations, nitrous oxide for supplemental analgesia is devoid of any consistently significant cardiac depression. Changes in cardiovascular performance secondary to nitrous oxide administration during sufentanil anesthesia are associated with decreased FIO_2 and a direct vasodilator action rather than a cardioselective depressant effect of nitrous oxide.

CONCLUSION

Under the conditions of this study, nitrous oxide and decreased FIO_2 affected cardiovascular performance in a similar fashion. Reduction in systolic pressure was related to both FIO_2 and nitrous oxide. We conclude that nitrous oxide can be used to supplement analgesia without risk of direct cardiac depression during a high dose of sufentanil anesthetic. The hemodynamic impact of nitrous oxide appears to be similar in both fentanyl- and sufentanil-treated patients.

REFERENCES

1. Lowenstein E, Philbin DM. Narcotic "anesthesia" in the eighties. Anesthesiology 1981;55:195–7.
2. Barash PG, Kopriva CJ. Narcotics and the circulation. In: LM Kitahata and JG Collins, eds. Narcotic analgesics in anesthesiology. Baltimore: Williams & Wilkins, 1982:91–132.
3. Lappas DG, Buckley MJ, Laver MB, Daggart WM, Lowenstein E. Left ventricular performance and pulmonary circulation following addition of nitrous oxide to morphine during coronary artery surgery. Anesthesiology 1975;43:61–9.
4. Stoelting RK, Gibbs P. Hemodynamic effects of morphine and morphine-nitrous oxide in valvular heart disease and coronary artery disease. Anesthesiology 1973;38:45–52.
5. McDermott RW, Stanley TH. The cardiovascular effects of low concentrations of nitrous oxide during morphine anesthesia. Anesthesiology 1974;41:89–91.
6. Stoelting RK, Gibbs PS, Creesser CW, Peterson C. Hemodynamic and ventilatory responses to fentanyl, fentanyl-droperidol and nitrous oxide in patients with acquired valvular heart disease. Anesthesiology 1975;42:319–24.
7. Lunn JK, Stanley TH, Eisele J, Webster L, Woodward A. High-dose fentanyl anesthesia for coronary artery surgery: plasma fentanyl concentrations and influence of nitrous oxide on cardiovascular responses. Anesth Analg (Cleve) 1979;58:390–5.
8. Balasaraswathi K, Kumar P, Rao T, El-Etr AA. Left ventricular end diastolic pressure as an index for nitrous oxide use during coronary artery surgery. Anesthesiology 1981;55:708–9.
9. Hilgenburg JC, McCammon RL, Stoelting RK. Pulmonary and systemic vascular responses to nitrous oxide in patients with mitral stenosis and pulmonary hypertension. Anesth Analg (Cleve) 1980;59:323–6.
10. Wynne J, Mann TFT, Alpert JS, Green LH, Grossman W. Hemodynamic effects of nitrous oxide administered during cardiac catheterization. JAMA 1980;243:1440–3.
11. Barash PB, Chen Y, Kitahata LM, Kopriva CJ. The hemodynamic tracking system: a method of data management and guide for cardiovascular therapy. Anesth Analg (Cleve) 1980;59:169–74.
12. Wong KC, Martin WE, Hornbein TF, Freund FG, Everett J. The cardiovascular effects of morphine sulfate with oxygen and with nitrous oxide in man. Anesthesiology 1973;38:542–9.
13. Eisele JH, Reitan JA, Massumi RA, Zelis RF, Miller RR. Myocardial performance and N_2O analgesia in coronary artery disease. Anesthesiology 1976;44:16–20.
14. Philbin DM, Foëx P, Lowenstein E, Ryder WA, Jones LA. Nitrous oxide causes myocardial dysfunction. Anesthesiology 1983;59:A80.
15. Moffitt EA, Scovil JE, Barker RA, et al. Myocardial metabolism and hemodynamics of nitrous oxide in fentanyl or enflurane anesthesia in coronary patients. Anesthesiology 1983;59:A31.
16. Michaels I, Kay H, Barash P. Does nitrous oxide or a reduced FIO_2 alter hemodynamic function during high-dose fentanyl anesthesia? Anesthesiology 1982;57:A44.
17. Sebel PS, Bovill JG, Wauquier A, Rog P. Effects of high-dose fentanyl anesthesia on the electroencephalogram. Anesthesiology 1981;55:203–11.

45 MYOCARDIAL DEPRESSION WITH NITROUS OXIDE ANESTHESIA

Daniel M. Philbin

Preliminary data collected during the past year at Oxford University suggest to us that nitrous oxide is a direct myocardial depressant. Using an open-chested preparation in dogs, similar to one previously reported [1], we created a critical stenosis of the left anterior descending coronary artery, defined as sufficient reduction in coronary flow to eliminate the hyperemic response to a 10-second occlusion but with no evidence of dysfunction prior to occlusion. Two pairs of ultrasonic piezoelectric crystals were implanted in the subendocardial myocardium. One pair was located in the distribution of the left circumflex coronary artery and the other in the area of distribution of the left anterior descending coronary artery distal to the stenosis.

Regional myocardial function was assessed by obtaining a continuous measurement of segment length between each pair of crystals. In the normal segment length, recording the distance between crystals is shortest at end-systole. With the development of myocardial depression and/or ischemia, the velocity and amount of systolic shortening is decreased and postsystolic shortening appears.

EFFECTS OF NITROUS OXIDE IN ANIMAL STUDIES

A series of dogs was anesthetized with an intravenous bolus of fentanyl, 100 μg per kilogram of body weight, followed by an infusion of 1 μg/kg/min. In the absence of critical stenosis, no evidence of regional dysfunction—that is, postsystolic shortening—was seen with or without nitrous oxide. Once critical stenosis was produced, however, the introduction of 66% nitrous oxide in place of nitrogen resulted in a significant decrease in systolic shortening and evidence of significant postsystolic shortening in the area of the left anterior descending coronary artery distribution [2]. This was not accompanied by any significant change in coronary blood flow, coronary vascular resistance, heart rate, or arterial oxygen tension. Function in the left circumflex distribution remained unimpaired. Elimination of nitrous oxide usually

261

(not always) resulted in a return to normal function.

CONCLUSION

These data demonstrate that fentanyl alone produces no evidence of regional myocardial dysfunction even in the presence of a significant reduction in coronary flow. In the presence of a critical stenosis, however, the addition of nitrous oxide results in marked deterioration in the area of compromised flow, which cannot be explained by an increase in demand. This suggests that nitrous oxide has a direct detrimental effect on regional myocardial function and that such an effect is not always reversible.

Supported in part by a Senior International Fellowship (Nuffield Department of Anaesthetics, Oxford) No. 1 FO6 TW00705-01, Fogarty International Center, NIH.

REFERENCES

1. Lowenstein E, Foëx P, Francis CM, Davies WL, Yusuf F, Ryder WA. Regional ventricular dysfunction in myocardium supplied by a narrowed coronary artery with increasing halothane concentration in the dog. Anesthesiology 1981;55:349–59.
2. Philbin DM, Foëx P, Lowenstein E, Ryder WA, Jones LA. Nitrous oxide causes myocardial dysfunction. Anesthesiology 1983;59:A80.

46 CHOICE OF RELAXANT WITH NARCOTIC-BASED ANESTHESIA

John J. Savarese

Judicious administration of narcotic and muscle relaxant drugs in combination allows us to manipulate a patient's physiologic state to achieve desired clinical effects. This potential has greatly enhanced our ability to provide safe and effective anesthesia in a wider range of clinical situations. This chapter briefly summarizes the pharmacologic properties of these classes of drugs and points up some considerations and cautions in their selection.

PHARMACOLOGIC PROPERTIES OF NARCOTICS AND MUSCLE RELAXANTS

The neuromuscular blocking agents currently in clinical use or soon to be released include the short-acting depolarizing agent succinylcholine, the intermediate-duration depolarizer decamethonium, and a group of nondepolarizing drugs with intermediate to long duration of activity. Metocurine, pancuronium, gallamine, alcuronium, and fazadinium are nondepolarizing agents of long duration; atracurium and vecuronium are of

intermediate duration. All these agents can be shown under proper experimental conditions to produce certain autonomic effects in experimental animals, ranging from histamine release and indirect sympathomimetic effects to muscarinic blockade. These effects are the basis for the cardiovascular actions of neuromuscular blockers in human beings, the most common being induction of hypertension or hypotension, tachycardia or bradycardia. The new relaxants atracurium and vecuronium are noteworthy for their lack of autonomic and cardiovascular effects. Table 46.1 summarizes the autonomic and cardiovascular actions of the neuromuscular blocking drugs.

The narcotic drugs morphine, meperidine, fentanyl, sufentanil, and alfentanil can induce hypotension, bradycardia, or tachycardia. These effects generally result from the vasodilatory and central sympathetic inhibitory action of the drugs when given in high doses. The significant cardiovascular effects to be expected when these agents are given as the sole anesthetic are summarized in Table 46.2.

CONSIDERATIONS ON A COMBINED ANESTHETIC TECHNIQUE

Table 46.3 lists typical conditions in which certain changes in heart rate or arterial pres-

sure might be desired that can be achieved with a combined anesthetic technique. The logical choices of narcotic and relaxant are indicated. A number of factors can influence their use.

TABLE 46.1. Cardiovascular and autonomic effects of the neuromuscular blocking drugs

Drug	Autonomic Effect	Clinical Cardiovascular Result (dose)
Succinylcholine (S-D)	Ganglionic (nicotinic receptor) stimulation [1]	Tachycardia, hypertension (1 mg/kg)
	Sinus node (muscarinic receptor) stimulation [2]	Bradycardia, hypotension
Decamethonium (I-D)	Very little [3]	Usually none; rare bradycardia (0.1 mg/kg)
d-Tubocurarine (L-ND)	Histamine release [4,5]	Skin flushing, hypotension, tachycardia, and bronchospasm rare (0.5 mg/kg)
Metocurine (L-ND)	Histamine release [4,6]	Skin-flushing, hypotension, tachycardia and bronchospasm all relatively rare (0.4 mg/kg)
Pancuronium (L-ND)	Muscarinic blockade— sinus node (vagolytic effect) [7,10]	Tachycardia (0.06–0.1 mg/kg or more)
	Indirect sympathomimetic effects [8,9]	Tachycardia, hypertension, arrhythmias (0.08–0.10 mg/kg or more)
Gallamine (L-ND)	Muscarinic blockade— sinus [10] node (vagolytic effect)	Tachycardia, more than with pancuronium, since vagolytic effect is stronger in the clinical dose range (0.5–4.0 mg/kg)
Alcuronium (L-ND)	Muscarinic blockade— sinus [10] node	Little or no cardiovascular effect, since mechanism probably occurs beyond the clinical dose range for neuromuscular blockade (0.5 mg/kg)
Fazadinium (L-ND)	Muscarinic blockade [10] (potent vagolytic effect)	Significant tachycardia (0.2–1.5 mg/kg)
	Ganglionic (nicotinic receptor) blockade [10]	Hypotension at large doses (1.0–2.0 mg/kg)
Atracurium (I-ND)	Very weak histamine release [6]	Few, but occasional mild flushing and brief fall in arterial pressure with very large doses given as rapid bolus (0.6 mg/kg or more)

TABLE 46.1.   *(continued)*

Drug	Autonomic Effect	Clinical Cardiovascular Result (dose)
Vecuronium (I-ND)	Muscarinic blockade—sinus [11] node (vagolytic effect)	Vagolytic effect 20 times weaker than that of pancuronium, therefore of theoretical interest only; no significant cardiovascular effect of vecuronium noted at dosage as high as 0.3 mg/kg, or 5 × the ED_{95} for neuromuscular blockade

S-D = short-acting depolarizer; I-D = intermediate-duration depolarizer; L-ND = long-duration nondepolarizer; I-ND = intermediate-duration nondepolarizer.

True drug interactions in which narcotics affect the magnitude or duration of neuromuscular blockade caused by depolarizing or nondepolarizing blocking drugs are virtually unknown, or at least not yet reported. It is a safe estimate, however, that approximately 1.5 to 2 times as much neuromuscular blocking drug will be required to produce a given degree of blockade under balanced anesthesia with a narcotic as under anesthesia with a potent anesthetic vapor.

Since the autonomic and cardiovascular effects of relaxants are dose related, more prominent side effects may be expected when narcotic-based anesthesia is used. This is especially true for pancuronium and gallamine, since the vagolytic and sympathomimetic effects of these drugs are unmodified or even accentuated by narcotic anesthesia.

Under narcotic anesthesia, baseline heart rates tend to be slower than in the absence of narcotics. In these cases, the percentage

TABLE 46.2.   Mechanisms and cardiovascular effects of high-dose narcotics

Drug	Cardiovascular Effect	Dose	Mechanism
Morphine	Flushing, hypotension, tachycardia	0.5–1.0 mg/kg	Histamine release [12,13], ?direct vasodilatation
Meperidine	Hypotension	10 mg/kg	Vasodilatation, ?histamine release, ?myocardial depression
	Tachycardia		?Vagolytic property; baroreflex
Fentanyl	Bradycardia	25–100 μg/kg	Central sympathetic inhibition, ?very weak vasodilation [14–16]
Sufentanil	Bradycardia	5–20 μg/kg	Central sympathetic inhibition, ?very weak vasodilation [17,18]
Alfentanil	Bradycardia, hypotension	100–300 μg/kg	Central sympathetic inhibition, ?very weak vasodilation [19,20]

TABLE 46.3. Cardiovascular effects of the narcotic and neuromuscular blocking drugs

Clinical Condition	Desired Cardiovascular Effect	Narcotic	Relaxant
Hypertension	Lowering of arterial pressure	Morphine	d-Tubocurarine
Bradycardia, moderate	Increased heart rate (moderate)	Meperidine	Pancuronium
Bradycardia, severe	Increased heart rate (dramatic)	Meperidine	Gallamine
Tachycardia	Heart rate slowing	Fentanyl	d-Tubocurarine or metocurine
Normal	Induced hypotension	Morphine	d-Tubocurarine
Coronary artery disease—no β blocker	Slowed heart rate	Fentanyl	Metocurine, atracurium, or vecuronium
Coronary artery disease—β blocker and/or Ca++ channel blocker	Maintained or slightly increased or decreased heart rate, no hypotension	Fentanyl, morphine with care	Metocurine with care, atracurium or vecuronium
Mitral valve stenosis with atrial fibrillation	Slowing of heart rate	Fentanyl, morphine, sufentanil	Metocurine, atracurium, or vecuronium
Aortic stenosis	No tachycardia, maintained diastolic pressure (severe bradycardia also undesirable)	Fentanyl, sufentanil	Vecuronium, atracurium, metocurine with care; pancuronium if slight heart rate increase is desirable

increase in heart rate caused by a given dose of pancuronium or gallamine would nearly always be greater than under inhalation anesthesia. On the other hand, because of the generalized cardiovascular depressant property of the anesthetic vapors, the hypotensive effect of d-tubocurarine and other histamine-releasing relaxants is generally enhanced.

Interactions in which the combination of certain relaxants with specific narcotics may result in unwanted cardiovascular effects are more common. For example, in patients with coronary artery disease who are being treated with β-adrenergic blockers, the combination of bolus succinylcholine with fentanyl anesthesia may result in severe bradycardia. In particularly sensitive individuals, the histamine-releasing properties of morphine and d-tubocurarine may be additive, such that moderate doses of each drug in combination may result in greater histamine release, and consequent hypotension, than would ordinarily be expected. In such situations, either prophylaxis or treatment with both H_1 and H_2 blockers (chlorpheniramine, 0.1 mg per kilogram of body weight, and cimetidine, 5 mg/kg) is useful in preventing or aborting the histamine-release response. If histamine release by morphine or d-tubocurarine occurs in patients receiving cimetidine or droperidol, the response may be somewhat exaggerated. This is because both drugs may inhibit histamine N-methyl transferase, the principal metabolic pathway for the inactivation of histamine (Moss J, unpublished observations, 1980).

In other clinical situations, the interaction of narcotic-induced bradycardia with relaxant cardiovascular effect may favor the use of vagolytic relaxants. This is especially true in patients with coronary artery disease who are receiving large doses of β-adrenergic blocking drugs. These subjects may require the vagolytic and indirect sympathomimetic properties of pancuronium, or even gallamine, to counteract narcotic-induced bradycardia and keep heart rate within the normal range. Furthermore, because of the vasoconstrictor properties of noncardioselective beta blockers such as propranolol, such patients may be somewhat more susceptible to the slight vasodilator properties of relaxants such as d-tubocurarine that release significant amounts of histamine.

CONCLUSION

A technique that exploits the autonomic properties of the muscle relaxant and narcotic agents in combination has proved to be a valuable addition to the practice of anesthesia. Proper drug selection is essential if the technique is to be applied successfully, and the synergistic effects of the drug interaction must be controlled so as to potentiate the desired results and avoid unwanted and possibly dangerous side effects.

REFERENCES

1. Paton WDM. The effects of muscle relaxants other than muscular relaxation. Anesthesiology 1959;20:453.
2. Thesleff S. Succinylcholine iodide: studies on its pharmacological properties and clinical use. Acta Physiol Scand [Suppl] 1953; 199:1.
3. Paton WDM, Zainis EJ. Methonium compounds. Pharmacol Rev 1952;4:219.
4. Savarese JJ. The autonomic margin of safety of metocurine and d-tubocurarine. Anesthesiology 1979;50:40–7.
5. Moss J, Rosow CE, Savarese JJ, et al. Role of histamine in the hypotensive action of d-tubocurarine in humans. Anesthesiology 1981;55:19–25.
6. Basta SJ, Savarese JJ, Ali HH, Moss J, Gionfriddo M. Histamine-releasing potencies of atracurium, dimethyltubocurarine and tubocurarine. Br J Anaesth 1983;55:105S–106S.
7. Bonta IL, Goorissen WM, Derkx FH. Inhibition of vagal receptors in the heart by pancuronium. Eur J Phamacol 1968;4:83–8.
8. Gardier RW, Tsevdos EJ, Jackson DB. Effects of gallamine and pancuronium on inhibitory transmission in cat sympathetic ganglia. J Pharmacol Exp Ther 1978;204:45–63.
9. Segarra Domenech J, Carlos Garcia R, Rodriguez Sasiain JM, et al. Pancuronium bromide: an indirect sympathomimetic agent. Br J Anaesth 1976;48:1143–8.
10. Hughes R, Chapple DJ. Effects of non-depolarizing neuromuscular blocking agents on peripheral autonomic mechanisms in cats. Br J Anaesth 1976;48:59–69.
11. Durant NN, Marshall IG, Savage DS, et al. The neuromuscular and autonomic blocking activities of pancuronium, ORG NC45 and other pancuronium analogues in the cat. J Pharm Pharmacol 1979;31:831–8.
12. Lowenstein E, Hallowell P, Levine FH, et al. Cardiovascular responses to large doses of intravenous morphine in man. N Engl J Med 1969;281:1389–96.
13. Philbin DM, Moss J, Akins C, Rosow CE. The use of H_1 and H_2 histamine antagonists with morphine anesthesia: a double-blind study. Anesthesiology 1981;55:292–8.
14. Stanley TH, Webster LR. Anesthetic requirements and cardiovascular effects of fentanyl-oxygen and fentanyl-diazepam-oxygen anesthetic in man. Anesth Analg (Cleve) 1978;57:411–6.
15. Lin WS, Bidwai AV, Stanley TH, et al. Cardiovascular dynamics after large doses of fentanyl and fentanyl plus N_2O in the dog. Anesth Analg (Cleve) 1976;55:168–72.
16. Gardocki JF, Yelnoski J. A study of some of the pharmacological actions of fentanyl citrate. Toxicol Appl Pharmacol 1964;6:48–54.
17. de Lange S, Boscoe MJ, Stanley TH, Pace N. Comparison of sufentanil-O_2 and fen-

tanyl-O_2 for coronary artery surgery. Anesthesiology 1982;56:112–8.

18. Sebel PS, Bovill JG. Cardiovascular effects of sufentanil anesthesia. Anesth Analg (Cleve) 1982;61:115–121.

19. de Lange S, Stanley TH, Boscoe MJ. Alfentanil-oxygen anaesthesia for coronary artery surgery. Br J Anaesth 1981;53:1291–7.

20. Nauta J, de Lange S, Koopman D, Spierdijk J, Van Kleef J, Stanley TH. Anesthetic induction with alfentanil: a new short-acting narcotic analgesic. Anesth Analg (Cleve) 1982;61:267–70.

47 NARCOTICS AND NEUROMUSCULAR BLOCKING DRUGS

Ronald D. Miller

EFFECT OF NARCOTICS AT THE NEUROMUSCULAR JUNCTION

The influence of fentanyl on the basic mechanisms of neuromuscular function has not been studied. Assuming that fentanyl has mechanisms of action at the neuromuscular junction similar to those of other narcotics, certain assumptions can be made. Although morphine has no postjunctional activity [1], it does impair release of acetylcholine from the motor nerve terminal, which in itself could augment a nondepolarizing neuromuscular blockade [2]. Specifically, meperidine and other narcotics probably locate on the inner surface of the muscle membrane associated with the sodium channel. Activation of the receptors located on the muscle membrane by narcotics probably interferes with the opening of the sodium channels in response to membrane depolarization [3]. This type of mechanism of action should augment a nondepolarizing neuromuscular blocking drug.

COMPARISON OF MUSCLE RELAXANT POTENCY DURING THE UNANESTHETIZED AND ANESTHETIZED STATE

Because of usual concomitant administration of nitrous oxide, it is difficult to ascertain the influence of narcotics themselves on the potency of neuromuscular blocking drugs. Independent of the anesthetic being used, however, the anesthetic state markedly decreases the amount of d-tubocurarine required for neuromuscular blockade. For example, Miller et al [4] found the ED_{50} (that dose of d-tubocurarine required for a 50% depression of twitch tension) in the awake patient to be 9.1 mg/m^3 (about 16 mg/70 kg). Yet, with nitrous oxide–narcotic anesthesia in which both meperidine and thiopental were used, the ED_{50} was decreased to 5.6 mg/m^3 (about 9.5 mg/70 kg).

COMPARISON OF MUSCLE RELAXANT POTENCY WITH DIFFERENT GENERAL ANESTHETICS

Inhaled anesthetics augment the neuromuscular block from nondepolarizing neuromuscular blocking drugs in a dose-dependent fashion. Of those anesthetics studied, inhaled anesthetics augment the neuromuscular blocking drugs in decreasing order—isoflurane and enflurane > halothane > nitrous oxide–barbiturate–narcotic anesthesia [5]. Basically, halothane shifts the d-tubocurarine dose-response curve to the left from the nitrous oxide–narcotic curve by a factor of approximately 50%. In other words, an average patient usually requires only half as much d-tubocurarine with halothane anesthesia as compared to nitrous oxide–narcotic anesthesia. Isoflurane and enflurane shift the curve even farther to the left. Specifically, a patient might require 60% to 80% less d-tubocurarine with isoflurane or enflurane than might be required with nitrous oxide-narcotic anesthesia. Thus if it is clinically desirable to use the least dose of neuromuscular blocking drug possible, the inhaled anesthetics (i.e., isoflurane, halothane, and enflurane) have clear advantages over the nitrous oxide–narcotic anesthetic technique.

COMPARATIVE INFLUENCE OF NARCOTICS ON THE PHARMACOKINETICS AND PHARMACODYNAMICS OF MUSCLE RELAXANTS

Although enflurane and halothane alter blood flow of the excretory organs (i.e., the kidney and liver), basically the pharmacokinetics of d-tubocurarine are identical during halothane anesthesia as compared to nitrous oxide–morphine anesthesia. The pharmacodynamics of the neuromuscular blocking drugs are markedly different between the two techniques, however [6]. A summary of the pharmacodynamics of d-

tubocurarine in patients anesthetized with nitrous oxide-morphine anesthesia versus those with halothane is presented in Figure 47.1. The $CP_{ss(50)}$ is that blood concentration of d-tubocurarine required to produce a 50% neuromuscular blockade. Specifically, the $CP_{ss(50)}$ in the nitrous oxide-morphine group was 0.6 μg/ml, while it was reduced to 0.36 μg/ml with halothane, 0.5% to 0.7%, and 0.22 μg/ml with halothane, 1.0% to 1.2%. It should be noted that the variability of response was much greater for the nitrous oxide–narcotic group than for the halothane group. I believe this is because the halothane anesthetic concentration was precisely controlled, whereas the narcotic concentration was impossible to control at a steady state.

CONCLUSION

Although the interaction of fentanyl with neuromuscular blocking drugs has not been specifically studied, I believe it is reasonable to take the conclusions reached with other narcotics and apply them to fentanyl. Nitrous oxide–narcotic anesthesia significantly enhances the response of neuromuscular blocking drugs as compared to the unanesthetized state. The response of nondepolarizing neuromuscular blocking drugs is much less and is more variable during nitrous oxide–narcotic anesthesia, however, compared to the response during inhalation anesthesia such as with halothane, isoflurane, or enflurane.

REFERENCES

1. Frederickson RCA, Pinsky C. Morphine impairs acetylcholine release but facilitates acetylcholine's action at a skeletal neuromuscular junction. Nature 1971;231:93–4.
2. Soteropoulos GC, Standaert FG. Neuromuscular effects of morphine and naloxone. J Pharmacol Exp Ther 1973;184:136–42.
3. Frank GB. Two mechanisms for the meperidine block of action potential production in

FIGURE 47.1. The values of the sensitivity variable of the pharmacodynamic model- $Cp_{ss(50)}$ (steady-state plasma concentration that produces a 50% effect). *From Stanski et al [6]. By permission.*

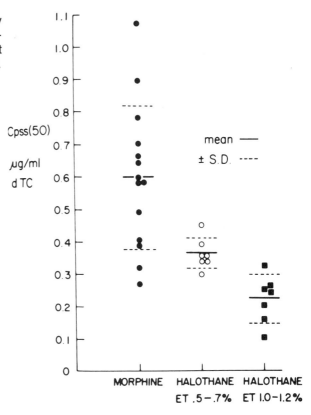

frogs' skeletal muscle: non-specific and opiate drug receptor mediated blockade. J Physiol (Lond) 1975;252:585–601.

4. Miller RD, Crique M, Eger EI II. Duration of halothane anesthesia in neuromuscular blockade with *d*-tubocurarine. Anesthesiology 1976;44:206–10.

5. Miller RD, Savarese JJ. Pharmacology of muscle relaxants, their antagonists and monitoring of neuromuscular function. In: Miller RD, ed. Anesthesia. New York: Churchill Livingstone, 1981;1:500–2.

6. Stanski DR, Ham J, Miller RD, Sheiner LB. Pharmacokinetics and pharmacodynamics of *d*-tubocurarine during nitrous oxide-narcotic and halothane anesthesia in man. Anesthesiology 1979;51:235–41.

48 CALCIUM CHANNEL BLOCKERS

Demetrios G. Lappas

For contractile proteins of the cardiac cells and of the vascular smooth muscle cells to become activated depends on an increase in calcium ion concentration of the cytoplasm. Recent work by Vanhoutte [1] has shown that free intracellular calcium increases through a combination of transmembrane calcium influx and simultaneous liberation of calcium from endoplasmic stores (sarcoplasmic reticulum, superficial binding sites, and mitochondria). The rise in concentration of activator ion triggers the contractile process. Calcium ions bind to protein and initiate excitation-contraction coupling through the splitting of adenosine triphosphate by calcium-dependent adenosine triphosphatase in the myofibrils. In this way, phosphate bond energy is transformed into mechanical work.

CONTRACTILITY

In the myocardial cell, calcium ion influx initiates and controls the degree of contraction. During activation of the cardiac cell, calcium rises markedly in the myocardial cytoplasm, where it binds with a regulatory protein, troponin. This process promotes a force-generating interaction between the myosin bridge and the thin actin filament, with consequent myocardial shortening and development of tension.

Activation of the contractile proteins of the vascular smooth muscle cells also depends on the concentration of calcium ions in the cytoplasm. The rise in cytoplasmic concentration of calcium, which leads to an increase of myogenic tone, can result from heightened permeability of the cell membrane to extracellular calcium, mobilization of calcium from cellular stores, or both mechanisms.

Fleckenstein's report that two new compounds, iproveratril and prenylamine, can block the excitation-contraction coupling of mammalian myocardium in vitro and in vivo first showed that these processes can be modified by pharmacologic means [2]. Recently it was demonstrated that the entry of calcium into cells can be inhibited by drugs with diverse molecular structures. Several drugs are presently available for treating a variety of cardiovascular disorders. Although they are classified as calcium entry blockers, marked variations among the compounds suggest that the blocking action of each is relatively specific for different tissues and that other actions may account for their heterogeneous effects. For example, no relationship between structure and effect on vascular tone has been found, nor has a single receptor been identified for these drugs, which differ in chemical structure and in their solubility in water or lipid. All, however, share a common effect of reducing the transport of extracellular calcium ions across the cell membrane. The relaxation of vascular smooth muscle produced by calcium channel blockers may result either directly, from inhibition of calcium-dependent contractility, or indirectly, from suppression of calcium-dependent membrane excitation.

THE CALCIUM ENTRY BLOCKERS

Verapamil, diltiazem, and nifedipine are the three calcium entry blockers presently available for clinical use [3]. Nifedipine and diltiazem have been shown to be primarily coronary vasodilators. Verapamil affects myocardial performance and cardiac pacemaker activity.

Verapamil inhibits excitation-contraction coupling primarily by interfering with the movement of calcium through slow membrane channels, and probably also by affecting its intracellular movement. Alteration in the concentration of activator ion leads to changes, first, in the amount of adenosine triphosphate consumed by the contractile system; second, in the magnitude of mechanical tension developed; and third, in the augmented oxygen uptake related to generation of the contractile force. Catecholamines and calcium antagonize the effect of verapamil on cardiac and vascular smooth muscle. Possibly β-adrenergic catecholamines, through formation of cyclic adenosine monophosphate, induce phosphorylation of sarcolemma membrane proteins, thus augmenting the number of binding sites that accumulate calcium.

Verapamil impairs cardiac pacemaker activity by greatly reducing the velocity of impulse propagation within the sinoatrial node, and especially through the atrioventricular node. Again, β-adrenergic catecholamines will restore impulse production and propagation in cardiac pacemaker tissues. Extra calcium is less suitable for restoring automaticity.

Excitation-contraction coupling of coronary smooth muscle is generally three to ten times more sensitive to calcium channel blockers than is that of other vascular beds. In cardiac cells, calcium blockers can inhibit the entry of calcium through the slow channels. For vascular smooth muscle such evidence is lacking. The effects of the calcium blockers correlate best with a reduction in the entry of calcium, probably due to change in membrane potential.

In the intact organism, the sympathetic nervous sytem is the most important determinant of vascular function. Norepinephrine released from the adrenergic nerve vesicles binds to an α-adrenergic receptor of the effector cell (postjunctional α-receptor). Thus, contraction is initiated. The relative contribution of the two sources of activator calcium ion—the inward movement and the intracellular mobilization of calcium—varies during α-adrenergic activation. In most arteries, in the arterioles, and in the splanchnic veins, calcium entry blockers curtail vasoconstrictor responses to sympathetic nerve stimulation and exogenous norepinephrine. This mechanism is important because in the smooth muscle cells of these blood vessels, catecholamines activate the contractile process primarily by increasing the permeability of the cell membrane to extracellular calcium. The mechanism is not well defined, but it has been suggested to result from opening of either the membrane potential–operated channels or the receptor-activated calcium channels.

Vascular tissue from hypertensive animals often shows significant differences in reactivity from normotensive controls, and it has been suggested that such differences may arise at least in part from alteration in calcium handling. Whether such alterations include changes in calcium channel function is not clear, but increased sensitivity to verapamil and nifedipine has been reported in aorta from hypertensive rats.

CLINICAL APPLICATIONS

Calcium ion flux plays a major role in the contraction of vascular smooth muscle, and its inhibition can lead to arterial vasodilation. Among the various systemic beds, the coronary arterial bed appears to be particularly sensitive to the action of calcium channel blockers. Recent studies suggest that the coronary circulation is more dynamic than previously thought and can contribute to myocardial ischemia when the arterial tone increases. Therefore, the use of calcium channel blockers can favorably influence myocardial oxygen supply and thus have a role in the treatment of angina pectoris.

Although coronary vascular effects are prominent with each of the calcium entry blockers, some appear to have other actions as well, including effects on the conduction system and on myocardial depression.

The chronic use of calcium entry blockers preoperatively has been reported to potentiate some of the hemodynamic effects of the drugs used during anesthesia. Hypotension and requirement for volume replacement during general anesthesia and surgery appear to be more common in patients taking calcium entry blockers. Finally, whether calcium entry blockade can potentiate and prolong the neuromuscular blockade produced clinically with muscle relaxant drugs is presently under investigation.

DRUG INTERACTIONS AND ADJUNCTIVE USES

Kapur and Flacke [4] have demonstrated some cardiodepressant interaction between verapamil and halothane in the dog. The mechanism for the negative inotropic effect of halothane may be related to slow channel blockade [5].

In a recently presented study [6] we found that patients receiving nifedipine and propranolol appeared to respond to large doses of fentanyl with a reduction in systemic arterial pressure due to decreased systemic vascular resistance. Whether this change is clinically significant is a question. Individual responses to large doses of narcotics or inhalation anesthetics have been reported to vary. Furthermore, several papers support the possibility that the preoperative medical regimen may affect the hemodynamic response to anesthetics. It is therefore possible for patients receiving chronic therapy with calcium entry blockers to have altered vascular tone and response.

Large doses of fentanyl are often used in cardiac surgery; an example is presented in Figure 48.1. Intravenous administration of fentanyl, 50 μg per kilogram of body weight, had minimal effect on the hemodynamic status of this patient, who had been scheduled for coronary artery bypass grafting. The patient was not taking calcium entry blockers. Measured hemodynamic stability is apparent. Figure 48.2 shows a tracing from another patient with coronary artery disease scheduled for myocardial revascularization who had been receiving nifedipine, 20 mg every 6 hours, and propranolol, 40 mg every 6 hours, preoperatively. Infusion of fentanyl resulted in a progressive decrease in systemic arterial pressure and heart rate. Cardiac output decreased but the stroke volume remained unchanged. Calculated systemic vascular resistance appeared to be low.

Recently, we evaluated the effect of calcium entry blockers in conjunction with inhalation anesthetic agents in animals. Chronically instrumented rats were studied over several days. On day 1, the catheters were inserted in the internal jugular vein and carotid artery. On the second day, initially verapamil was administered intravenously and later calcium was added in awake animals to reverse the decrease in arterial pressure that resulted from the calcium entry blocker. On the third day, verapamil and calcium were given to the same animals, which were anesthetized with either halothane, enflurane, or isoflurane.

We found that verapamil caused a mild decrease in arterial pressure when administered in the awake state. Administration of calcium chloride partially reversed this ef-

FIGURE 48.1.   Hemodynamic response to fentanyl in a patient with severe coronary artery disease undergoing triple coronary artery bypass grafting. Administration of 50 μg/kg of fentanyl intravenously had minimal effect on pulmonary arterial (PAP), pulmonary capillary wedge (PCWP), right atrial (RAP) and systemic arterial (SAP) pressures, heart rate (HR), and cardiac output (CO). The patient was not taking calcium entry blockers. An intraaortic balloon assist device was inserted preoperatively.

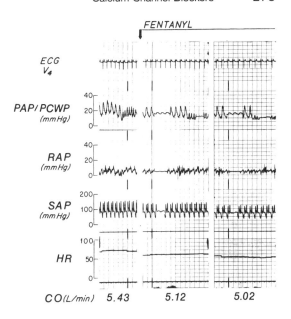

fect. When verapamil was given to anesthetized animals, however, the hypotension was severe. Again, administration of calcium chloride partially restored the arterial pressure. These observations, although not conclusive, indicate that calcium blockers administered during anesthesia may cause hypotension.

FIGURE 48.2.   Hemodynamic response to fentanyl infusion in a patient with severe coronary artery disease receiving nifedipine, 20 mg, and propranolol, 40 mg, at 6-hour intervals preoperatively. (Abbreviations are the same as in Figure 48.1).

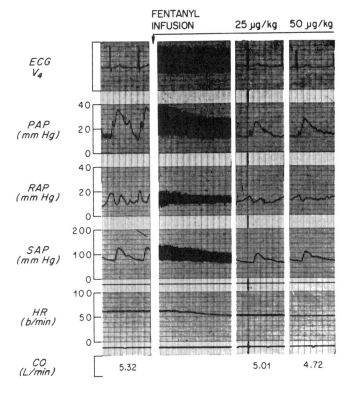

CONCLUSION

Calcium channel blockers are widely used in patients with severe coronary artery disease. Recent clinical and experimental data support the possibility that the preoperative administration of these drugs may affect the hemodynamic response to anesthetics. It is therefore possible for patients on chronic therapy with calcium entry blockers to have altered vascular tone and reactivity to drugs. In addition, possible hormonal and autonomic nervous system alterations may result from the use of these drugs. These need to be studied. Finally, if a calcium entry blocker can modify the hemodynamic effect of fentanyl or any other anesthetic, should we discontinue the drug prior to surgery?

REFERENCES

1. Vanhoutte PM. Calcium-entry blockers and vascular smooth muscle. Circulation 1982; 65(suppl I):11–19.
2. Fleckenstein A. Specific pharmacology of calcium in myocardium, cardiac pacemakers and vascular smooth muscle. Annu Rev Pharmacol Toxicol 1977;17:149–66.
3. Braunwald E. Mechanism of action of calcium-channel-blocking agents. N Engl J Med 1982;307:1618–27.
4. Kapur PA, Flacke WE. Verapamil-halothane: epinephrine arrhythmias and cardiovascular function. Anesthesiology 1980; 53:S132.
5. Lynch C, Vogel S, Speralakis N. Halothane depresses cardiac slow action potentials. Anesthesiology 1980;53:S420.
6. Freis E, Lappas DG. Chronic administration of calcium entry blockers and the cardiovascular responses to high doses of fentanyl. Anesthesiology 1982;57:A295.

49 CALCIUM BLOCKERS AS ADJUVANTS TO OPIOID ANESTHESIA

Patricia A. Kapur

The calcium channel-blocking drugs were released for clinical use in the United States with very little work published concerning interactions with anesthetic agents. Published work to 1983 has mainly reported interactions of calcium channel blockers with inhalation anesthetics. This chapter summarizes that work and evaluates the available data about interactions of these drugs with narcotics.

Our own studies of the effects of the continuous infusion of verapamil during either enflurane or isoflurane anesthesia in dogs demonstrated dose-dependent decreases in mean arterial pressure, cardiac output, and rate of rise of left ventricular pressure (dP/dt). The only difference in effects between isoflurane and enflurane was that the 50% depression of blood pressure was achieved with lower plasma verapamil levels in animals given enflurane than it was in those given isoflurane, and higher degrees of heart block were achieved with lower plasma verapamil levels in the presence of enflurane compared with isoflurane [1]. We were able to show, in halothane-anesthetized dogs given intravenous bolus doses of verapamil, that the amount of depression of cardiovascular function is related to the rate of verapamil administration [2]. For example, if we gave 0.2 mg of verapamil per kilogram of body weight over 30 seconds, we could achieve 40 mm Hg depression of mean arterial blood pressure. When we gave the same dose over 10 minutes, there was only 10 mm Hg decrease in mean arterial blood pressure.

Dr. Reves and colleagues [3] have shown additive depressant hemodynamic effects with nifedipine and inhalation anesthetics. Kates et al [4] demonstrated that the combined depression of verapamil and isoflurane was related not only to the plasma verapamil level but also to the concentration of isoflurane. Zaggy and colleagues [5] have now reported that diltiazem has additive depressant effects when combined with inhalation agents.

What can be said about narcotic anesthetics and calcium channel blockers? Zimpfer et al [6] gave a bolus of verapamil during neuroleptanesthesia in healthy patients and observed decreased systemic vascular resistance and mean arterial blood pressure, maintenance of cardiac output, and no change in pulmonary artery pressure. Kates and Kaplan [7] gave 0.075 mg/kg verapamil immediately prior to cardiopulmonary bypass to coronary artery surgery patients anesthetized with morphine. The investigators observed decreases in systemic vascular resistance and mean arterial pressure with no untoward clinical consequences. The patients had negligible verapamil levels at the end of bypass.

This chapter considers what effects the long-term administration of calcium channel blockers may have on anesthetic management, as well as a theoretical rationale for some possible narcotic interactions with such extended use.

INTERACTION OF CALCIUM CHANNEL BLOCKERS AND NARCOTIC ANESTHETICS

Undoubtedly, calcium channel blockers have therapeutic benefit for patients in whom narcotic anesthesia may be planned. Not only might it be deleterious to withdraw their drugs before surgery, but potential benefits to patients in the perioperative period, including coronary vasodilation, antiarrhythmic effects, and myocardial protection during cardiopulmonary bypass, would be lost. We need data to substantiate whether proposed interactions, such as those reported by Freis and Lappas [8], that nifedipine-treated patients have blood pressure difficulties during high-dose fentanyl administration, are reproducibly observed. If indeed, there are reproducible interactions of narcotics in patients who are receiving long-term calcium channel blocker therapy, we need to know if we can modify these interactions by altering our anesthetic techniques so that patients are not deprived of therapeutically useful agents.

One of the possible rationales for such an interaction derives from the observation that slow channel blockade results in vasodilation and direct myocardial depression in vitro, with nifedipine being the most depressant, in vitro, of the presently available slow channel inhibitors. This vasodilation, though, is thought to induce autonomic compensatory reflexes, which work to counteract the vasodilation and the direct myocardial depression. Thus patients who have autonomic dys-

function, whether on a physiologic, anatomic, or pharmacologic basis, may have interference with these compensatory reflexes and may be at risk for experiencing the direct depressant effects of the drug. Perhaps high-dose narcotics, by their sympatholytic actions, also put patients at risk by unmasking the direct depressant effects of calcium channel blockers.

COMPARISON OF RESPONSES TO ACUTE AND EXTENDED ADMINISTRATION OF CALCIUM CHANNEL BLOCKERS

A distinction must be made, however, between reflex responses to the short- and long-term effects of administering these drugs. With regard to Freis and Lappas's work [8], we can consider what is known about acute compared to extended administration of nifedipine.

In a study of the acute oral adminisration of nifedipine, Lederballe Pedersen et al [9] documented decreased peripheral resistance and blood pressure with increased heart rate in hypertensive patients, a group that is known to have more marked responses to vasoactive drugs. The normotensive patients in the same study also had rises in heart rate, although less marked. This was presumably the reflex compensation after acute administration of nifedipine. In another study, Aoki et al [10] again noted the rise in heart rate after acute administration of nifedipine to a hypertensive group, with a smaller rise in a normotensive group, that was dose related when 10 mg was compared with 30 mg of nifedipine. The rise in heart rate was abolished by simultaneous administration of propranolol.

Lederballe Pedersen et al [9] observed a rise in plasma norepinephrine upon acute administration of nifedipine in both normotensive and hypertensive patients. In a study in which the acute administration of nifedipine was used to reduce the afterload in patients with congestive heart failure, Corea et al [11] observed that both the rise in norepinephrine and the drop in total peripheral resistance were correlated with rises in cardiac index and with improvement in the preejection period to left ventricular ejection time ratio. They therefore speculated that nifedipine not only reduced the afterload of the heart but resulted in improved myocardial function per se, because of adrenergic activation.

EFFECT OF NARCOTICS COMBINED WITH CALCIUM CHANNEL BLOCKERS ON CIRCULATING NOREPINEPHRINE LEVELS

Flacke et al [12] showed that the baseline plasma norepinephrine level in dogs was correlated with the drop in mean arterial pressure that follows administration of high doses of fentanyl. Combining data from patients as well as animals, Flacke and Flacke [13] found that the baseline plasma norepinephrine level was also correlated with the decrease in plasma norepinephrine upon high-dose fentanyl administration. We might have a situation in which patients, after receiving nifedipine acutely, may have high catecholamine levels and therefore could be expected to have large decreases in blood pressure when their catecholamine levels fall after fentanyl administration.

Sustained elevations in norepinephrine levels have not always been observed in patients receiving long-term nifedipine therapy, however. Lederballe Pedersen et al [14] studied patients who received nifedipine for six weeks. The mean arterial pressure was decreased from 133 to 113 mm Hg; the mean heart rate was increased slightly from 82 to 91. Body weights were similar. After extended administration of nifedipine, however, these investigators could not show any difference in plasma renin activity, aldosterone levels, or norepinephrine levels compared to values before nifedipine was started. Thus one might postulate that there may be different mechanisms of control and compensation with extended compared to acute

administration of nifedipine. Another study, reported by Corea et al [15], included patients who had received nifedipine acutely as well as patients who had taken it for three weeks. While normotensive and hypertensive patients both had rises in norepinephrine levels after acute administration, levels in hypertensive patients were still elevated compared to baseline after three weeks of nifedipine therapy. Thus the consensus is less clear on the effects of long-term nifedipine administration on peripheral norepinephrine levels.

Although the data were not specifically gathered for the purpose of investigating this point, Dr. Joan Flacke of the UCLA Department of Anesthesiology was kind enough to let me review some of her catecholamine results because we do not withdraw patients from nifedipine before cardiac surgery in our institution. Of 32 cardiac surgery patients in whom she had measured catecholamine levels, 13 were taking calcium blockers (12 nifedipine, 1 diltiazem) while 19 were not. There was no statistically significant difference in the preanesthetic norepinephrine levels. In fact, the mean ± SEM level of patients taking calcium channel blockers was 274 ± 49 pg/ml, while for those not taking calcium channel blockers it was 266 ± 41 pg/ ml. An interesting thing we found when going over Dr. Flacke's data was that while the 32 cardiac surgery patients had a mean norepinephrine level of 269 ± 31 pg/ml when taken together, 44 general surgery patients had a significantly lower mean norepinephrine level as well as lower mean epinephrine level immediately prior to anesthetic induction. For a variety of reasons, patients undergoing cardiac surgery may very well have higher catecholamine levels, which may be associated with more marked responses upon administration of high doses of fentanyl, whether or not they are taking nifedipine.

CONCLUSION

Careful hemodynamic monitoring and titration of any anesthetic technique to the desired clinical effect should allow patients to enjoy not only the benefits derived from calcium channel blockade but the benefits to be gained from application of the latest developments in the field of anesthetic agents and adjuvants.

REFERENCES

1. Kapur PA, Flacke WE, Olewine SK. Comparison of effects of isoflurane versus enflurane on cardiovascular and catecholamine responses to verapamil in dogs. Anesth Analg (Cleve) 1982;61:193–4.
2. Kapur PA, Flacke WE. Epinephrine-induced arrhythmias and cardiovascular function after verapamil during halothane anesthesia in the dog. Anesthesiology 1981; 55:218–25.
3. Marshall AG, Kissin I, Reves JG, Bradley EL Jr, Blackstone EH. Interaction between negative inotropic effects of halothane and nifedipine in the isolated rat heart. J Cardiovasc Pharmacol 1983;5:592–7.
4. Kates RA, Kaplan JA, Guyton RA, Dorsey L, Hug CC Jr, Hatcher CR. Hemodynamic interactions of verapamil and isoflurane. Anesthesiology 1983;59:132–8.
5. Zaggy AP, Kates RA, Norfleet EA, Mueller RA, Heath KR. The comparative cardiovascular effects of verapamil, nifedipine, and diltiazem during halothane anesthesia. Anesthesiology 1983;59:A44.
6. Zimpfer M, Fitzal S, Tonczar L. Verapamil as a hypotensive agent during neuroleptanaesthesia. Br J Anaesth 1981;53:885–9.
7. Kates RA, Kaplan JA. Cardiovascular responses to verapamil during coronary artery bypass graft surgery. Anesth Analg (Cleve) 1983;62:821–6.
8. Freis ES, Lappas DG. Chronic administration of calcium entry blockers and the cardiovascular responses to high doses of fentanyl in man. Anesthesiology 1982;57:A295.
9. Lederballe Pedersen O, Christensen NJ, Ramsch KD. Comparison of acute effects of nifedipine in normotensive and hypertensive man. J Cardiovasc Pharmacol 1980; 2:357–366.
10. Aoki K, Kondo S, Mochizuki A, et al. Antihypertensive effect of cardiovascular Ca^{2+}-antagonist in hypertensive patients in the absence and presence of beta-adrenergic blockade. Am Heart J 1978;96:218–26.
11. Corea L, Bentivoglio M, Cosmi F, Alunni G. Catecholamines plasma levels and haemodynamic changes induced by nifedipine in chronic severe heart failure. Cur Ther Res 1981;30:698–707.
12. Flacke JW, Flacke WE, Bloor BC, Olewine S. Effects of fentanyl, naloxone, and clonidine on hemodynamics and plasma catecholamine levels in dogs. Anesth Analg (NY) 1983;62:305–13.
13. Flacke WE, Flacke JW. Cardiovascular physiology and circulatory control. Semin Anesth 1982;1:185–95.
14. Lederballe Pedersen O, Mikkelsen E, Christensen NJ, Kornerup HJ, Pedersen EB. Effect of nifedipine on plasma renin, aldosterone and catecholamines in arterial hypertension. Eur J Clin Pharmacol 1979;15:235–40.
15. Corea L, Miele N, Bentivoglio M, Boschetti E, Agabiti-Rosei E, Muisan G. Acute and chronic effects of nifedipine on plasma renin activity and plasma adrenaline and noradrenaline in controls and hypertensive patients. Clin Sci 1979;57:115s–17s.

Part VII DISCUSSION

DR. FAWZY G. ESTAFANOUS: I have two comments about calcium channel blockers. Dr. Tarazi and his group used different doses to block the calcium channels of rats and tested the response to norepinephrine. The animals that were totally blocked did not respond adequately even to very high doses of norepinephrine, and the response was dose related to the degree of block. Hypotension complicating the use of calcium channel blockers does not respond to even large quantities of catecholamines, nor is it altered by calcium. In our experience in the operating room, the only drug we have found that adequately controlled this hypotension was Neo-Synephrine in very large doses.

Clinically, the hypotension in patients receiving large doses of calcium channel blockers has mainly followed cardiopulmonary bypass. It is extremely rare during induction of anesthesia, occurring in about 1 in every 300 to 400 cases. This hypotension, when it happens, is very severe. It is associated with peripheral vasodilatation and increased cardiac output. Unless the peripheral vascular resistance can be adjusted, it is very difficult to maintain adequate perfusion pressure. In our early experience with these drugs over two years ago, we encountered a patient with an impaired ventricle and low perfusion pressure secondary to the vasodilatation. Ischemia was inevitable. Since then we have been very aware of the problem and have adjusted the systemic vascular resistance at an early stage to maintain perfusion pressure by any means. Unlike the mistake we made with propranolol, we do not recommend discontinuation of the drug before surgery. But we do emphasize recognition of a very rare but potential problem.

DR. WILLIAM HAMILTON: Does anyone want to comment on what Dr. Estafanous has said? I think he just confirmed that what our two experts on calcium channel blockers warned might occur actually did happen in his experience.

DR. PATRICIA A. KAPUR: I am in the middle of a new study with a high-dose fentanyl anesthetic that includes patients receiving nifedipine. The catecholamine levels we measured in the subjects receiving long-term nifedipine therapy were actually slightly lower than in the patients not taking nifedipine. Baseline hemodynamic values were similar in the two groups, and the changes observed after the anesthetic induction were much the same. These patients were also given pancuronium and diazepam, so I should clarify that this was a response to fentanyl, pancuronium, and diazepam.

In my study, I was looking at subsequent effects of verapamil and the anesthetic induction was incidental. I was replacing volume as necessary to maintain constant filling pressures, which ties into a point Dr. Lappas has made in the past concerning differences in volume requirements in these patients. Perhaps it was because I was very attentive to keeping the filling pressure constant, but I did not have difficulty inducing anesthesia with fentanyl in these patients. I don't know whether Dr. Estafanous was using inhalation agents when he had his problems.

DR. ESTAFANOUS: We use inhalation agents in many of our patients. After our first experience two years ago with calcium channel blockers, we collected data on 300 consecutive patients receiving these drugs. We had no problems with either narcotic anesthesia or inhalation agents until the day we stopped collecting data, when one patient developed severe hypotension. I have to emphasize that, following bypass, hemodilution and rewarming contribute to the decreases in systemic vascular resistance with calcium channel blockers. So, as I say, the complication is very rare, and it is manageable. Clinically, it is not related so much to the anesthetic as to the arteriole-dilating effect of the calcium channel blockers.

DR. PAUL R. HICKEY: Dr. Lappas begged a question during his presentation and I would like to give him the opportunity to answer it. Do you think, Dr. Lappas, that nifedipine should be discontinued prior to surgery?

DR. DEMETRIOS G. LAPPAS: The question whether or not to discontinue one drug starts with the indication why the drug is given in the first place. Nifedipine, a new drug, is given now in almost every patient with coronary artery disease. But it has a specific indication, and that is for vasospasm, which is common in myocardial ischemic disease, and as an adjunct to nitrates in patients with unstable angina. Nifedipine should be continued and given to these patients on the day of surgery. In patients with exertional angina, it is not necessary to continue the drug. In general, we prefer to administer nifedipine until the day of surgery and be prepared to treat low blood pressure by administering volume and phenyl-ephrine as required. In a patient receiving nife-dipine and propranolol, large doses of fentanyl were given and metubine was used as a muscle relaxant. The induction of anesthesia was un-eventful and the patient was hemodynamically quite stable.

In some instances, discontinuation of the drug may precipitate vasospasm and severe ischemia. An example was a patient undergoing coronary artery bypass grafting who experienced 17 myo-cardial ischemic episodes after nifedipine was dis-continued preoperatively.

DR. DAVID A. DAVIS: Dr. Lappas alluded to sev-eral instances of vasospasm. Another type of spasm is related to calcium metabolism or activ-ity, and it is much more common than most of us realize. This is a skeletal muscle spasm induced by hyperventilation. I would like to ask you, Dr. Lappas, if you think hyperventilation influences the activity or effects of the calcium channel blockers.

DR. LAPPAS: If I heard you correctly, you men-tioned hyperventilation as a cause of coronary vasospasm. One of our earlier discussants also mentioned hypoxemia or hypercapnia during anesthesia as a cause of hemodynamic changes. I think this is very true, particularly in patients with coronary vasospasm. I think changes in carbon dioxide may contribute to that.

DR. CARL E. ROSOW: I'd like to comment on our study that Dr. Reves presented. The interaction between diazepam and fentanyl may well be dose dependent. We can't say a great deal about this from our study, since at the lowest dose of diaze-pam tested, 0.125 mg/kg, the effect was maximal. It may well be that at lower doses there is less effect. I wonder, philosophically, if a predictable drug interaction is necessarily a bad thing. It pro-duces vasodilatation, and we can treat that. I have a nagging suspicion that each drug we add to a narcotic-oxygen regimen somehow completes the anesthetic. I think that's what is happening with diazepam: it puts the patient (or at least his me-dulla) to sleep and thereby lowers the central sympathetic tone. The question is, does this in-teraction vitiate the purpose of high-dose narcotic anesthesia, or is it a good thing?

DR. HAMILTON: Over the years we have seen pharmacologic effects from a combined anes-thetic regimen that are not evident when we ad-minister one drug alone. The barbiturates and nitrous oxide are an early example.

DR. PAUL DAUCHOT: In his presentation I think Dr. Reves omitted a very important study con-ducted by Dr. Hempelmann and his group in 1974. Hempelmann gave 0.3 mg of diazepam intrave-nously to patients undergoing coronary artery by-pass surgery and found substantial decreases in right and left atrial pressure as well as in peak dP/dt. His conclusion was that the decrease in peak dP/dt was not related to diminished con-tractility but rather to vasodilation. In the early 1970s Côté and his group (Montreal, Canada) gave diazepam during cardiac catheterization and found substantial reductions in left ventricular end-diastolic pressure (LVEDP). Two years later they did a similar study in patients with increased end-diastolic pressure and again found marked reductions in LVEDP with diazepam. They never compared the two groups—they probably could not—but from looking at the data it is evident that diazepam was much more effective in reduc-ing preload (LVEDP) in patients with elevated end-diastolic pressures.

Therefore we studied diazepam in two groups of patients scheduled for coronary artery bypass grafting. One group had low (<15 mm Hg) and one had higher (≥15 mm Hg) LVEDP. We found that a total dose of 120 µg/kg intravenously re-sulted in much more hypotension and a greatly prolonged preejection period in the group with preexisting high end-diastolic pressure. There-fore I think we should consider patients' LVEDP before talking about the effects of diazepam.

Dr. Reves, you have not mentioned that di-azepam can work by decreasing preload rather than by decreasing contractility. Is this a negli-gible mechanism, or is it a real one?

DR. J. G. REVES: The work you refer to by Dr. Côté's group, (*Circulation* 1979;50:1210) showing that diazepam is much like nitroglycerine in its effects is what led us to give diazepam as an in-duction agent for patients with ischemic heart dis-ease. They showed an increase in coronary blood flow, a decrease in filling pressure, and no change in cardiac output. This may be similar to what occurs after fentanyl administration, but since we wanted to put patients to sleep in a hurry, we chose a benzodiazepine because we could achieve a more rapid induction. So to answer your ques-tion, we have seen and documented decreased preload with diazepam. Furthermore, both mid-azolam and diazepam decrease pulmonary artery wedge pressures, though I don't know the mech-anism (*Anesth Analg* [Cleve] 1981;60:802). Pul-monary artery wedge pressure, as you know, is a composite of a number of factors, contractility being one, venous return being another.

In the laboratory we found very interesting changes in venous return associated with midazolam (*Anesth Analg* [Cleve] 1983;62:135). Initially a decrease occurs and the blood seems to be sequestered in the hepatic circulation. That circulation is difficult to measure, but the portal venous blood flow initially decreases; then, as a compensatory response to the concomitant hypotension, blood ultimately enters from the hepatic circulation. Portal blood flow increases and compensates for reduced preload, which can be maintained to ensure adequate cardiac contractility.

A hypothesis that I lacked the time to mention during my presentation is that when we combine benzodiazepines with narcotics or calcium blockers, perhaps even some of the other drugs, we may somehow be paralyzing the compensatory response of the venous circulation. I postulate that these profound decreases in cardiac output may result from the diminished venous return. I'm not certain if that is true, because the effect is hard to measure, but we do have some evidence to suggest it.

I agree that we have to be careful about filling pressures when administering the benzodiazepines. Their effects may be augmented when they are combined with other agents, and this may account for the reduction in filling pressure.

DR. GUNTER HEMPELMANN: Based on our investigations, which were performed some years ago (*Anaesthesist* 1978;27:357 and 1977;26:245), we think vasodilatation is the primary hemodynamic effect of the benzodiazepines. We administered these agents at three points during operation: for induction of anesthesia; after sternotomy, with left ventricular function being measured; and during extracorporeal perfusion. When the drug is added during perfusion, measurement of volume loss in the oxygenator and of arterial pressure can indicate whether vasodilation is occurring in the arterial or the venous circulation.

We found that arterial pressure decreased about 30% to 40%. Our investigations were performed with midazolam, flunitrazepam, and diazepam. Diazepam and flunitrazepam produced similar effects when they were given at a ratio of 1 to 10. The effect of midazolam was less. We were able to demonstrate that the benzodiazepines are very strong vasodilating drugs on the arterial as well as the venous side. They have less effect on contractility.

DR. REVES: Dr. Samuelson and I published a paper on this very point of arterial versus venous effects (*Arzneim Forsch* 1981;12a:2268). I don't know how valid our findings were since so many things, including enormous elevations in catecholamines, are going on during cardiopulmonary bypass. As I recall, though, we found a minimal vasodilatory effect on the arterial side and an appreciable effect in the venous reservoir. Midazolam is more of a venodilator, which fits with our findings in dogs. I think when midazolam—which is a benzodiazepine, not a narcotic—becomes available, we will have to be careful when we administer it, because it does have profound venous effects.

DR. JOAN W. FLACKE: I have a question for Dr. Miller. Are the signs of inadequate anesthesia any different in patients anesthetized with an inhalation agent and muscle relaxants than in those receiving a narcotic? What signs do you yourself use to determine whether anesthesia is adequate when your patient is paralyzed?

DR. RONALD D. MILLER: That is an excellent question. Basically, we have to judge more by the drug concentrations than by the patient's signs. With the inhalation anesthetics, most of us have enough experience to know what concentrations are required to prevent movement and memory, and we measure the concentrations either directly or indirectly.

The key is being able to measure the anesthetic concentration, and this is not as easy with narcotics as with inhalation agents. When a narcotic is given as a large bolus dose, we really don't know what the drug level is in the middle of the procedure. So unless a narcotic is given by infusion, we can't determine the depth of anesthesia or the potency of the anesthetic concentration.

DR. DAVIS: Dr. Savarese, would you comment very briefly on the relationship between hyperventilation and dosage of a skeletal muscle relaxant?

DR. JOHN J. SAVARESE: Several studies have been conducted with all the muscle relaxants to investigate the effect on neuromuscular blockade of hyperventilation with lowered P_{CO_2} and elevated pH. To summarize this work, at present *d*-tubocurarine is the drug most significantly affected by hyperventilation because of the tertiary amine. Its potency weakens if pH is elevated. However, atracurium may be affected even more because higher pH augments the Hoffmann elimination. Aside from these two drugs, I don't think pH changes significantly affect the duration or depth of blockade produced by neuromuscular blocking agents, so I don't pay much attention to hyperventilation. Acidosis, though, is a different story.

DR. DONALD STANSKI: Dr. Eger and his colleagues have shown that muscle relaxants change the requirement for inhalational anesthetics as measured by MAC. Do we have any evidence that muscle relaxants change the anesthetic requirement for narcotics?

DR. SAVARESE: Not that I know of.

DR. C. J. HULL: I'd like to ask Dr. Miller a question. We've heard several speakers describe anesthetic techniques in which preanesthetic doses of nondepolarizing muscle relaxants were given to prevent the muscle rigidity associated with a narcotic with which they optimistically proposed to anesthetize a patient. With the variation in response to neuromuscular blocking agents in mind, do you think this technique is kind to patients, or that it even approaches being a good idea?

DR. MILLER: I'm really not the right person to say whether it's a good idea to prevent narcotic-induced rigidity, because the way I practice anesthesia I don't see rigidity. On your other question, the evidence is overwhelming that the technique is not unkind.

DR. HULL: I don't think it's a problem either, because I don't produce rigidity, but I *do* think it's unkind.

DR. HAMILTON: The only time in my practice that I absolutely do not give nitrous oxide is during open heart surgery once the intravascular instrumentation begins. I base this on the assumption that some of these patients may have a degree of intravascular gas embolism. Dr. Philbin, are you certain there is no possibility that gas emboli could be playing a role in your model?

DR. DANIEL M. PHILBIN: Yes, about as certain as I can be, particularly given the time course of our studies. They extend over a five- to six-hour period, so toward the end we were about seven hours past all the instrumentation that was done. I find it hard to believe that an air phenomenon could be a problem at such a late stage.

DR. TONY L. YAKSH: This meeting has really brought home to me how little we know about the mechanisms at work during anesthesia. Three thoughts come to mind. First, we have been talking about the effects of opiates on catecholamine release and the stress response. Opiates can have central effects on catecholamine release, as in blocking the peripheral spinal sympathetic reflexes, or they may occur directly in the adrenal medulla or in the pituitary. Two, the question of muscle relaxation is important. I was expecting to find some answers but, in fact, we are not really certain whether it is a central or a peripheral effect, although from animal studies it appears to be central. The third issue concerns the mechanisms of the opiate effect on the EEG. We know some correlation exists between the EEG and opiate activity, but we don't know whether it is causal or corollary. These questions suggest a number of animal and clinical experiments that may shed light on some of the problems affecting our practice of anesthesia.

VIII OPIOID ANESTHESIA AND POSTOPERATIVE CARE

50 POSTOPERATIVE VENTILATORY CONTROL AFTER ANESTHESIA WITH FENTANYL, ALFENTANIL, AND SUFENTANIL

Nathan L. Pace

Narcotics such as fentanyl are used by themselves or with adjuvants (nitrous oxide, volatile inhalational agents, sedative-hypnotics) to provide surgical anesthesia. Two new analogs of fentanyl, alfentanil and sufentanil, are currently undergoing clinical trials in the United States. Alfentanil is one-third to one-fourth as potent as fentanyl and is shorter acting; sufentanil is five to ten times as potent and is shorter acting than fentanyl. It is known that ventilatory control is depressed immediately after fentanyl–nitrous oxide anesthesia [1–3]. Will the more rapid elimination of these new drugs produce less postoperative respiratory depression than current anesthetics?

COMPARISON OF EFFECTS OF THE THREE AGENTS

We investigated ventilatory control before and immediately after anesthesia. In three studies we evaluated (a) comparable doses of alfentanil and thiopental used for induction of anesthesia; (b) comparable doses of alfentanil and fentanyl given by bolus injection for maintenance of anesthesia; and (c) comparable doses by bolus injection of sufentanil and fentanyl administered for maintenance of anesthesia. As a measure of drug effect on control of ventilation, we determined inspiratory occlusion pressure at 100 msec (P100) and minute ventilation during carbon dioxide rebreathing before and 30 and 60 minutes after anesthesia.

Thirty healthy patients scheduled to undergo general, orthopedic, and gynecologic surgery were entered into each of the three trials. In the induction study, anesthesia was induced with either thiopental sodium, 3 to 5 mg per kilogram of body weight, or alfentanil, 200 to 250 μg/kg, intravenously as a bolus; halothane was then given to maintain anesthesia. In the studies of drugs used for maintenance of anesthesia, induction was done with thiopental sodium, 3 to 5 mg/kg intravenously. Then fentanyl, 7 μg/kg, alfentanil, 20 to 30 μg/kg, or sufentanil, 1.0 μg/kg, was given intravenously over one minute. In all three studies, ventilation was mechanically controlled with 60% nitrous oxide–40% oxygen.

Ventilatory control was measured by the Read carbon dioxide rebreathing method [4]. The P100 values were determined as suggested by Whitelaw et al [5]. Ventilatory control was studied on the morning of surgery prior to anesthesia and 30 and 60 minutes after arrival in the recovery room.

Before each rebreathing challenge, the patient was accustomed to the mouthpiece for several minutes and the resting end-tidal partial pressure of carbon dioxide (end-tidal PCO_2) was determined. Comparisons of ven-

tilatory control were done by contrasting resting end-tidal PCO_2, the slope of minute ventilation versus end-tidal PCO_2, and the slope of P100 versus end-tidal PCO_2. A smaller slope of minute ventilation or P100 versus end-tidal PCO_2 indicated less ventilatory response to carbon dioxide rebreathing, that is, ventilatory depression.

There were no significant differences in patient characteristics or operative events between the treatment subgroups within each of the three studies. Drowsiness, pain, and nausea prevented many patients from completing rebreathing challenges in the recovery room.

Resting end-tidal PCO_2 values were always normal or low before and after anesthesia (Table 50.1). In the induction study, end-tidal PCO_2 levels following alfentanil were

TABLE 50.1. Values for end-tidal partial pressure of carbon dioxide in the resting state

Study	Control	30 Minute	60 Minute	Significance of Group Differences
Induction				
Thiopental	34.5 ± 0.6 (N = 14)	36.0 ± 1.2 (N = 4) †	35.6 ± 1.2 (N = 9) *	} p = 0.004
Alfentanil	31.8 ± 0.6 (N = 13)	41.8 ± 1.5 (N = 10)	39.8 ± 1.8 (N = 11)	
Alfentanil maintenance				
Fentanyl	33.1 ± 1.0 (N = 13)	36.7 ± 1.3 (N = 12)	38.9 ± 1.3 (N = 10)	} NS
Alfentanil	29.0 ± 1.0 (N = 13)	33.9 ± 1.4 (N = 9)	34.3 ± 1.0 (N = 8)	
Sufentanil maintenance				
Fentanyl	32.3 ± 0.7 (N = 15)	35.8 ± 1.7 (N = 9)	36.7 ± 1.1 (N = 10)	} NS
Sufentanil	32.8 ± 1.2 (N = 13)	37.6 ± 1.8 (N = 7)	38.8 ± 1.8 (N = 11)	

Values are means ± SEM, mm Hg. Comparisons of group differences are: *<0.05; †<0.01. NS: not statistically significant.

higher than after thiopental at 30 and 60 minutes. In the study of maintenance anesthesia, resting end-tidal P_{CO_2} was not significantly different in the patients given fentanyl than in those given alfentanil. Similarly, there was no difference in resting end-tidal P_{CO_2} between the treatment subgroups in the sufentanil maintenance study.

A general minor reduction in the slope of minute ventilation versus end-tidal P_{CO_2} occurred after anesthesia (Table 50.2). There was a statistically significant difference between the subgroups of the alfentanil maintenance study, with the slope of minute ventilation versus end-tidal P_{CO_2} being lower for alfentanil than for fentanyl at 60 minutes.

The slope of P100 versus end-tidal P_{CO_2} showed some reduction postoperatively (Table 50.3). No subgroup differences were found in any of the three studies for this slope.

PATIENT RESULTS

The methods we used to assess the control of ventilation are well established [6]. We used three determinations—resting end-tidal P_{CO_2} and the slopes of minute ventilation and P100 versus end-tidal P_{CO_2}—to seek differences between drug subgroups. The slopes of minute ventilation and P100 to end-tidal P_{CO_2} were determined by a non-steady-state carbon dioxide rebreathing challenge. The P100 versus end-tidal P_{CO_2} slope is a measurement of neuromuscular output that is considered to be unaffected by respiratory system mechanics which might be altered by surgery. Decreases in either slope indicate respiratory depression.

Alfentanil and sufentanil are two new fentanyl analogs. Alfentanil is eliminated more rapidly than fentanyl [7]; it is also less potent than fentanyl. Sufentanil, less well studied,

TABLE 50.2. Slopes for minute ventilation versus end-tidal P_{CO_2}

Study	Control	30 Minute	60 Minute	Significance of Group Differences
Induction				
Thiopental	1.95 ± 0.21 (N = 14)	1.51 ± 0.23 (N = 3)	1.65 ± 0.34 (N = 8)	NS
Alfentanil	2.62 ± 0.77 (N = 13)	1.58 ± 0.29 (N = 9)	1.65 ± 0.34 (N = 10)	
Alfentanil maintenance				
Fentanyl	1.39 ± 0.23 (N = 13)	0.96 ± 0.21 (N = 12)	1.70 ± 0.32 (N = 11)	p = 0.02
Alfentanil	1.87 ± 0.32 (N = 13)	1.00 ± 0.24 (N = 9)	0.68 ± 0.17 * (N = 8)	
Sufentanil maintenance				
Fentanyl	1.59 ± 0.30 (N = 15)	0.28 ± 0.23 (N = 9)	0.58 ± 0.18 (N = 10)	NS
Sufentanil	1.10 ± 0.18 (N = 14)	0.77 ± 0.15 (N = 7)	0.97 ± 0.18 (N = 12)	

Values are means ± SEM. Slope is in L/min/mm Hg. Comparisons of group differences are: *<0.05. NS: not statistically significant.

TABLE 50.3. Slopes for inspiratory occlusion pressure at 100 msec versus end-tidal P_{CO_2}

Study	Control	30 Minute	60 Minute	Significance of Group Differences
Alfentanil induction				
Thiopental	0.21 ± 0.04 (N = 13)	0.20 ± 0.03 (N = 3)	0.16 ± 0.05 (N = 8)	
				NS
Alfentanil	0.39 ± 0.20 (N = 13)	0.16 ± 0.04 (N = 10)	0.14 ± 0.02 (N = 11)	
Alfentanil maintenance				
Fentanyl	0.38 ± 0.21 (N = 13)	0.17 ± 0.05 (N = 12)	0.18 ± 0.03 (N = 11)	
				NS
Alfentanil	0.29 ± 0.04 (N = 13)	0.15 ± 0.04 (N = 9)	0.13 ± 0.05 (N = 9)	
Sufentanil maintenance				
Fentanyl	0.19 ± 0.03 (N = 15)	0.02 ± 0.07 (N = 9)	0.07 ± 0.06 (N = 10)	
				NS
Sufentanil	0.07 ± 0.02 (N = 14)	0.38 ± 0.20 (N = 7)	0.08 ± 0.02 (N = 12)	

Values are means ± SEM. Slope is in cm H_2O/mm Hg. NS: not statistically significant.

is more potent and somewhat more rapidly eliminated than fentanyl [8]. As both alfentanil and sufentanil are pure narcotic agonists, increasing respiratory depression accompanies increasing doses [6]. When used during balanced narcotic–nitrous oxide anesthesia, severe respiratory depression is expected. Yet the actual postoperative ventilatory control is a balance between residual narcotic effects on the one hand and pain and awareness on the other. Thus how and when these drugs are given during anesthesia are important determinants of postanesthetic breathing. Stanski and Hug [7] predicted that if a steady-state plasma level sufficient to supplement inhalational anesthesia is established, it will take two half-lives (3 hours for alfentanil and 7.2 hours for fentanyl) for plasma concentrations to decay sufficiently for return of spontaneous ventilation ade-

quate to assure normal arterial blood gas tensions. A similar prediction contrasting fentanyl and sufentanil is not possible, as the therapeutic plasma level for sufentanil is not known; however, the more rapid elimination of sufentanil makes it unlikely that adequate spontaneous ventilation will return later than after fentanyl [8].

In spite of the shorter half-lives of alfentanil and sufentanil compared to fentanyl, there was little difference in ventilatory control 30 and 60 minutes after surgery with respect to the narcotics used for maintenance of anesthesia. The greater depression in the slope of minute ventilation versus end-tidal P_{CO_2} in patients given alfentanil was not confirmed by differences in the slope of P100 versus end-tidal P_{CO_2}. Similarly, there were no differences between the sufentanil and fentanyl subgroups in the sufentanil maintenance study. The modest respiratory depression seen postoperatively certainly suggests that the intraoperative administration of drugs (fentanyl, alfentanil, and sufentanil) was accompanied by postoperative plasma levels in the threshold range suggested by Stanski and Hug as being necessary for adequate spontaneous ventilation [7]. As plasma levels were not determined, possible effects of differences in pharmacokinetics cannot be quantified.

When alfentanil was compared to thiopental for induction of anesthesia, the postoperative differences in ventilatory control were trivial and probably artifactual. Patients given thiopental required higher concentrations of halothane and were thus much less arousable postoperatively. In fact, at 30 minutes only three of the patients given thiopental could attempt the rebreathing test. As the duration of surgery in patients given alfentanil for induction averaged 1.7 hours and patients received only an induction dose of the study drug, rapid redistribution of alfentanil should have been associated with very low plasma levels at the time ventilation measurements were made postoperatively. Any ventilatory depression would most likely have been due to residual halothane.

Respiratory measurements in the immediate postoperative period are very difficult as ventilatory control of breathing is so easily perturbed by pain, discomfort, environmental stimuli, and sleep, all known to affect resting end-tidal P_{CO_2} and the slopes of minute ventilation or P100 versus end-tidal P_{CO_2} [6]. In spite of our best efforts, some of the variability of our results is certainly due to random differences in pain, discomfort, and sleep among our patients.

Nevertheless, our values for resting end-tidal P_{CO_2} and the minute ventilation versus end-tidal P_{CO_2} slope preoperatively and postoperatively are in reasonable agreement with previous studies [1–3], although we found less respiratory depression. To our knowledge, this is the first report using P100 values in the immediate postanesthetic period. Although Becker et al [1] observed a

biphasic respiratory depression after fentanyl–nitrous oxide anesthesia, other investigators have not been able to confirm it [2,3]. For this and other reasons, especially logistic constraints, we did not extend our respiratory measurements past 60 minutes. When narcotics were used in the manner we gave them, little ventilatory depression was evident 60 minutes after anesthesia by any measure. This lack of depression after anesthetic doses of narcotics is most likely the result of summation of the effects of low plasma levels of the narcotics and of pain and awareness following major surgery.

CONCLUSION

Are the three measures we chose able to predict problems? We used standard techniques to study ventilatory control. Our results show adequate function immediately postoperatively. Unfortunately, an apparatus such as ours of itself affects ventilatory control [6]. In addition, the apparatus is cumbersome, and observations are extended into the first postoperative night only with the greatest difficulty. The standard techniques we used are therefore of limited value except under controlled experimental conditions. Perhaps the recent advent of methods for sleep studies, including noninvasive, accurate oximetry and respiratory impedance plethysmography, may offer new ways to continue observations into the postoperative period that will prove applicable to more ready evaluation of postanesthetic ventilatory control. Until then, traditional rebreathing studies such as ours must suffice.

REFERENCES

1. Becker LD, Paulson BA, Miller RD, Severinghaus JS, Eger EI II. Biphasic respiratory depression after fentanyl-droperidol or fentanyl alone used to supplement nitrous oxide anesthesia. Anesthesiology 1976; 44:291–6.

2. Vejlsted H, Hansen M, Jacobsen E. Post-operative ventilatory response to carbon dioxide following neurolept anaesthesia. Acta Anaesthesiol Scand 1977;21:529–33.

3. Smedstad KG, Rigg JRA. Control of breathing after fentanyl and innovar anaesthesia. Br J Anaesth 1982;54:599–604.

4. Read DJC. A clinical method for assessing the ventilatory response to carbon dioxide. Australas Ann Med 1967;16:20–32.

5. Whitelaw WA, Derenne JP, Milic-Emili J. Occlusion pressure as a measure of respiratory center output in conscious man. Respir Physiol 1975;23:181–99.

6. Jordan D. Assessment of the effects of drugs on respiration. Br J Anaesth 1982;54:763–82.

7. Stanski DR, Hug CC Jr. Alfentanil—a kinetically predictable narcotic analgesic. Anesthesiology 1982;57:435–8.

8. Bovill JG, Sebel PS, Blackburn MB, Heykants J. Kinetics of alfentanil and sufentanil: a comparison. Anesthesiology 1981;55:A174.

51 MORPHINE AND THE NEW NARCOTICS IN POSTOPERATIVE VENTILATORY CONTROL

Norig Ellison

This chapter expresses a personal bias concerning the reason morphine anesthesia has now joined ether as being primarily of historical interest.

THE PLACE OF MORPHINE ANESTHESIA

In 1972 we presented a paper on plasma levels of morphine [1]. In five patients undergoing open heart surgery, plasma morphine levels after a single 10-mg intravenous dose were determined at 1-minute intervals for 5 minutes. The remainder of the induction dose (average, 1.08 mg/kg; range, 0.50 to 1.40) was then given over approximately 20 minutes. Induction was considered complete when the patient would not open his eyes on command. Twenty additional minutes were allowed to elapse without further morphine administration. At the end of this time, another plasma morphine level was determined, 10 mg more morphine was given intravenously, and plasma morphine levels were obtained at 2 and 5 minutes. The re-

sults are depicted in Figure 51.1. The 1-minute peak level of plasma morphine after a single 10-mg intravenous dose was not surprising; however, the degree to which the initial plasma peak exceeded the level 20 minutes after the much larger total induction dose was startling.

To study the dynamics of cerebral uptake, healthy volunteers undergoing cerebral blood flow studies were given a single 10-mg intravenous dose of morphine. Arterial plasma levels were determined 30 seconds and 1, 2, and 3 minutes after the injection, and levels in the jugular bulb at 1, 2, and 3 minutes. Rapid cerebral uptake is demonstrated in Figure 51.2 for one subject in whom the jugular bulb morphine level was below the arterial level at 1 minute and then higher at 2, 3, and 5 minutes. The arterial line shows the concentration being presented to the brain and the jugular bulb the concentration being drained from the brain. At any time when arterial concentration is less than venous concentration, the brain is already giving up morphine.

293

FIGURE 51.1. Plasma morphine levels in five patients undergoing cardiac surgery. See text.

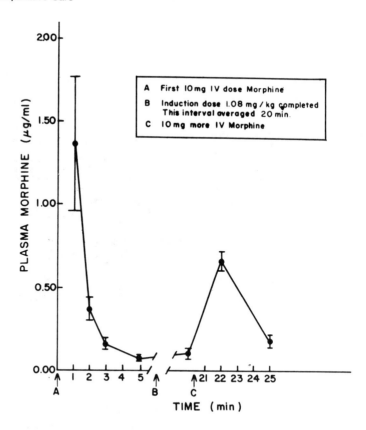

A   First 10mg IV dose Morphine

B   Induction dose 1.08 mg / kg completed
     This interval averaged 20 min.

C   10mg more IV Morphine

On the basis of these data we offered two tentative conclusions:

1. The data may explain the clinical observation that small doses of morphine given rapidly often cause more hypotension than large doses given slowly.
2. The data further suggest that circulatory response to expected painful stimuli may better be prevented by a well-timed small dose than by increasing the induction dose many minutes earlier.

With the benefit of ten years' hindsight, I would like to suggest that a third conclusion should have been offered in 1972:

3. A more rapid-acting narcotic with a short duration of action is needed for use in the management of patients undergoing both cardiac and noncardiac surgery.

LIMITATIONS OF MORPHINE ANESTHESIA

One of the major advantages of morphine anesthesia that made it so popular in 1972 was that it permitted a transition to elective postoperative ventilatory support by endotracheal tube. In 1972, the practice of cardiac anesthesia and surgery was considerably different than it is today. At that time most patients had valvular heart disease, many with associated lung disease, and overnight mechanical ventilation was the rule rather than the exception. Morphine anesthesia made this much easier. Furthermore, the assist devices on the mechanical ventilators of that day were inadequate when compared to today's models, and intermittent mandatory ventilation had not yet been described.

At the same time, the fact that patients had received the morphine anesthetic dictated overnight mechanical ventilation. Over

FIGURE 51.2. Arterial and jugular bulb plasma morphine levels in a volunteer subject. See text.

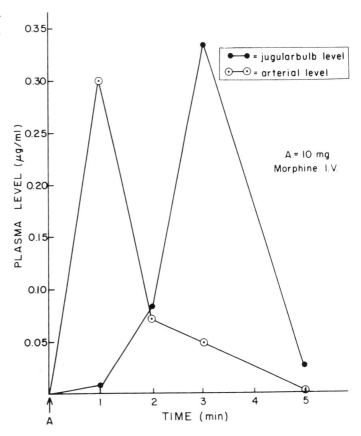

the next five years, the explosive growth in coronary artery surgery radically altered the practice of cardiac anesthesia and surgery. In 1977 my colleagues compared two groups of patients cared for in the same months in 1972 and 1977 [2]. In contrast to 1972, most of the patients in 1977 had coronary artery disease with good left ventricular function, and in comparing these two groups it was concluded that early extubation of patients whose postoperative courses were otherwise uncomplicated after cardiac surgery allowed more rapid mobilization and progress to the intermediate care areas without introducing undesirable sequelae. Since morphine anesthesia precluded early extubation, we shifted initially to volatile anesthetics and later to fentanyl in order to permit earlier extubation than was heretofore possible. Table 51.1 demonstrates this change in the patient population and in the anesthetic agents used.

CONCLUSION

It is fortunate that others developed the more rapid-acting narcotic analgesics with shorter duration of action that we failed to call for in 1972. Their availability has not only facilitated intraoperative management, but has made postoperative respiratory care, especially early extubation, a real possibility.

REFERENCES

1.   Ellison N, Behar MG. Plasma morphine levels in patients and volunteers. Abstracts of Scientific Papers, 1972 ASA Annual Meeting, 269–70.

2.   Klineberg PL, Geer RT, Hirsh RA, Aukburg SJ. Early extubation after coronary artery bypass graft surgery. Crit Care Med 1977;5:272–4.

TABLE 51.1. Summary of the cardiac anesthesia and surgery experience at the Hospital of the University of Pennsylvania, 1972–1982*

Year:	1972	1973	1974	1975	1976	1977	1978	1979	1980	1981	1982
Total cases	189	212	253	385	512	660	669	530	675	719	737
Types of cases (number)											
1. CABG	69	85	119	195	288	374	381	315	408	463	481
2. CABG + additional	5	10	13	20	29	42	50	39	49	48	67
1 + 2 = % of total	39%	45%	52%	56%	62%	63%	64%	67%	68%	71%	74%
3. Valves	87	83	92	129	163	174	156	105	106	120	111
4. Other	28	34	29	41	32	70	82	51	112	88	78
Anesthetic agents used (%)											
Halothane	52.3	41.0	64.8	85.5	96.6	95.0	87.3	75.1	65.3	58.0	47.6
Enflurane	0	1.9	1.2	9.4	1.8	1.2	1.3	6.6	1.5	1.8	2.0
Isoflurane	0	0	0	0	0	0	0	0	2.7	11.3	14.8
Morphine	46.6	56.1	32.8	4.2	1.4	2.0	2.2	1.3	2.1	0.3	0.5
Fentanyl	0	0	0	0	0	0	3.0	13.0	27.3	26.6	34.3
Other	1.1	1.0	1.2	0.9	0.2	1.8	6.2	4.0	1.1	2.0	0.8

*The upper half lists the types of cases by number and illustrates the marked growth in coronary artery surgery between 1972 and 1982. The lower half lists the percentage of cases anesthetized using each agent and illustrates the disappearance of morphine as an agent and the growth of both fentanyl and isoflurane.

52 OPIOID REVERSAL AND POSTOPERATIVE NARCOTIC ANALGESIA

Theodore C. Smith

Opioid antagonist drugs have been known since the early 1900s and clinically employed for overdose since 1950 [1], but not for opioid-supplemented anesthesia for three reasons: available drugs had unpleasant side effects, the antagonism was incomplete at best, and emerging reliable respiratory support (equipment and practitioners) made longlasting analgesia and respiratory depression desirable. In the 1970s, the potent opioids morphine and fentanyl were increasingly used in a balanced cardiac anesthetic technique. That decade also saw the study and introduction of two pure antagonists: naloxone and naltrexone. Their interactions with opioids fit the pharmacologic notion of drug receptors so well that the inescapable postulation of a morphine-like endogenous substance and its receptor led directly to the identification of such substances in mammalian central nervous systems [2]. It occurred to many that these new drugs could be used to end opioid anesthesia. Several groups reported just such studies, with variable results [3–9]. Other studies were aborted or not published.

Antagonism of a potent drug effect is an acceptable and useful technique in medicine generally and anesthesia particularly. The ubiquity of paralyzant reversal makes it useful to explore the reasons for its acceptability. Five classes of arguments favor the practical use of drug antagonists:

The pharmacodynamic argument: dose-response relationships
The pharmacokinetic argument: time course relationships
The pathophysiologic argument: variability in disease
The clinical argument: evidence of effect
The etymologic argument: subliminally pleasant terminology

The arguments are examined here for curare and then for opioid antagonists.

ARGUMENTS FOR REVERSAL OF NEUROMUSCULAR BLOCK

The pharmacodynamic argument states that a dose of antagonist can be prescribed that will produce the desired effect without confounding effects. After neuromuscular block, one wants respiratory muscle strength without bronchorrhea or bradycardia. Vital capacity is less affected by curare than is grip strength, for example [10], and if atropine is given to full effect a small overdose is of no consequence. Despite the "substantial pharmacologic objections" to selection of a single fixed dose of anticholinesterasecum-atropine [11], a fixed dose regardless of relaxant regimen simplifies the workload of the anesthesiologist at a task-intensive time, emergence from anesthesia.

The pharmacokinetic argument states that the duration of action of the antagonist should be of the same order as the agonist. Anticholinesterases have substantially the same half-life as the commonly used relaxants [12, pp 97–136]. Clinically, "recurarization" has been searched for and not found. The clinician feels secure that after a single reversing dose and a few distribution half-lives (15 or 20 minutes), the patient with adequate strength will "stay reversed."

The pathophysiologic argument claims that even uncommon states do not negate the two preceding arguments. Temperature, acid-base status, electrolyte and albumin concentrations, renal function, drug interactions, and metabolic degradation rates do little to unbalance relaxant and reversant [12]. In experiment and in practice, the one-dose algorithm is satisfactory still.

The clinical argument for practical antagonism of neuromuscular blockade is the clincher. Relatively simple signs exist as guides. Clinicians feel that with grip strength and head lift using Kallos's sign [13], they can assure their patients' safety. Furthermore, the neuromuscular stimulators with display of current delivered are rugged, simple, flexible, and cheap. The signs associated with various receptor occupancy levels are widely published and unambiguous. There is no clinical problem distinguishing adequate from borderline efficacy of cholinesterase inhibition.

The final argument is etymologic: we tend to give good words to things we like and that work well. Consider that we give relaxants, not paralyzants, and that we reverse, not antagonize, the effect at the end. Clearly, we are satisfied with these neuromuscular drugs.

THE PROBLEMS WITH REVERSAL OF OPIOID ANESTHESIA

The reversal of opioid-agonist effects is efficacious and specific with naloxone and naltrexone. It is, in my opinion, not a useful clinical routine, however, for reasons given by the five arguments: there is not a single response effect to restore to normal, there is imbalance in time course of agonist and antagonist, there are pathophysiologic considerations counseling caution, there are inadequate clinical assurances to guide the therapist, and our vocabulary is cast in harsh and alerting words.

The human response to opioids includes two major effects: analgesia and respiratory depression. Dose-response curves show complete overlap [14,15]. Furthermore, total analgesia may promote sleep. Severe depression of ventilation follows the combination of sleep and morphine [16]. Numerous mixtures of opioids and antagonists have been advocated for analgesia without respiratory depression, but none has withstood critical examination [17,18]. Small doses of morphine for premedication and for postoperative analgesia are prescribed far more commonly now than in years past, despite marginal analgesic efficacy. Fear of respiratory depression overshadows evidence that adequate analgesia permits better cough, sigh, and breathing pattern. Even for patients supervised by good recovery room staff, anesthetists elect less-than-comfortable patients rather than depressed respiration. But achieving a nice balance of responsiveness to pain and to carbon dioxide is difficult to prescribe [19]. It requires moment-to-moment titrations.

Once achieved, a desired balance does not stay achieved. The time course of naloxone is very short. Perhaps naltrexone and alfentanil are a matched pair, but with currently available drug pairs, renarcotization after

initial recovery is real and regularly reproducible. Agonists and antagonists have dissimilar kinetics [20]. Kaufman et al [15] in
an elegant study calculated a 20-minute elimination half-life for naloxone. Smith [21]
found that single doses of naloxone and naltrexone have effective half-lives of 12 to 15
minutes and 20 to 25 minutes respectively
during isohypercapnia. Under similar conditions a single analgesic dose of fentanyl has
a half-life of upwards of an hour [22,23].
Similarly, the clearance of naloxone is ap-
preciably faster than that of fentanyl [12].
Finally, the clinical duration of fentanyl is
grossly prolonged with the newer high-dose
induction regimens of 50 to 150 μg per kilogram of body weight. The redistribution of
these doses results in blood and brain concentrations sufficient to produce major retention of carbon dioxide, which wanes with
the prolonged half-life of elimination, not redistribution.

The pathophysiologic argument is in large
part unexplored for the pairing of opioid agonist and antagonist. In small doses the very
lipid soluble drugs such as fentanyl might not
have as extended half-lives in the face of liver
disease as morphine might. But reversal of
anesthesia in recently operated patients may
put severe burdens on compromised patients. Flacke et al [24] reported one such
case where reversal of anesthesia in a compromised, fluid-loaded patient caused near-
fatal pulmonary edema that required renarcotization. The injection of naloxone often
causes intense pruritus, copious diuresis, and
even major episodes of nausea and emesis.
We do not know the variability of dose and
response, or of time course, that results from
major alterations of renal, hepatic, and central nervous system function.

The clinical argument sums up the clinician's uncertainty about the foregoing three
arguments. Many authors have searched for
a protocol that will effectively and satisfactorily permit routine prescription of narcotic
reversal regimens [3–9]. None has met ac-
claim or wide acceptance. A major problem
is lack of a single definitive observation to
guide therapy. Simple respiratory rate has
too many variable inputs to accept. Multiple
blood gas measurements are expensive and
questionable if an arterial catheter has not
been placed for another reason. Pain will not
do: all of us have been called to prescribe
analgesia and found a sleeping patient. We
distrust nurses' judgment, as evidenced by
orders for tiny doses as needed, widely
spaced in time even in husky young adults.

The final argument rests on the words we
use. To my ears, the word *antagonist* itself
is harsh and unpleasant. The word *narcotic*
has changed in meaning from Winterstein's
use of altered sensation to one with conno-
tations of abuse and illegality. We "block"
with these drugs, recalling the rib-crushing
image of a pulling guard or blocking half-
back, or the frustration of a mental block.

Do these arguments mean there is no way
to use narcotic analgesics for anesthesia and
to assure adequate level of consciousness and
respiratory control soon postoperatively?
Perhaps, but not quite. First, one could in
suitable circumstances, using almost the same
kind of moment-to-moment observation and
care characteristic of our intraoperative
practice, follow patients in emergence, administering antagonists and even agonists as
needed. This is expensive of personnel time
and rarely justifiable to third-party reimbur-
sers. Second, newer partial agonists such as
nalbuphine or butorphanol may well be useful [25,26]. It would require major retraining
of some to accept an arterial carbon dioxide
tension above 40, but techniques of respiratory care can help assure safety with alveolar hypoventilation. Third, one can use
other analgesic techniques for postoperative
relief of pain. Major nerve blocks, long-acting local anesthetics, and continuous catheter techniques for epidural and plexus block
have been demonstrably effective in practiced hands. Finally, one may capitalize on
the rapidity of onset and reversibly competitive nature of the agonist/antagonist interaction. Self-administered (demand) analgesia is an effective therapy. Patient demand
could trigger interruption of an infusion of

short-acting antagonist. A resurgence of studies on dose and regimen for analgesic therapy is overdue.

In considering postoperative analgesia, one should also put epidural or spinal opioids in perspective. This initially appealing concept had given birth to well over 200 publications by 1982, with perhaps two to four times that number of unpublished or in-progress studies extant. Considerable clinical confusion comprises the current climate. Some dose-response studies find 2 or 4 mg efficacious, while others find 5 mg partially ineffective or inadequate. Usually, dose and volume injected are selected without regard to the site of injection and to the segment in which pain is relayed to higher centers. The specter of delayed respiratory depression or apnea looms irregularly and unpredictably. In spinal anesthesia, intrathecal injection of large doses of long-acting local anesthetics do not reach the brain and produce convulsions, but epidural injections of small doses of morphine are alleged to reach the fourth ventricle or surface of the medulla and to halt breathing. There is much yet to learn here.

CONCLUSION

The future of improved patient analgesia with safer techniques seems assured. Pharmacology is one of the newest of the basic sciences and anesthesiology one of the newest of the clinical sciences. Although anesthesiologists pride themselves on their knowledge of pharmacology, the quantitative tools of dynamics and kinetics are only recently finding application in our work. Given the present state of knowledge, I feel comfortable in stating categorically that high-dose narcotic anesthesia is not a technique to be followed by pharmacologic reversal. It cannot be done safely with our current tools and training. On the other hand, our tools and training are rapidly changing. We owe our patients safe anesthesia, and modern narcotic-based balanced anesthesia has many applications in

that regard. We owe our patients adequate and safe postoperative analgesia, and we are continually learning ways to improve that. Achieving both goals in the same patient is a conceivable as well as a desirable ambition.

REFERENCES

1. Eckenhoff JE, Elder JD, King BD. N-Allylnormorphine in the treatment of morphine or Demerol narcosis. Am J Med Sci 1952;223:191–7.
2. Goldstein, A. Opioid peptides. Science 1976;193:1081–8.
3. Foldes FF, Lunn JN, Moore J, Brown IM. N-Allyl noroxymorphine: a new potent narcotic antagonist. Am J Med Sci 1963;245:23–30.
4. Hasbrouck JD. The antagonism of morphine anesthesia by naloxone. Anesth Analg (Cleve) 1971;50:954–8.
5. Longnecker DE, Grazis PA, Eggers GWN. Naloxone for antagonism of morphine-induced depression. Anesth Analg (Cleve) 1973;52:447–52.
6. Heisterkamp DV, Cohen PJ. The use of naloxone to antagonize large doses of opiates administered during nitrous oxide anesthesia. Anesth Analg (Cleve) 1974;53:12–18.
7. Johnstone RE, Jobes DR, Kennell EM, Behar MG, Smith TC. Reversal of morphine anesthesia with naloxone. Anesthesiology 1974;41:361–7.
8. Kripke BJ, Finck AJ, Shah NK, Snow JC. Naloxone antagonism after narcotic-supplemented anesthesia. Anesth Analg (Cleve) 1976;55:800–5.
9. Drummond GB, Davie IT, Scott DB. Naloxone: dose-dependent antagonism of respiratory depression by fentanyl in anaesthetized patients. Br J Anaesth 1977;49:151–4.
10. Gal TJ, Smith TC. Partial paralysis with d-tubocurarine and the ventilatory response to CO_2. Anesthesiology 1976;45:22–8.
11. Kitz RJ. Pharmacology of cholinesterase inhibitors. ASA refresher course lectures, 1981:223–4.
12. Stanski DR, Watkins WD. Drug disposition in anesthesia. New York: Grune & Stratton, 1982.

13. Kallos T. Open-mouth head lifting, a sign of incomplete reversal of neuromuscular blockade. Anesthesiology 1972;37:650–2.

14. Girvan CB, Dundee JW. Alterations in response to somatic pain associated with anaesthesia. Br J Anaesth 1976;48:463–8.

15. Kaufman RD, Gabathuler ML, Bellville JW. Potency, duration of action and pA2 in man of intravenous naloxone. J Pharmacol Exp Ther 1981;219:156–62.

16. Forrest WH, Bellville JW. The effect of sleep plus morphine on the respiratory response to carbon dioxide. Anesthesiology 1964; 25:137–41.

17. Rouge JC, Banner MP, Smith TC. Interactions of levallorphan and meperidine. Clin Pharmacol Ther 1969;10:643–54.

18. Girvan CB, Moore J, Dundee JW. Pethidine compared with pethidine-naloxone administered during labour. Br J Anaesth 1976;48:563–9.

19. Hug CC Jr. Improving analgesic therapy. Anesthesiology 1980;53:441–3.

20. Kosterlitz HW, Watt AJ. Kinetic parameters of narcotic agonists and antagonists. Br J Pharmacol Chemother 1968;33:266–76.

21. Smith TC. Comparison of naltrexone and naloxone in man. Anesthesiology 1979; 51:S373.

22. Kaufman RD, Aqleh KA, Bellvilk JW. Relative potencies and durations of action with respect to respiratory depression of intravenous meperidine, fentanyl and alphaprodine in man. J Pharmacol Exp Ther 1979; 208:73–9.

23. Downs JJ, Kemp RA, Lambertsen CJ. The magnitude and duration of respiratory depression due to fentanyl and meperidine in man. J Pharmacol Exp Ther 1967; 158:416–21.

24. Flacke JW, Flacke WE, Williams GD. Acute pulmonary edema following naloxone reversal of high-dose morphine anesthesia. Anesthesiology 1977;47:376–8.

25. DiFazio CA, Moscicki JC, Magruder MR. Anesthetic potency of nalbuphine and interacted with morphine in rats. Anesth Analg (Cleve) 1981;60:629–30.

26. Hug CC Jr. New narcotic analgesics and antagonists in anesthesia. Semin Anesth 1982;1:14–20.

53 POSTOPERATIVE OPIOID REVERSAL AND ANALGESIA AFTER OPEN HEART SURGERY

Michael B. Howie

It is becoming increasingly clear that high doses of narcotics provide a much more secure and technically convenient method of anesthesia then was heretofore available for all types of patients with heart disease. Together with the application of modern cardiac physiology, this form of anesthesia has turned what was a mystical religious ceremony into an ordinary event. Thus it is in the area of the recovery from anesthesia after such large doses of narcotics, especially when they have been administered after open heart surgery, that real gains can be made in morbidity and mortality rates.

EXTUBATION

With respect to the technique used for anesthesia, I believe that all patients should be transported from the operating room to the intensive care unit with the endotracheal tube in place. Assessment of whether extubation should be performed should only be carried out after the patient has experienced a pe-

riod of stable hemodynamics and the routine of intensive care for that patient has been established. There are many reasons for allowing a period of pulmonary and cardiac stabilization. The purpose of the heart operation is to improve the patient's chance to return to a somewhat normal life; therefore the quality of myocardial preservation must be carried into the postoperative period. All consideration should thus be given first to the patient's heart, and then his lungs. The desire for early extubation seems to disregard the heart and concentrate on rapid, independent respiration as the mark of success, perhaps at the expense of stress on the cardiovascular system.

Many patients experience multiple organ failure, and the initial cause is often inadequacy of organ perfusion because of low cardiac output. Concentrating on protecting and enhancing myocardial function in the early hours postoperatively will allow a recovered heart to withstand the stress of weaning more easily. Sudden, stressful events just after the operation can only reverse the anticipated benefits of a cardiac operation.

Undoubtedly, any of the dosage regimens for fentanyl, whether 50 µg per kilogram of body weight supplemented with other anesthetics or 100 µg/kg with oxygen, will produce drug levels above the threshold for normal carbon dioxide response, and then at least 17 hours will be needed to allow these levels to decline to concentrations that are low enough to begin weaning [1].

In the seriously compromised myocardium, there are definite intraoperative advantages to this simple technique. Are any advantages found in these patients postoperatively? The occurrence of hypertension and tachycardia, though not differing with various doses of fentanyl, is reasonably easy to control in the postoperative period. Patients who have had a predominantly inhalational technique require significant amounts of sedation and analgesia to stabilize rises in blood pressure because of pain and anxiety in the postoperative period. The administration of morphine sulfate in amounts greater than 45 mg is commonly reported [2]. This period of postoperative stress is the area in which we will continue to improve our results, and one of the methods for contributing to the reduction of morbidity is to protect the myocardium by increasing the patient's comfort.

The very ill patient with cardiac and pulmonary problems should be in a separate category from the relatively healthy patient undergoing myocardial revascularization. Conservative postoperative ventilation in the ill patient allows us to concentrate on one system at a time; thus introduction of weaning and the work of breathing can be delayed until the cardiac problem has been stabilized.

Before we consider whether we should extubate early in any patient, we should review several characteristics.

1. The type of surgery is an important consideration. For example, the left internal mammary artery graft has special problems and a different pulmonary morbidity when compared to simple saphenous vein bypass grafting. Similarly, multiple valve replacement carries a different risk than simple aortic valve insertion.

2. Age and nutritional state have an influence on the ability of the patient to face immediate weaning.

3. If severe myocardial damage exists, it seems wise to allow the heart to recover for several hours.

4. Does the patient need to undergo reoperation for bleeding that is excessive or not reversible with correction of an abnormal coagulation profile. If there is any possibility, then the endotracheal tube should be left in place.

5. Removing the work of breathing reduces the onset of other organ failure in a precarious circulatory state.

6. The anesthetic technique includes muscle relaxation and the reversal of relaxant.

The amount of narcotic or benzodiazepines given should be considered as well. A period of patience on the part of the anesthesiologist may be of more benefit to the patient than full pharmacologic reversal as soon as he enters the intensive care unit.

Numerous self-evident reasons exist not to initiate weaning. Severe arrhythmias should not be aggravated by a sudden stressful weaning process. Mitral valve patients with pulmonary hypertension and congestion may benefit with elective ventilatory help. Corrections of volume status and bleeding, including the optimizing of cardiac output, seem obvious steps to take.

ANALGESIA AND STRESS AVOIDANCE

With the newer narcotics we have seen even more stable postoperative courses. Although sufentanil possesses a shorter time to recovery than fentanyl, the number of hours the patient is intubated is still comparatively long. Excellent hemodynamic stability with normal cardiac output and systemic vascular resistance has been our experience in this period, however. These results are surely of some benefit in preserving the integrity of the myocardium and ensuring good organ performance. Very few of our patients who received sufentanil required further analgesic or sedative drugs in the postoperative period. The consistently normal cardiac outputs in our trials of sufentanil with a group of patients undergoing coronary artery bypass make it difficult not to give some credit for this stability to the continued state of analgesia associated with the plasma concentrations of the drug [3].

What do we gain from reversal of the narcotic? It is doubtful that the monitored security of an intensive care unit should be exchanged for a not-so-well monitored ward. Anesthesiologists must not assume that their reversal regimen is complete and thus relax their observations. They require the same or increased observation with narcotic reversal and must be prepared to institute additional vasodilator intervention.

Perhaps we should look to a reduced narcotic dose supplemented with inhalational agents in the healthier patient. This technique would be one way to decrease postoperative respiratory depression and improve the chances for narcotic reversal. Balanced anesthesia intraoperatively would introduce more interventive therapy, and the postoperative period would carry the risk of longer and higher hypertensive episodes. Extra sedation would have to be given, which could preclude early postoperative weaning.

Achieving independent respiratory status by an opiate antagonist means risking sudden precipitation of severe pain and possible circulatory consequences ranging from pulmonary edema to ventricular fibrillation [4]. The severe stress may damage a myocardium beyond repair and reverse the benefit of the operation. Sudden awakening may be even more stressful in patients who have been deeply narcoticized. Gradual decline in plasma concentrations of narcotics allows a more comfortable accommodation to awakening.

Although theoretically better physiology is produced by early spontaneous respiration, there are no real differences in the requirements of these patients for intensive care therapy. The discharge hour is about the same, and the frequency of pulmonary complications is related to the type of surgery and the preexisting lung disease. Arrhythmias are far more frequent in the second and third postoperative days than in the first 24 hours.

There is uncertainty about the optimal dose of narcotic antagonist. A certain dose in one patient may be far too much in another, causing sudden severe pain and hypertension in the hyperalgesic patient.

The ability of a patient to recognize his surroundings and participate in the weaning process does not correlate closely with residual narcotic concentrations for the response to carbon dioxide [5]. The relationship between early weaning and relatively high narcotic levels could be a major problem in clinical judgment of the weaning process. If this problem were combined with old age and a generally decreased ability to respond to high carbon dioxide levels and hypoxia, even in a non-narcotized patient, the overall weaning process and evaluation could be dangerously clouded.

Unpredictable and sudden cardiac events can take place with acute reversal of narcotics by naloxone and even some of the newer agents. Reports of pulmonary edema, massive increases in afterload, and ventricular arrhythmias leading to fibrillation with as little as 0.1 mg of naloxone show that the unnecessary dangers for the cardiac patient far outweigh any possible benefits [6]. The duration of the effects of naloxone, compared to most of the currently used narcotics, indicates that at any time beyond 60 minutes, remorphinization can occur. The increased duration of effect of naltrexone and the 6-oxo analog of oxilorphan S-20682 may alleviate this duration problem, but careful postoperative observation will still be necessary [7].

The exaggerated hemodynamic response

with narcotic reversal in the patient who has right ventricular stress and failure may precipitate irrecoverable right ventricular dilatation and pulmonary hypertension. What are the alternatives? Because of its shorter half-life, alfentanil may have a very important place either as a basal narcotic or as a continuous infusion for pain. A second alternative may be to use one of the partial antagonist/agonists for slower reversal, allowing the properties of one of these agents to protect and compensate for the sudden withdrawal of analgesia while still permitting respiratory exchange to become spontaneous [8]. The final alternative is to abandon all but the smallest doses of narcotics as part of a cardiac anesthetic technique, denying the patient the benefit of a valuable and safe method of anesthesia.

REFERENCES

1. Bovill JG, Sebel PS. Pharmacokinetics of high-dose fentanyl: a study in patients undergoing cardiac surgery. Br J Anaesth 1980;52:795–801.

2. Wallach R, Karp RB, Reves JG, Opani S, Smith LR, James TN. Pathogenesis of paroxysmal hypertension developing during and after coronary bypass surgery: a study of hemodynamic and humoral factors. Am J Cardiol 1980;46:559–65.

3. Howie MB, Reitz J, Reilley TE, Harrington K, Smith D, Dasta JF. Does sufentanil's shorter half-life have any clinical significance? Anesthesiology 1983;59:A146.

4. Andree RA. Sudden death following naloxone administration. Anesth Analg (Cleve) 1980;59:782–4.

5. Heisterkamp DV, Cohen PJ. The use of naloxone to antagonise large doses of opiates administered during nitrous oxide anesthesia. Anesth Analg (Cleve) 1974;53:12–18.

6. Michaelis LL, Hickey PR, Clark TA, Dixon WM. Ventricular irritability associated with the use of naloxone hydrochloride. Ann Thorac Surg 1974;18:608–14.

7. Freye E, Hartung F, Kaliebe S. Prevention of late fentanyl-induced respiratory depression after injection of opiate antagonists naloxone and S-20682: comparison with naloxone. Br J Anaesth 1983;53:71–8.

8. Magruder MR, Delaney RD, Difayio CA. Reversal of narcotic-induced respiratory depression with nalbuphine hydrochloride. Anesthesiol Rev 1982;9:32–7.

DR. CARL C. HUG, JR.: This symposium has dealt with a number of problems as well as benefits associated with anesthetic agents. I hope I can be forgiven for interjecting a somber note, but the narcotic analgesics, like the inhalational anesthetics, pose the problem of abuse. We know that this occupational risk may have reached epidemic levels. I will not go into particulars about what the problems are nor will I try to offer solutions, but I ask that the problem be recognized in this symposium.

We need to acknowledge that we in anesthesiology are particularly liable to this hazard. Ours is a stressful occupation, and we have easy access to large quantities of drugs that are poorly controlled. Many young people coming into our training programs have a tolerant attitude toward drugs. We're all human, and occasionally some of us show poor judgment. The important point is to look at the drug issue realistically and to hold ourselves accountable by being alert to problems among our colleagues and knowing what to do when they occur.

The American Society of Anesthesiologists is focusing its attention on the problem of drug misuse. The 1983 meeting featured a plenary session on physician impairment, presented by the Committee on Occupational Health of Operating Room Personnel. The committee is also compiling information on programs available throughout the United States for dealing with the impaired physician. These activities underscore the seriousness with which we should view the potential for abuse of the agents we work with so closely in our practice.

I apologize for inserting this issue into the program, but I think we need to be every bit as concerned about the abuse potential of narcotic agents as we are about environmental pollution from the inhalational agents. Perhaps the issue could be addressed at our next symposium.

DR. EDMOND I. EGER II: I have a question for Dr. Pace relating to data from his narcotic studies. Dr. Pace, you examined various indices of respiratory depression at 30 and 60 minutes following administration of the agents. In some cases you cited figures that showed more depression at 60 minutes than at 30 minutes. Were any of those changes significant, and were there many patients who showed more depression at 60 than at 30 minutes? If so, how do you explain it?

DR. NATHAN L. PACE: I don't recall that we actually saw more respiratory depression at 60 than at 30 minutes. The problem with the data we collected is that the standard errors were so large that there was no statistical significance in the differences you referred to.

DR. THEODORE C. SMITH: I'd like to reemphasize what Dr. Pace has just said: the large standard error, and thus the large standard deviation, means that some patients had a very flat response curve. Another point is that the ventilatory response to carbon dioxide is expressed by a straight line that has two parameters—not just a slope, but something that describes displacement. After doses of an opioid, a nearly normal slope is possible in a ventilatory response curve that is shifted markedly to the right. This can be attained by doing what the Scandinavians have done for years to manage overdoses: give 'em black coffee, slap 'em in the face, get 'em up, and walk 'em around. As long as the patient is aroused, the slope of the curve may be very steep, but it may fall as soon as those external stimuli are stopped. The result will look like a diphasic response, a renarcotization or something of the sort. It doesn't happen with every patient, but it is frequent enough to be worth looking for.

DR. PACE: Dr. Ellison has reminded me that my original manuscript showed statistically significant differences for some groups with greater respiratory depression at 60 than at 30 minutes. I would explain it on the basis of what Dr. Smith has just described: changes in the patient's level of arousal or sleepiness happening by chance in the recovery room. I would not attribute it to a difference in pharmacokinetics, that is, the blood level of a drug increasing from 30 to 60 minutes.

DR. EGER: Did you in fact treat your patients differently at 60 as opposed to 30 minutes? Were they stimulated more?

DR. PACE: We tried to maintain a constant level of care.

DR. EGER: I'd like to ask Dr. Smith about his terminology, if I may. I wonder how someone from Mars would react to "We test for head lift with a closed mouth."

DR. SMITH: Let me explain. Normally a person can very easily lift his head with the teeth clenched. For someone who is partially paralyzed, though, very often the mouth will fall open when he tries to raise his head from the mattress. If a patient is able to raise his head, he probably still has 60% to 70% receptor binding. I should credit Dr. Tamos Kallos for describing this test.

DR. CARL E. ROSOW: The point has been made that agonist/antagonists can be used to reverse fentanyl or morphine anesthesia. The technique is called sequential analgesia, and the Europeans have been doing it for some time. I have real doubts and concerns about sequential anesthesia, though. For example, how do we know that using a partial agonist is going to prevent too much reversal, or hypertension and arrhythmias, and the like?

DR. SMITH: Most surgery in most institutions is not cardiac, and hypertension and tachycardia are not the major problems. The main difficulty is getting the patient out of the recovery room so that the bill doesn't get horrendous. For these patients one might consider accepting a small amount of respiratory depression, say a PCO_2 in the very high 40s, with supplemental oxygen and reasonably good nursing care in some kind of intensive or immediate care unit. However, in the case of cardiac surgery, I strongly agree that the endotracheal tube must be left in place until the patient's condition is stable.

DR. WILLIAM HAMILTON: A statement was made that challenges whether anesthesia can be done as well with anything other than the current opiate techniques. I don't have any more data than the person who made that statement, but I would be glad to challenge his assertion. I can assure you that the very sickest of patients and the very sickest of hearts can be managed most satisfactorily without the use of high-dose opiate or narcotic anesthesia. There are no data to suggest otherwise. I think it's wrong to say that one technique or one approach is better than the other. A statement like that should not be made.

DR. MICHAEL B. HOWIE: I could start with a compliment and say there are probably anesthetists who can do anything with any drug. But we don't have to look far to realize that opiates are used on the majority of sick hearts in this country at this time. They are chosen because they are safer and more convenient, and I believe that, except in certain institutions, the sicker patients are now predominantly managed with narcotic technique.

DR. NORIG ELLISON: In his review of the literature comparing inhalational and narcotic anesthesia, Dr. Howie concluded with a statement very close to what is frequently said at our morbidity and mortality conferences: that it's the anesthetist and not the anesthetic that counts, and someone who knows what he is doing can use Harry Wollman's IV glue and get away with it.

DR. FAWZY ESTAFANOUS: We really should not promote one technique and call it the only way. I appreciate what narcotics have contributed to anesthesia—that is why we convened this symposium—but there is not a single technique we can apply in every case. Each patient is individual, each has different hemodynamics, and every operation presents a different situation.

DR. HOWIE: I can reply to that. I trained on halothane anesthesia and used it for all my pediatric cardiac cases. I don't dispute that inhalational agents have their place and I've never claimed there is only one technique, but at this time, narcotic anesthesia is the most convenient technique and it is used in the majority of cases.

DR. ADEL ABADIR: I'd like to move to another topic and hope it does not cause as much controversy. All of us who have large residency training programs are faced with the problem of substance abuse that Dr. Hug raised. Given that large-dose narcotics are never complete anesthetics, should we continue to use these drugs, or should we switch to the agonist/antagonist group, which probably will do 99% of what we need without our having to keep large quantities of narcotics available? Also, has anybody noticed that there is less misuse of the newer drugs—fentanyl and its derivatives—than of the older narcotics such as morphine? Should we consider taking morphine and meperidine off the shelves and restrict our choices to drugs that have less potential to be misused?

DR. HUG: I don't think we can do with agonist/antagonists what we are able to do now with pure agonists. These drugs are limited in their efficacy. Like several other researchers, we at Emory have attempted to anesthetize patients as well as dogs with butorphenol and with nalbuphine, and we can't do it. These drugs simply are not adequate substitutes for pure agonists such as fentanyl, alfentanil, and sufentanil.

Can we relieve the problem by removing some of the drugs? Probably not, although we might reduce the incidence, and to the extent that we might be able to control things better, maybe this is something to consider. But I don't believe the answer to the problem lies in limiting the availability of one drug or another. We must learn to deal with the overall problem, which has social as well as professional implications.

DR. CRAIG MOLDENHAUER: I'd like to respond to Dr. Rosow's question about sequential analgesia. As Dr. Hug mentioned, we have looked at nalbuphine, or Nubain, for reversing high-dose fentanyl anesthesia in a group of patients who had undergone coronary artery bypass (Roach GW, Moldenauer CC, Finlayson DC, et al. Nalbuphine reversal of respiratory depression following high-dose fentanyl anesthesia. Abstracts of the Fifth Annual Meeting of the Society of Cardiovascular Anesthesiologists, San Diego, 1983; pp. 140–144). The technique works and can be done safely, but we are certainly not ready to advocate it for routine clinical care. There is great safety in mechanically ventilating patients overnight. If one titrates the dose of nalbuphine, it does seem to be acceptable, at least in our small group of patients.

Our study was divided into two parts. First we studied patients who were late being extubated the morning after surgery. We gave 15-mg/kg doses of nalbuphine, which is about 1 or 2 mg. After one or two doses, these patients were able to maintain a Pco_2 of 48 mm Hg and a pH of 7.32 or greater. They were then extubated, and except for some hypertension that did not exceed their preoperative range of blood pressures, side effects were minimal.

We then became more courageous and tried to extubate people on the day of surgery. We waited until patients had warmed and were hemodynamically stable with no bleeding, and then administered nalbuphine incrementally in doses of 15 μg/kg. After one to three doses, 9 of 10 patients were able to maintain their Pco_2 at 48 mm Hg or less, and were extubated. However, there were side effects. Three patients became renarcotized, but were easily treated with additional doses of nalbuphine. One patient also became hypertensive after the first dose of nalbuphine and required treatment with nitroprusside. He became renarcotized, was redosed, and again became hypertensive. Because of the possibility of these side effects, this is not a technique to be handled as a routine order to the ICU or recovery room nurses. The dose must be titrated and the patient must be carefully monitored.

The technique raises some interesting points. For example, we had patients who complained of pain after the first dose of nalbuphine. With additional drug, the pain was controlled or eliminated, and we were able to extubate them. So respiratory depression and analgesia appeared to

be separated, but not in a very clear manner. Finally, we had one patient who continued to complain of pain after extubation despite additional doses of nalbuphine. Morphine, 16 mg, controlled his pain somewhat; however, he continued to complain of pain throughout his hospital stay despite treatment with morphine and codeine. I'm not sure why his analgesic requirements were so great.

DR. ROSOW: Were the dynamics of these mixed drugs studied? Does the antagonist effect have a shorter duration than the agonist effect?

DR. MOLDENHAUER: We have created a very complex interaction here. I'm not sure what the precise relationship between these two effects is, but I agree it would be an advantage if we could identify it.

DR. HUG: Dr. Smith has demonstrated the dose-response interaction that one can theoretically predict with agonist/antagonists, so these drugs are following established principles of drug-receptor interaction.

DR. MOLDENHAUER: Yes, but that was a theoretical curve that he showed.

DR. HUG: He had actual data.

DR. SMITH: A group of myths arose shortly after Eckenhoff introduced nalorphine for overdose. People said that the drugs would not work unless the antagonist was given before the agonist, or after it, or that they had to be given together, and all sorts of other things. To my knowledge, no quantitative work has yet dissociated, in time or dose response, the analgesic from the respiratory effect for the drugs we have available clinically. If we think in terms of the displacement of a more efficacious drug by one less efficacious at a receptor, we can explain every observation that has been made.

DR. EGER: It seems to me that we have paid homage to our artistic as well as our scientific capacities when we say that it is much more important to consider the administration of these drugs than the qualities of the drugs themselves. We say that we could give a good anesthetic with glue, or—as Ralph Waters did—with carbon dioxide; or even, I'm told, with ethyl gasoline.

I think this has to be contrasted with the fact that we have come to this symposium primarily to learn about the comparative effects of the newer narcotics, which we hope might be better than the old ones. There is no question that the way we give anesthesia and the way we monitor our patients have important, vital, and perhaps preeminent effects on the patients' survival and on morbidity. But we can't ignore the fact that some drugs are better than others and that we can do our best work with better drugs. We have dropped anesthetics like chloroform for good reason, for even though chloroform may have been an excellent anesthetic in its time and could be safe when used properly, we have safer agents available today.

SUMMATION

DR. THEODORE H. STANLEY: We have only to think back to the early 1970s to remember the enormous enthusiasm that existed for morphine at that time. It is interesting to reflect on how that enthusiasm changed and became very much tempered over the years. It is equally interesting to think back to the fall of 1979, when a number of investigators were beginning to use the high-dose fentanyl technique. Some of the annoyances and problems they experienced appear to have become less important over the last three or four years.

A number of speakers described for us their varied experiences with alfentanil. Some suggested it is a very good drug; others seemed to think it really did not differ from the drugs already available. We heard that experience with sufentanil has been somewhat more positive. Nevertheless, there still are difficulties, and several speakers, including myself, expressed some doubts or suggested that there is room for improvement.

I wonder what we will think five years from now. Sufentanil, as we know, is very similar to fentanyl; the only real difference is its potency. Therefore it is easy to substitute sufentanil for fentanyl in virtually any anesthetic technique we are familiar with. Alfentanil is another matter. Its onset of action is very fast and its duration very short. It is a narcotic with qualities we have never experienced before.

In 1979 Dr. de Lange and I visited Dr. de Castro to learn about his experience with sufentanil and alfentanil. We were cocky when we got back to Leiden—we thought we would become experts in a few weeks and then go on to better things. Well, it was easy with sufentanil, but when we started working with alfentanil, I remember Dr. de Lange's reaction at the end of one week. I won't use his exact words, but it was in effect,

"My God!" I still hear those words, and I've heard them during our sessions at this conference.

If I might project ahead, I think sufentanil is going to be welcomed and will prove easy to use. Alfentanil may take longer to learn to apply. It's a kind of drug we have not had experience with, and it has unique characteristics. However, we are beginning to obtain good data and more than a casual experience with the drug. We simply must learn to use these data and gain additional experience. The process will be interesting. Dr. Estafanous is planning another meeting in three years to see what our views are at that point.

DR. CARL C. HUG: It is appropriate that one of Dr. Smith's slides showed a receptor illustrated in three dimensions. That is really where Dr. Paul Janssen began one of his projects that led to the development of fentanyl. Beckett and Casey, in the late 1950s in England, had described that structure as a kind of mirror image of the chemical structures that were known at that time to have narcotic analgesic potency. One of the tenets of their hypothesis was that compounds underwent N-demethylation when they affixed to that receptor. Dr. Janssen started his work by proving their hypothesis: he made a compound that could be N-demethylated faster than pethidine or meperidine, and from that work he realized he could make other compounds in their place that would not be N-demethylated. One of the compounds he made, of course, was phenoperidine, which does not undergo N-demethylation and is many times more potent than meperidine.

I describe this process to suggest that over the next ten years, pharmacologists and medicinal chemists will continue to create compounds that we will be able to review. For, despite great progress, we are still faced with several problems.

310

We've heard some of them during this conference. We still cannot separate analgesia from respiratory depression, nor can we antagonize one without antagonizing the other. Moreover, we have not yet been able to make a potent analgesic that has no potential for inducing dependence.

The active search for improvement in these areas has been going on for some fifty years now. In the mid-1930s, when concern about drug dependence was developing in this country, some key contributions were made by people who are not recognized today because most of us have forgotten about them. Himmelsbach and Eddy described in great detail the pharmacology and effects of narcotic drugs and began to quantify them in much the same ways that we are struggling with now; they were doing it by clinical signs. And Lyndon Small at the University of Virginia set out to make a number of derivatives, trying to find the chemical compound that would have fewer drug dependence inducing properties and provide better analgesia.

When the two-volume work *Pharmacology of the opium alkaloids* was produced by the group at Michigan in 1939, they summarized the world literature and presented more than 10,000 references. We now have well over 100,000 citations dealing just with narcotic analgesics, and some of the same problems are still with us. So there is work to be done. We have not yet reached the ideal state with these drugs, but I hope that bringing people together in a symposium such as this to allow a free exchange of ideas and biases will lead us into asking some of the important questions that remain to be answered.

DR. FAWZY G. ESTAFANOUS: I have enjoyed every minute of this meeting, as I enjoyed the challenge of organizing it, and I am glad both the clinicians and the researchers had the opportunity for a fair exchange of experiences and ideas. I would emphasize, as I have repeatedly over the years, that while research results published in the literature are legitimate, true, and honest, they are the outcome of studies done under strict, controlled circumstances, even in the clinical setting. When these results are applied in everyday practice, we may be faced with completely different findings. But when we amalgamate research and clinical experience, as we have during this meeting, we can reach some very beneficial conclusions.

Several points have particularly impressed me during this meeting. I think it's worth repeating Dr. Stanley's reminder that every patient is an individual, and that our techniques and drugs must be adjusted according to the way the patient reacts. There really is no bible or any one right way to give narcotic anesthesia, and I am glad this is becoming more and more clear. Another thing that impressed me was the discussion about stress response and hormones. We are seeing more attention paid in clinical practice to evaluating heart rate, blood pressure, signs of ischemia, and the like, as they occur.

The discussion was extensive and informative, and we have learned many new things about opioid receptors. But we discovered that we are far from understanding everything about these receptors. I liked Dr. Vandam's comment that we are now at the same stage we were with the catecholamine receptors a few years ago. Perhaps as we understand more about opioid receptors with these very potent, highly specific narcotics, we may be able to eliminate some of the side effects such as addiction and respiratory depression.

From the discussion about calcium channel blockers and the muscle relaxants, it is clear that many of the effects we see are not due to the narcotic or the inhalational agent alone. The combination of drugs used and the way the anesthesia is conducted contribute to the effect. We can probably add a new title to our literature now: "Drug interaction among narcotics and other agents used in everyday practice." Adjuvant agents are always available for fine adjustments.

Let me take this opportunity to thank all of you for being here, and for your efforts and your contribution to the science of anesthesiology.

DR. LEROY VANDAM: This symposium has amply fulfilled its purpose. I had great pleasure listening to the American and European investigators who have been using the new opioids, even though we have had a biased sample of people concerned with cardiac anesthesia.

My comments are based on the information presented at this conference, and perhaps the first thing I would say is that history repeats itself. There is a place in anesthesiology for a variety of opioids, old and new, in all kinds of operations and for the treatment of pain. As with the older agents, the choice among the newer opioids must rest logically upon their pharmacokinetic properties. Let me emphasize two points.

First, the opioids cannot be classified as anesthetics. They form part of the fabric of balanced anesthesia, and balanced anesthesia is designed to approach several goals, including mental obtundation of a sort, freedom from harmful reflexes, and muscle relaxation when necessary. Second, balanced anesthesia is rarely, if ever, a prescribed, undeviating method, no matter the combination of intravenous, inhalation, or regional technique used. The balance must always depend upon clinical judgment, the particular patient, the disease, the patient's other therapeutically prescribed drugs and their interactions with anesthetics, the interaction among anesthetics per se, and finally, upon the kind of operation, its duration, and its anticipated complications.

Problems with most of the opioids used in anesthesia include lack of precision, lack of reliable clinical indicators, and the need for some sort of concept, such as the MAC BAR, that can correlate clinical and biochemical effects. An additional problem is awareness. Frankly, I doubt that the electroencephalogram will ever solve this question. I look upon the electroencephalogram as if I were listening to a phonograph record for the first time and had never seen an orchestra: I wouldn't know what the sounds meant or where they came from.

We also have problems of chest wall spasm and rigidity, respiratory depression and its reversal, somnolence, and minor difficulties such as seizures, nausea, vomiting, and bronchospasm. There is the question of the meaning of stress during anesthesia. Probably it is a survival mechanism, and I suspect that a little stress might be a good thing. However, this is a different matter from the major stress of massive trauma, hemorrhage, or prolonged mental stress. I suppose that in the long run we should also consider the economic cost of anesthetic techniques.

To me, the opioids have not quite lived up to expectations. In fact, their most useful function so far might lie in the role they have played in increasing our knowledge of a variety of receptors throughout the body. Perhaps knowledge of these receptors will help us to develop more selective anesthetic compounds.

DR. WILLIAM HAMILTON: I am continually impressed—or perhaps I should say depressed—by the fact that the anesthesia community still tends to view decreases in blood pressure, cardiac output, and cardiac index as completely negative events. Certainly we would all agree that severe decreases are harmful, but I think the importance of declines in these indicators has been overemphasized in clinical practice.

I would like to add some perspective to Dr. Eger's statement that "we can do better with better drugs." That is an operational statement with which no one can seriously disagree. But to determine, define, and measure "better" is a difficult thing. We have been trying for a long time and have not yet succeeded.

During my career I've seen nitrous oxide–Demerol, the technique with which I started anesthesia, disappear. Similarly, cyclopropane, fluroxene, diethyl ether, vinothene, and a number of other drugs have fallen from use. Nearly all were greeted with the same initial enthusiasm and claimed to have the same "logical support" as our current favorites. Anesthesia is more than a century old, and I would plead that we conduct ourselves like members of a mature specialty. We must recognize that while these may be fine, interesting, thought-provoking drugs that we are discussing at this meeting, we should not embrace them based on superficial evidence and without considering what may happen later on.

I would also like to echo what Dr. Hug mentioned earlier about the social problem with narcotics. During my 25 years as a program director in anesthesia, I've had seven residents that I know of who became addicted to drugs. With one exception, they were detected through our record keeping and not because of their performance, which suggests to me that many more may have been clever enough not to get caught. Of the seven, two died. This is a mortality figure we absolutely cannot take lightly. This is a tremendous problem, and I suspect it will become worse.

DR. AZMY BOUTROS: Let me conclude the summation by saying that I have learned a great deal during this conference, although I think we created more questions than we have answered.

I would like to make a prediction. With the increasing impact of government on the medical profession in the United States, I think one of two things will happen: either the drug companies will lower the cost of anesthetic agents to make them competitive with the less expensive drugs, or the anesthesia profession will be forced to determine which is the best drug to use and then ask if its cost can be justified. I suggest that at the next meeting we will have to look at the overall results and the expense for all the drugs we use.

I thank all of you for attending the meeting and for your participation.

Index